Skin Care Practices
and Clinical Protocols

A Professional's Guide to Success

in Any Environment

Skin Care Practices and Clinical Protocols

A Professional's Guide to Success

in Any Environment

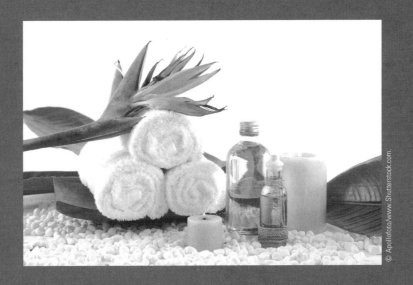

© Apollofoto/www.Shutterstock.com.

SALLIE DEITZ, LE

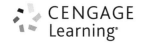

Skin Care Practices and Clinical Protocols: A Professional's Guide to Success in Any Environment
Sallie Deitz, LE

Vice President, Milady & Learning Solutions Strategy, Professional: Dawn Gerrain

Director of Content & Business Development, Milady: Sandra Bruce

Acquisitions Editor: Martine Edwards

Editorial Assistant: Sarah Prediletto

Director, Marketing & Training: Gerard McAvey

Associate Marketing Manager: Matthew McGuire

Senior Production Director: Wendy Troeger

Production Manager: Sherondra Thedford

Design and Project Management: PreMediaGlobal

Cover Image: Bio-Therapeutic, Inc.

For product information and technology assistance, contact us at
Cengage Learning Customer & Sales Support, 1-800-354-9706

For permission to use material from this text or product, submit all requests online at **www.cengage.com/permissions**
Further permissions questions can be e-mailed to
permissionrequest@cengage.com

Library of Congress Control Number: 2012939006

ISBN-13: 978-1-111-54239-9

ISBN-10: 1-111-54239-2

Milady
5 Maxwell Drive
Clifton Park, NY 12065-2919
USA

Cengage Learning is a leading provider of customized learning solutions with office locations around the globe, including Singapore, the United Kingdom, Australia, Mexico, Brazil, and Japan. Locate your local office at **international.cengage.com/region**

Cengage Learning products are represented in Canada by Nelson Education, Ltd.

For your lifelong learning solutions, visit **milady.cengage.com**

Purchase any of our products at your local college store or at our preferred online store **www.cengagebrain.com**

Visit our corporate website at **www.cengage.com**

Printed in the United States of America
1 2 3 4 5 6 7 16 15 14 13 12

Table of Contents

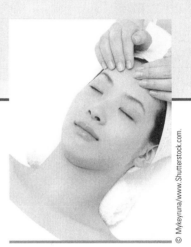

© Mykeyruna/www.Shutterstock.com.

Chapter 2

Chapter 3

Chapter 8

Foreword

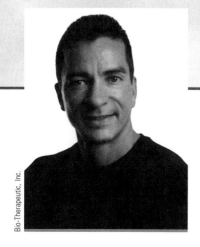

By David Suzuki

President, Bio-Therapeutic, Inc.

Today's world of skin care is evolving at lightning speed, with new technology, science, and efficacy sprinting forward with a magnificent evolution of options for us to choose from. The growth of age defying solutions is endless, and our culture is aligned with healthy, sustainable, noninvasive pathways to achieve its objectives—all of which are relative to you, the skin therapist.

Your journey will begin with basic skin care and transverse the wide scope of professional services, using the most forward-thinking technology and ingredients available. Never before have we had so many exciting opportunities and ways to reach our objectives. All the while, we must remember that embracing the fundamentals is necessary to build infrastructure and mastery and will ultimately allow you the freedom to create unique skin care solutions for every client.

This book is a comprehensive compilation that will take you from the essentials of self-preservation, to the most complex layered technology services available to the skin therapist today, and everything in between. Never before has this level of detailed, relevant information been captured in one publication. This is truly a gem of a book that will add value at multiple levels to every business owner and skin therapist who embraces the ideas within.

As important as the content of this book is the author who is sharing her knowledge. Sallie Deitz is a seasoned clinical esthetician, magnificent educator, talented author, and team member of Bio-Therapeutic, Inc. located in Seattle, Washington. She is an integral member of our product and development team, heads our education development department, and oversees the management of our flagship spa: The Bio-Therapeutic Anti-Aging Skin Spa. This book represents more than two decades of hands-on experience that has been beautifully captured in an easy-to-read, logical format.

I have been blessed to know Sallie professionally and personally and cannot say that I have ever met a more inspiring, positive, and uplifting individual. I think you will feel her passion for our industry in the pages of this book as well as her optimism and love of life.

Remember, you are more than a purveyor of skin care product and technology. You are a dynamic individual who will use your education, knowledge, experience, and intuition to change lives. You are a skin therapist!

Preface

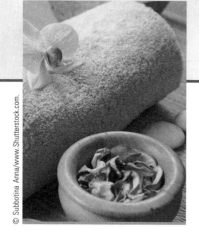

HOW CAN THIS BOOK HELP YOU, THE ESTHETIC PROFESSIONAL?

This book can help the esthetic professional by offering step-by-step protocols of esthetic treatments as well as those that border the medical and clinical realms, such as laser hair removal. At the end of each chapter, you will find biographies of practicing estheticians from around the globe who share their inspiring and highly informative experiences, wisdom, and training with us. This is an excellent book for seasoned professionals who are retooling and looking to bring something new to their skin care menus or for those in need of a refresher in knowledge. New estheticians and students will benefit from this book: it will prepare any learner for the next step into the workplace by providing color photographs of treatments and services, authors' experiences, and a level-headed approach to working as a skin care professional in today's world in any venue.

This book explores the following topics:

- Self-care and the importance of building a strong support system and eliminating distractions and negative forces in one's practice
- Education, learning, and skin care associations and networks
- Step-by-step protocols for chemical peels, with pre- and post-treatment care
- Step-by-step protocols for technology facials, with pre- and post-treatment care
- Physician-directed esthetic services and treatments provided by estheticians, such as laser hair removal and IPL, with protocols and pre- and post-treatment care

- Common procedures as performed by physicians such as rhytidectomy (facelift), blepharoplasty (eye lift), laser resurfacing; injectables, such as neurotoxins and soft-tissue fillers, with pre- and post-operative care as facilitated by the esthetician
- Business practices, uncomplicated business planning, and handling risk management
- Product positioning and the importance of retailing skin care products in your practice; the options, challenges, and solutions for carrying a single line, multiple product lines, private labeling, and exclusive medical products
- The lives and practices of dedicated estheticians practicing today in a variety of venues and global locations

 ## HOW THIS BOOK CAME TO BE

This book is the result of the author's 27 years of experience as a licensed esthetician, 12 years of service as a clinical esthetician and patient and client educator, and her current position with Bio-Therapeutic, Inc., where she serves in product and spa development and as the education director. The author wishes to continue to learn and to help others grow and flourish in the skin care industry, where there is truly no limit to what an individual may be able to do with a good attitude, a passion for helping people, and applying learned skills in an effective and ethical manner. It is a privilege and a labor of love to help others feel better about their skin, and as we know, this improves their self-esteem. They feel better about themselves and return the favor to someone else as they grow and their lives are enriched.

 ## HOW TO USE THIS BOOK

As with most books, it is a good idea to look over the table of contents for items that may be of initial interest; a topic may trigger a desire for an immediate, closer look. Then start with the first chapter. Allow yourself to think about you. You right now, in this time and place. Ask yourself a few questions, such as "Am I where I want to be?" "Is my life working the way I want it to?" "Am I in the right place for me?" "What sort of changes do I want to make?" "What changes do I need to make?"

Whether you have been practicing for 30 years and have an accomplished practice, or are just beginning esthetic courses, your self-care is the most important detail that you will attend to in your life or out of the treatment room. Make sure that you are growing and stay true to yourself. Look again at Chapter 1.

Chapter 2 reminds us that education that has a lifetime focus is the foundation of all success, be it monetary or for personal knowledge. If you feel that you have gone as far as your esthetic's license will take you, get a bachelor's degree, a master's degree, or a doctorate. If you are working in a medical office as an esthetician, and have reached a peak, set the bar higher. Obtain a higher level of education by perhaps earning an LPN (licensed practical nurse), RN (registered nurse), ARNP (advanced registered nurse practitioner), PA-C (physician's assistant certified), or MD (medical doctor) degree. Or, if you love teaching clients and patients, consider the teaching arts by obtaining your teaching credentials.

Chapter 3 leads with new concepts in infection control. If it has been a while since you have updated your knowledge of infection control methods, spend some time on Chapter 3. If you are new to esthetics, this chapter will support what you are learning in prevention and infection control in all settings in or out of your practice.

Chapters 4, 5, and 6 are devoted to procedures and protocols in peels, technology facials, and in pre- and post-operative phases performed by the esthetician. Chapter 4 is an overview of peels ranging from enzymes to chemical peels; and from single applications to layering peels to peel cocktails. There are instructions for every step of the protocol, and an easy-to-use table that describes the pre- and post-peel care at a glance. Chapter 5 provides a brief overview of technology facials, including wet/dry microdermabrasion, oxygen therapy, microcurrent, and LED (light-emitting diode); this is followed with procedural notations on how to apply the technology in a single service; and then culminates in using technologies together in a layered facial. Chapter 6 is excellent information for anyone working in a medical setting, where the esthetician is supporting a physician in pre- and post-operative stages. This section includes extensive details on in-office treatments, home care protocols, and patient compliance.

Chapter 7 is all about business. Straightforward business planning and the ability to create a plan for success is a huge opportunity for us as estheticians. Many estheticians have been in practice for years but are barely meeting their obligations at the end of each fiscal year. Chapter 7 offers support to set a real plan; it is a plan that is easy to stick to when challenges arrive (as we know they will). Business planning is an excellent tool to keep the positive momentum going in a practice, and help estheticians stay on track when things become a little too challenging.

Chapter 8, the final chapter in the book, offers information on the importance of retailing products. It covers the pros and cons of (and solutions for) offering single- or multiple-line products; private-label options, with your name on them, generic skin care lines; or medical-focused skin care lines—and gives a sound rationale for offering each line. If you have been a long-term esthetician and are well known in your community and market, it may be time for you to create your own private-label line.

About the Author

Sallie Deitz

Sallie Deitz is the education director for Bio Therapeutic, Inc., in Seattle, WA. There, she serves in product development and oversees the Bio-Therapeutic Anti-Aging Skin Spa. Deitz has been a licensed esthetician since 1985. She has 12 years of clinical esthetic experience and is the author of *The Clinical Esthetician: An Insider's Guide to Succeeding in a Medical Office* (Milady Publishing, 2004); and *Amazing Skin: A Girl's Guide to Naturally Beautiful Skin* (Drummond Publishing Group, 2005). Deitz is a contributing author to *Milady's Standard Comprehensive Training for Estheticians* (2004); *Milady's Standard Esthetics Fundamentals,* 10th and 11th editions (2009, 2012); *Skin Care Beyond the Basics: Student Workbook*, 3rd edition (Mark Lees, 2007); and *Milady's Standard Esthetics Advanced,* 1st and 2nd editions (Milady/Cengage Learning, 2009, 2012).

Deitz speaks at various esthetic tradeshows, hosts webinars, and presents at select seminars. She is an advisory board member with the Northwest Aestheticians' Guild, Seattle, WA; an advisory board member for The Salon Professional Academy, Tacoma, WA; and has served as a committee member in test development for NIC (National Interstate Council of State Board of Cosmetology Esthetics Division), and is an NCEA (National Coalition of Estheticians, Manufacturers/Distributors & Associations) member.

Deitz lives with her husband Gary and their Boston Terrier Ike near Seattle, Washington, where she loves to write, work, beach walk, and kayak.

Acknowledgments

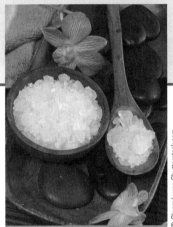

Thank you to the staff at Milady Publishing and Cengage Learning for all they have done in the making of this book.

Martine Edwards, Acquisitions Director

Sandra Bruce, Director of Content and Business Development

Jessica Mahoney, Senior Project Manager

Gerard McAvey, Director of Marketing and Training

Sarah Prediletto, Editorial Assistant

Alyssa Hardy, Editorial Intern

A special thank you to the staff at Bio-Therapeutic, Inc., in Seattle, WA, for all they have done in the making of this volume. Thank you for showing me the way every day.

David Suzuki, President

Dena Suzuki, Vice President

Patrick Conrardy, Art Director

Terrance Luke, Controller, Model

Rose Marshall, LE, Account Manager, Model

Beth McCoy, Event and Education Coordinator

Edgar Juarez, Account Manager, Educator Latin America

Debra Oster Clinton, LE, Account Manager

Linda Porter, Account Processing

David Yamamoto, Operations Director, Model

Art Ma, Sales Manager, IT, Model

Sierra Burnett, Spa Operations

Tom Every, Customer Service

Cami Martlin, LE, Educator

Meghan Kelly, LE, Educator

Nancy Lisac, LE, Educator

Joyce McFarlane, LE, Educator

Franciska Fokkinga, LE, Educator

Kayla Peterson, LE, Esthetician and Technologist

Seretta Soule-MS, LMP, Massage Therapist, Educator, and Body Technologist

Jesus Juarez-Production and Sales

Kristie Djang-Adminstrative

Keth Nget-Production and Repair

James Suzuki-Product Development

🔘 A Special Thank You in Memoriam:

To Jan McKinney, LE, educator: In memory of your bright light in the world and your willingness to gently and steadily train us to be our best; we honor you and your work as you tirelessly focused on improving our industry. We miss you and know that you are at peace.

Thank you to the subject matter experts who have given of their time, knowledge, and experiences:

Samantha Tradelius, Strickler Insurance

Paul Tradelius, Jr., Commercial

Brenda Rogers, Wellness, Life and Fitness Coach

Mark Lees, PhD, LE, CIDESCO, Mark Lees Skin Care, Educator

Garnis Armbruster-Ollivierre, LE, CIDESCO, Educator

Janet D'Angelo, LE, Educator, Author

Jesse Cormier, Executive Director, Associated Skin Care Professionals (ASCP)

Katie Armitage, President, Associated Skin Care Professionals (ASCP)

Debbie Higdon, Associated Skin Care Professionals (ASCP)

Thank you to the team at Bellingham Ear, Nose and Throat & Facial Plastic Surgery and the Hecht Aesthetic Center, Bellingham, WA:

Amy Classen, LE

Jason Lichtenberger, MD

Emil Hecht, MD

Marji Lykke, Clinic Administrator

Jean Hurlbert, LPN

Susan Lichtenberger

Cheryl Hindman

Luanne Bass

Thank you to the owners, educators, and students at The Salon Professional Academy, Tacoma, WA, for giving so generously of their time and facility. Thank you for asking me to serve on your advisory board and for having me speak to your students. It has been a blessing!

Michael Shea, Owner

Karen Shea, Owner

Katherine Morgason, MA, LE, Educator

Brionna Jennings, LE, Student, TSPA

Tristan Steele, LE, Student, TSPA

Tiffany Craig, LE, Student, TSPA

Jacqueline Perry, LE, Student, Model, TSPA

Ryane Bensley, LE, Student, Model, TSPA

Christiane Northrup, MD: Thank you for keeping women and men abreast of women's health issues for so many years and for leading the mind, body, spirit movement as a physician and a metaphysician.

Howard Gardner, PhD: Thank you for taking the time to respond to my e-mails about the theory of multiple intelligences.

Pamela Hill, RN: Thank you for helping our industry with your writing, support, and training throughout the last few years. You have been a catalyst for positive change in our industry. Always with a kind approach, you have guided us along our new path in uncharted territory.

Thank you to the following physicians who have done so much to help skin therapists and estheticians worldwide and in the arts and sciences for the professional esthetician. We appreciate all of your lectures, articles, books, and workshops.

Peter Pugliese, MD

Steven Dayan, MD

Carl Thornfeldt, MD

A special thank you to all the subjects of our esthetician profiles. You truly are testaments to success with your compassion for helping others and in raising the level of professionalism in our industry. We appreciate all that you do!

Suzanne Greene, LE

Melissa Siedlicki, LE, CIDESCO

Anne Martin, LA, CIDESCO

Louise Gray, RN, Beauty Therapist

Pamela Springer, LE

Jane Mann, LE

Debbie Caddell, RE, LE, CLS, CPE

Michelle D'Allaird-Brenner, LE, CIDESCO

Alex Cole, Beauty Therapist

Alex Leeder, LE

Gaynor Farmer, LE, CIBTAC

Terri Wojak, LE

Krista Bourne Rambow, LE

Ivana Querella, Beauty Therapist, Manicurist

I would also like to thank the Aesthetic Science Institute and the models who participated in the photo shoots.

Reviewers

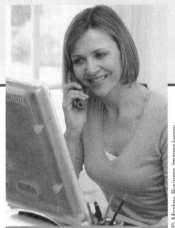

The author and publisher would like to thank the following professionals for their assistance and expertise in the preparation of the final product.

Stephanie Decosta, Skin Therapist/Education Leader, Paul Mitchell the School; Costa Mesa, CA

Ashley Duckworth, Head Educator, Paul Mitchell the School, Arlington, TX

Nichole Fox, Paramedical Esthetician, Assistant Instructor, Florida College of Natural Health, Coral Springs, FL

Larissa Harlbert, Esthetician and Lead Instructor, Bellus Academy, San Diego, CA

Lisa Ryan, Co-Owner, DermMania Inc., IL

Jasmine Sandhu, Esthetics Educator and Medical Educator, Medical Spa Owner, NV

Melissa Siedlicki, Esthetician, Esthetics/Medical Esthetics Instructor, Tacoma, WA

Madeline Udod, Esthetician, Bellport, NY

MILADY INFECTION CONTROL ADVISORY PANEL REVIEWERS

Barbara Acello, MS, RN, Denton, TX

Mike Kennamer, EdD, Director of Workforce Development & Skills Training, Northeast Alabama Community College

Leslie Roste, RN, National Director of Education & Market Development, King Research, Barbicide, WI

David Vidra, CLPN, WCC, MA, President

Dedication

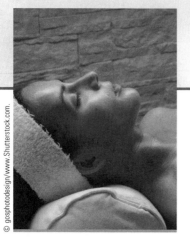

This book is dedicated to estheticians and skin therapists worldwide, as you are the "angels on Earth" who make a positive impact on the lives of those you serve every day.
Many blessings!

To my mother, Barbara Jean Howe Strickler:
Your love, wisdom, courage, and strength have allowed me to believe in my dreams and to make them come true.
God bless!

To my husband, Gary Deitz:
Thank you for your unrelenting love, support, and humor during the times of great rewards and the many challenging times, which have always provided great opportunities.
You are my hero!

Introduction

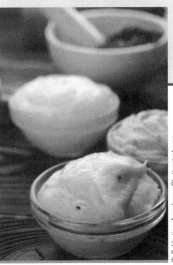

The state of affairs of esthetics and the esthetician has never been more interesting. We now have a paradox that has manifested over the last 10 years. We have a distinct vantage point today because of advanced technologies. We have more respect, more earning power, and more opportunities than we have had before. Advancements in technologies have required more education, knowledge, and technical ability—and of this we can be proud. The irony lies within the reality that we may not be able to use our education and training, as current state licensures may not allow the use of some technologies in states. As a call-out to all estheticians, we must continue to further our education. Those who are interested must serve on state boards and advisory committees in order to become involved in directing our future. It is imperative that we comply with our state licensing requirements and that we remain in compliance. We have a long way to go to standardize our education and training and become a united force. Our livelihood depends upon dedicated professionals' continuing to apply their knowledge, experience, and training to improve our industry and expand it beyond our current limitations.

Self-Care

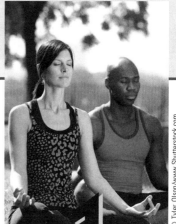

© Tyler Olson/www.Shutterstock.com.

> "Liken yourself to a beautiful, unique flower, delighting the world with your beauty and energy. A strong root system and water must be present in order to thrive. Therefore, we must connect daily with that refreshing, nurturing center, to pray, meditate, or visualize as this supports our life. This is the way that we discover our true essence and spread our light and energy in the world!"
>
> –*Brenda Lee Rogers, Wellness Trainer*

Chapter

Chapter Capture

After completing this chapter, you will be able to:

- Understand how much you matter.
- Recognize types of stress and stressors.
- Recognize how to manage stress.
- Manage your emotions.
- Understand how to flourish in your life.

SELF-CARE AS A TOP PRIORITY

While the topic of self-care should be at the top of our to-do lists, many estheticians and skin therapists often put it at the bottom. This is why this topic introduces the chapters in this book. We recommend the idea of self-care on a daily basis to our clients, yet at times we wait for certain symptoms before our attention to our own self-care becomes a priority (Figure 1–1).

As we have evolved on many levels in the past 20 years as professionals, it is interesting that many of us still engage in habits that plague us: not eating well, living with fear and anxiety, smoking, drinking too much, and definitely working too hard. Moreover, we are often the conduit that holds everything together in our lives. Unfortunately, many of us have people around us who drain us dry, whether financially, emotionally, or spiritually. The paradox lies in the fact that most of us have deep compassion for others and love to help people, yet often do not have our own needs met. This causes stress, resentments, and often burnout.

We have all experienced burnout on occasion. We are still trying to figure out how to let go of the systems, practices, processes, and people that no longer serve our best interests. This can be especially disheartening considering that when we try to make a move, we often jump back into the vortex from which we are trying to remove ourselves. "They won't let me go," we often hear in our heads. This may be true. Many of us stay in jobs, relationships, and conditions too long, which can be detrimental to our health. It is at a minimum a conditioned response. People need us, and we need to feel needed. It is an

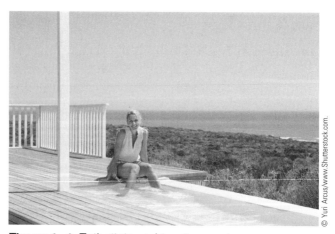

Figure 1–1 Esthetician taking time out.

enticing aspect to our psyche, and it can feed into our professional lives as well. We may also be attracting clients and people into our lives with problems that we cannot solve. This in turn may increase our stress levels and ability to cope.

TYPES OF STRESS AND STRESSORS

When we look at the concept of stress, we often think of it as a negative condition that depends upon our present circumstances, triggers, and stressors in our lives. Technically, there are two different types of stress. There is good stress, known as **eustress**, and bad stress, called **distress**. Eustress culminates in a positive result and its effects are often short term. We experience eustress when we prepare to make a speech, ask an employer for a raise, or experience the days leading up to our wedding. Eustress can enhance productivity, can increase a sense of well-being, and supply us with motivation needed to complete our goals in life. Distress, on the other hand, is the type of stress that we usually associate with generalized stress, which has a negative and cumulative effect. It tends to be chronic, and can pose health concerns that can lead to serious illness and death. Stress from a divorce, the death of a loved one, excessive weight gain, the abuse of alcohol and drugs are examples of conditions that can lead to distress.

Experts say that stress is a response to an event or perceived situation that ignites a reaction. A stressor is the trigger in the situation, which creates the stress response. There is a direct cause and effect relationship between the two. The stressor is the cause, and the stress is the effect. This explains why we may overeat or drink too much if we feel an abundance of stressors, which can trigger the response of stress itself.

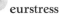 **eurstress**
Stress that culminates in a positive result is often short term. Eustress can enhance productivity, increase a sense of well-being, and supply the necessary motivation to complete goals in life.

distress
Associated with generalized stress, which tends to be chronic; can pose health concerns and has a negative and cumulative effect.

HOW TO MANAGE STRESS

In the text *Stress Management for Life, a Research-Based, Experiential Approach* (Cengage Learning, 2010), authors Michael Olpin and Margie Hesson ask us to look at perception in relationship to stress. They ask us to examine how much of our stress lies in our thinking or individual interpretation of an event. They suggest that it may be our own perception of the event or trigger that causes us to feel stressed. For example, how is it that one individual loves to make a presentation at an

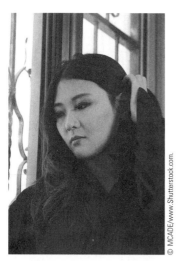

Figure 1–2 Certain events can create a certain level of stress.

esthetic conference while another feels stressed while trying to find a seat in the back row of a meeting at that same conference?

Science tells us that all facets of our personality, background, and early life experiences provide the training ground for how we interpret events, both positively and negatively. All of these factors shape how we deal with stress throughout lives. Much is known today about our ability to change how we perceive information and thus stop the progression of our stress becoming out of control.

Certainly, there are events that happen that can create an acute level of stress in one's life, such as suffering a horrible accident or being a victim of a crime (Figure 1–2). However, most of our day-to-day lives are often spent accumulating undue amounts of stress by reacting to perceived threats, which can trigger our emergency flight or fight mechanisms. These mechanisms date back to our early human needs for survival. These survival needs today are not as they were when we ran from wild animals, yet we retain the same stress responses as when we were in a constant fight for our existence. Stress begins to build in our minds and bodies if we have no release or strategy in place to reduce the build-up from responses. The key to reducing stress reactions and responses is to prevent them when possible.

Creating New Perceptions

The moment that we feel fear or a stress response, it is important to choose to mitigate the reaction by intervening with a redirect of the perception. Impacted by our own perceptions and self-talk, stress responses grow unless we make our self-talk positive or at least neutralize the negative.

Tips on how to redirect perceptions and interpretations of stressors appear in Table 1–1.

Keeping a Stress Journal

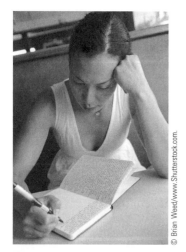

Figure 1–3 Keep a daily stress journal.

One of the ways to learn about your own stress triggers is to keep a daily journal of how your perceptions in life are affecting your stress levels (Figure 1–3). This will help you identify which type of stress you are dealing with on a regular basis. You will also be able to determine what type of support plan you need, whether it is for eustress (short term) or distress (long term and chronic). The latter may indicate a need for professional help with diet, exercise, or even therapy. Once you are able to recognize habitual stressors, you can make a

Table 1–1 Perceptions and Interpretations of Stressors

Stressor	My Stress Perception	Redirecting My Perception
A new esthetician is hired in the spa.	I might lose a client.	I am excited to get to know our new team member. Maybe we can refer clients to each other.
My new employee does not seem to be catching on fast enough.	I may have made a hiring mistake.	What do I need to give him or her in the way of support or training?
An educator has asked me to speak at their annual sales meeting.	I do not know this group; maybe I will not be well received.	I am going to ask a few questions about what he or she would like me to cover in my talk and share a couple of ideas with the educator to see if I am on target with my talk.
In a meeting, a colleague made a comment about my project being behind schedule and wondered if I needed help.	This seems like criticism; I am doing the best I can.	Perhaps the delivery of my project affects that individual's project ETA. Maybe we should have a separate meeting on this, just the two of us, and work it out.
I notice that one of the other estheticians seems to get all of the business in the salon.	It really makes me upset that I cannot seem to capture some of the clients that come in. Maybe I am just not cut out for this. I do work hard at it.	I am going to watch her more closely and see what she does that works for her. Maybe I can learn something. I am good at what I do but am still learning.
Our physician continues to ignore my requests for sending referrals my way in the clinic.	I think he is trying to keep all of the patients from me. This makes no sense, as I work for him.	Perhaps the doctor just gets busy and forgets that I can help him. I am going to ask him how I can be of more help with the patients so that we can retain them as clients for skin care and treatments.
A nurse in the medi-spa is especially abrupt and aggressive and seems to ignore me on purpose.	I feel so uncomfortable working with this woman. Every day is a struggle.	Maybe she has not figured out what my gifts are. Perhaps I should give her the benefit of the doubt and treat her to a facial. I can also ask her if she can give me tips to improve patient support.

© Milady, a part of Cengage Learning.

plan to remedy your responses to stress and redirect your perceptions. For example, if you find that every time a certain client comes in for service, you get angry or anxious or begin to shut down and feel sad, there may be a reason this is occurring. Your daily journal writing will give you valuable cues for helping yourself in your particular situation, and allow you to focus your energy on specific areas of concern.

You may not think that you have time to write or observe your thoughts, perceptions, and actions, but spending time feeling stressed out can rob you of valuable time as well. Give it a go.

Activity

Daily Stress Journal

Keep a daily stressor journal for one month. It need not be a long, drawn-out accounting of what you perceive to have stressed you out every day. Just spend 5 to 10 minutes answering these questions as objectively as possible. Look for patterns and commonalities in your documentation.

1. Where were you when you began to feel the stress?
2. What were your physical responses to the stressor? (i.e., rapid heartbeat, stomachache, dizziness, etc.)
3. Who or what was the cause of your stress?
4. How did you feel emotionally when the stress began?
5. What did you do to redirect your perception of the stressor?

Review your daily stress journal after one month. You will begin to see how you cope with your stressors and learn to prevent them from affecting your life.

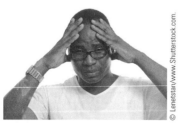

Figure 1–4 Worried about worrying.

STRESS AND WORK

How we think about things really affects our stress levels. For example, if you have outgrown an environment and feel that there is no chance to grow as an individual or professionally, it might be time to access your skills, update your résumé, and give yourself the gift of letting go and finding something new. Do keep in mind, however, that stressors and your response to them will exist at the next workplace, so do your homework. Determine what your triggers are and choose to prevent your own negative stress responses. Remember: we are everywhere we go.

Managing Emotions

Emotional stress has been written about and discussed since the beginning of modern times. This is specifically the stress that arises in response to worry, anger, fear, and anxiety. Worriers tell us that they cannot stop worrying, and many feel that worrying is hereditary. They worry about worrying (Figure 1–4). We often hear from worriers that their mothers, fathers, grandmothers, and other family members are all worriers too. Is worrying a learned condition (environmental) or hereditary?

The answer may lie somewhere in the middle. Genetics may play a role in the "worry gene," although it may not be fate. Just as those exposed to chronic worriers may exhibit characteristics of a worrier, their challenges with worrying, fretting, and thus feelings of anxiety can be redirected. Many of us feel a sense of control when we worry. We feel that if we worry about something that we are afraid of, we may be able to control it from existing, either internally or externally. The payoff in the worry cycle is that there is a physiological response to worry. **Fight or Flight responses** are activated when we worry and become anxious. This process stimulates a release of hormones such as cortisol. Cortisol is responsible for blood pressure regulation, immune function, and glucose metabolism which temporarily heightens our senses and provides a quick burst of energy. This energy gives us a false sense of action or control: we feel we can act upon a situation by either fighting or running. The problem is that neither fighting nor fleeing is necessary or appropriate, as worry is an abstraction in thought and has no basis for reality.

Chronic worry becomes a bad habit, and a default mechanism that we leap to when we sense a trigger—whether it comes from within or outside ourselves. By-products of worry become anger, fear, and ultimately anxiety as we move along the worry cycle. From anxiety, we can develop clinical conditions such as depression, phobias, and obsessive–compulsive disorders that may require more in-depth therapies to address, manage, and heal.

Anger, Fear, and Anxiety

Anger, fear, and anxiety are all fodder for emotional stress; they can be generated greatly by worry, and in some cases may be by-products of worry. The key to handling worrying and its by-products is to know that when we decide to worry, we remove ourselves from the present moment—which is where the power to change is located—and we deny the potential of a positive outcome. There are ways to manage and mitigate the effects of worrying. We can balance our lives by using the following methods:

- Creativity
- Education
- Mentorship/coaching/therapy
- Meaningful relationships
- Exercise
- Rest
- Vacations

Creativity

We are all born with creativity. It is not measured by societal standards, such as the representations of creativity that we see on the Internet, in magazines, at the theater, or in museums, but rather our own particular way of doing even the most routine things. It comes in many forms, such as the way we relate to another person, the colors and scents that we choose to apply both therapeutically and strategically in the treatment room, flower arrangements, cooking, or our own particular form of art. When we are in the state of creating, we connect to our intuition and spirituality, to our mental and emotional processes, and, of course, to our physical beings (Figure 1–5).

We need not look far to see creativity working as a healing agent. Breast cancer survivors relate stories of the creative expressions that helped them through the process from diagnosis to recovery: they wrote books, sang songs, and shared stories while dealing with their therapies. Others creatively help their families and friends cope with their illness through humor, kindness, and leadership. Evelyn Lauder of Estée Lauder and *Self* magazine can be credited for creative expression and support through their use of a pink ribbon to raise awareness and funding for breast cancer research; this has been expanded upon and still lives on today.

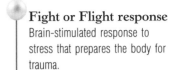

Fight or Flight response
Brain-stimulated response to stress that prepares the body for trauma.

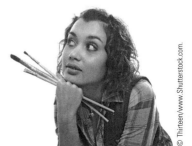

Figure 1–5 Find ways to express your creativity.

© Thirteen/www.Shutterstock.com.

Creativity is necessary for our mental and emotional health. By unlocking our creative energy, we allow flexibility, ingenuity, and adaptation into lives that may otherwise may be rigid, lackluster, and vacuous. Our problem-solving ability is fueled by creative expression just by the inherent nature of creating; we are always more open-minded when in a state of creating. When we allow our creativity to flourish, we are less apt to feel that the success of any one task, project, or experience determines our worth. While we are engaged in creating, matters resolve naturally, in an ebb and flow, like a cycle or season.

Education

Education is a fundamental aspect of caring for our mental health. If we think in terms of comprehensive education, we need to look at the entire picture, not just a few accents that will take us through the next season, or create a flurry of activity in our practices. We need to add the necessary components to our knowledge that will increase the value of what we know; for example, one idea might be to run some case studies on a new device or product that you have acquired, and take before and after photos along the way. Once you have obtained permission to use them from your client, you can share them with newer clients and have the case study published in a trade journal or magazine. This gives you more credibility in your work and demonstrates your knowledge and abilities as a practitioner. You will learn and teach in the process. The application of the education that we receive is vital for growth, and we become more in the process. (For more on education, review Chapter 2.)

Mentorship/Coaching/Therapy

We all need mentors. We often feel that we need to handle everything alone, or the hard way, but the truth is, until we are properly mentored, we do not have a sense of connectedness to a world larger than that of our own self-interest. Self-interest will carry us only so far and may be fraught with anxiety and self doubt. Ultimately, we need to view others and ourselves as connected and serving with intention and purpose for the greater good of all. This connectedness is found in both giving and receiving mentorship.

Finding an open-hearted, well-meaning life coach or therapist can prove to be beneficial on many levels, the least of which is in gaining a new perspective. For some, disappointments and unrealized goals may be a matter of focus and outlook. A trained support person in your life can assist in removing roadblocks and self-sabotaging habits and behaviors. Friends are wonderful for companionship; however, without the proper training; it can be difficult for a friend to offer the healthy support that we need.

Meaningful Relationships

Meaningful relationships are vital to the mental health of all estheticians. We deal with appearance, and self-esteem issues with our clients on a regular basis, and it is important to be able to step back and look at the world through a broader lens. Further, we know there is more to life than dealing with the latest moisturizing product, or obsessing about the lack of business last week. It is good to have friendships with others who are not related to the industry and who have a completely different orientation to work, and to surround ourselves with happy people. Happy can be a great choice in meaningful relationships.

Exercise

Exercise will increase our overall wellness and sense of well-being. This is due to the release of endorphins, our "feeling good" neurotransmitters that reduce the impact of stressors. The American Heart Association recommends 150 minutes of moderate exercise a week, which equals about 30 minutes a day, five days a week. You can break this up into 10- to 15-minute periods if that works out better with your schedule. The idea is to move the body and burn calories; this creates an aerobic environment, which increases oxygenation and respiration, and which is excellent for reducing stress and increasing stamina. By increasing stamina, we reduce tension and anxiety, which in turn supports our ability to rest and sleep. Ultimately, we are calmer (Figure 1–6).

Rest

Restful sleep can be challenging in the 24/7 lifestyle of today. Many of us are texting and/or passively or actively participating in some type of dialogue online well into the late hours of the evening. This activates the mind, which can disrupt the body's ability to operate with its

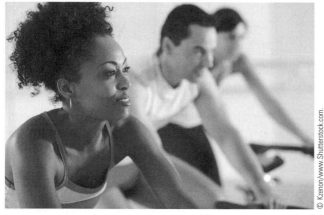

Figure 1–6 Exercise to maintain a healthy life.

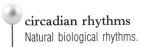

circadian rhythms
Natural biological rhythms.

natural **circadian rhythms** (natural biological rhythms), which it uses for rest and relaxation. Depending upon the individual need in terms of age, hormonal stage, and physical and mental condition, we require a consistent amount of sleep each night, which brings about the slowing of the physiological being and its systems. For decades, it has been recommended that we get at least eight hours of sleep for rest and rejuvenation; however, many of us are lucky to get five or six. A lack of sleep can contribute to the following health problems:

- Weight gain
- Lack of ability to concentrate
- Vulnerability to colds and the flu
- Lack of creativity and problem-solving ability
- Anxiousness, irritability, and lack of focus
- Increased risk of diseases, such as heart disease and diabetes
- Paranoia and other more serious mental health problems

If you have trouble getting to sleep, make certain that you share this with your physician or health care provider. Make certain to set the stage for a restful, peaceful sleep by applying these simple techniques to fall into a deep slumber:

- Sleep in a dark room (cover or remove all lights on electrical devices present in the room)
- Turn off the TV, computer, or cell phone
- Set a specific time for sleeping and awakening (the body loves routine)
- Avoid intense, emotional debates prior to going to bed
- Know that issues that have not been resolved today can be reviewed again tomorrow
- Avoid caffeine, alcohol, smoking, and **high-glycemic** (higher levels of sugar substances being absorbed into the bloodstream) foods prior to going to bed
- Make certain to exercise earlier in the day, not right before bedtime
- Meditate, pray, or journal write to lessen the "worry talk" right before bed

high-glycemic
Higher levels of sugar substances being absorbed into the bloodstream.

Remember to make appointments with yourself. Allowing enough sleep and rest is vital for a healthy, flourishing life. With all that you do for others, claim the best for yourself as well. If need be, make appointments for you, whether it be for rest, lunch, quiet time, exercise, or any other need that must be met. There is an old adage that states, "If it's to be, it's up to me." It truly is up to us to make it happen.

Vacations

Vacations are necessary. Take one! That means time away from work, home life, daily problems, money worries, everything. We do not need an expensive getaway, but we do need time for recharging and restoring our energy reserves. By not taking time away from routine practices, we can increase a burnout factor, and we can become less effective in all areas.

When planning a vacation, make certain to plan the type of vacation that you need. If you are in a highly competitive environment and need a break from it all, do not select a vacation with groups that value highly competitive sports and activities. Break it up with a nice beach walk, or take some alone time to read and be quiet. Look for a vacation that resonates as a respite, rather than time away where you will be taking care of someone or a group. This is your time; there will be plenty of time to share your wonderful gift of serving others.

WEB RESOURCES

For excellent, current health information, go to:
http://health.harvard.edu
www.health.discovery.com
www.webmd.com

 # FLOURISHING: YOUR BIRTHRIGHT

Famous physician, women's wellness advocate, and fabulous human being Christiane Northrup, M.D., describes in her book *Women's Bodies, Women's Wisdom* (3rd ed., Bantam Books, 2010) the importance of flourishing by imagining your future with a powerful vision, one which includes the inner guidance of body, mind, and spirit. She further states that our cells continue to replace and recycle everyday—which we estheticians and skin therapists know—and reminds us that we have completely new bodies every seven years. This brings new meaning to the idea of renewal, as our bodies want us to thrive. Within the notion of renewal comes flourishing. When we care for ourselves, we flourish. When we flourish, others flourish. Flourishing is one of the best gifts that we can give to the world.

How Do We Flourish?

The next most logical step is for us to think about what it takes to flourish, from a practical aspect. The term **flourishing** is defined in general as prospering, growing well, thriving, being successful, and being productive. We may think that we are all of these things and yet have resisted for some reason truly flourishing. Having a realistic and positive sense of self, along with confidence and self-esteem, are also congruent with flourishing. You have it within you to flourish.

To flourish, we often need to let go of old, limiting thoughts and behaviors that may have us captive. As with the stress information stated earlier, some of the reactions that we have to stressors may serve as indicators for what we need to do and clear up as we move forward. As we are growing and developing, the process is often two

 flourishing
Prospering, growing well, thriving, being successful and productive.

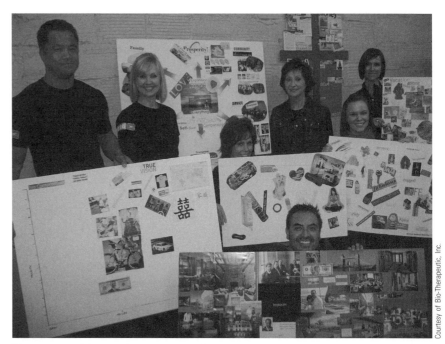

Figure 1–7 Team sharing vision boards.

steps forward and half a step back. This can happen at every age. Wise people and sages will tell us that it is normal to experience advancement and then mini or even major setbacks along the way. They are correct: we know that change in any realm and on all levels can take time. We share that human experience.

A straightforward, practical step toward flourishing is to envision your future. Take some time to create the ideal plan without any of the judgments that you have had in the past. Allow yourself to dream and imagine what is next in your life. Figure 1–7 presents an idea.

Build or Update a Vision Board

vision board
A visual accounting of ideas, hopes, and dreams of what we would like to have happen in our lives.

A **vision board** is a visual accounting of the ideas, hopes, and dreams of what we would like to see manifested in our life (Figure 1–8). We may think that we are too old, too sophisticated, or too beyond the need for a vision board. It is well known and documented, however, that creating a vision board with powerful words; imagery in the way of photos, sketches and artwork; charts and graphics, and even fabrics can draw us closer to the dreams, desires, and aspirations of both our conscious and unconscious mind. Another exciting aspect of building a vision board is that it may reveal an unconscious or hidden desire that you

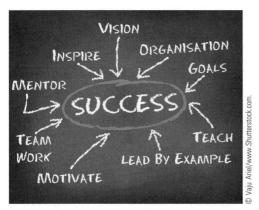

Figure 1–8 Create a vision board for success.

have that could take you onto an undiscovered trail leading to a new career path, lifestyle, or an unrealized talent. This is very exciting.

It is important to build a vision board in steps. To begin, find images, pictures, paintings, words, colors, fabrics, scents, poems, and other items that you may want to use. Cut them out of magazines or books, print them from Web sites, or look at other sources that yield interesting objects that have a profound effect on you when you look at them. The items that you use must stimulate an emotional response; otherwise, they will not generate a powerful result on your board. If an item gives you a ho-hum response, let it go. Find something that really moves you. Weed out a few of these items a week or two later if they are no longer relevant. Then begin to assemble and apply the items to your board. The size of the board can be of your choosing. Put your vision board in a space where you can see it easily every day, such as in your office or in a special place in your home. Remember: this is not just an exercise. Do it with gusto and you will be surprised at what it may bring to your life.

Vision Boarding

We recently developed a vision board for a women's conference for 200 women: the Northwest Women's Conference Healthy, Wealthy, and Wise. By conference standards, it was small; however, it was very personal and intimate. We selected a venue by the sea; it was a hotel with waterfront views from every room, catering capabilities, and an adjacent spa. We arranged for a high-end, local furniture store to bring in their luxurious furnishings and set up vignettes of furniture settings detailed to the point of including a perfectly coordinated throw and pillow for each chair or sofa.

The conference featured speakers from the health industry, financial services, and education. Vendors included skin care professionals, hair stylists, cosmetic surgeons, dentists, writers groups, fitness groups, yoga instructors, spa directors, dietitians, the Arthritis Foundation, educators, and a mammography center with breast education models.

Life coaches discussed courage, loss, and empowerment; financial planners discussed various personal and business-oriented financial planning options; educators spoke about lifelong learning; and home design specialists shared information about living well in your home. Not only was the event a sellout, but the women did not want to leave. During several speeches, there was not a dry eye in the space. We believed the success of the day was due to our conceptualizing of the event: we had built a vision board before we attempted to put our plan in place.

Give Thanks

We often do not give thanks to ourselves for all that we have accomplished in a day, week, month, or year. It is vitally important to acknowledge all of the planning, hard work, and execution that we have put into a task or realized goal. Make a plan to celebrate its completion with a reward, such as updating your wedding ring (restyling, getting a new one, adding a diamond or two), taking a day to be alone, or inviting friends over for a glass of champagne or tea in celebration of your accomplishment. Mark it in some way that is meaningful to you, without making it yet another task to accomplish.

When we rush from one project to another without giving proper gratitude, we can very easily become overwhelmed. The truth is, when projects begin to run together, we do not feel a sense of closure, and we begin all over again. This leads to burnout and dissatisfaction, both personally and professionally.

Give Thanks to the Staff

Gather your staff together to have a celebratory lunch, and give each staff member a hearty thank-you and a round of applause (Figure 1–9). Invite a vocalist to come sing a favorite ballad, or at holiday time to sing a few special songs. Tell your staff what they mean to you. Too often today, we see competitive environments in the workplace, which operate out of scarcity and fear. Healthy competition is good and natural, but when it takes over every meeting and conversation, it can be debilitating. Work to keep a positive and healthy attitude between yourself and your staff.

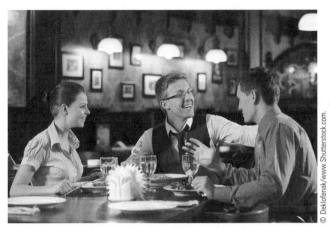

Figure 1–9 Take your staff out for lunch.

If you are a sole practitioner, make certain that your needs are met in ways that fuel your passion and give you the motivation and the accolades that you deserve for meeting your goals and running a successful business. Change your schedule one day a week so that you may have a morning off or can leave early on a typically lighter day. Clients will adjust, and as newer clients come in to your practice, they will pick up the difference if others cannot work it out.

Four-Day Workweek

While this might not seem like a good idea to some, it can be an excellent strategy for many. Many of us are interested in using extra day for education, or working one day as a volunteer to help expand our knowledge base and give back to our community. Serving in another capacity in a noncompetitive type of practice can be a great change. For example, if you are in a salon for four days, you could work in a clinic for one day. We have a staff member who works in a gift shop on an alternate day in order to add fun and variety to her life. Many of us enjoy the diversity; it keeps the passion alive, and we learn something to bring back into our primary position, whether it is new technique or a new customer service practice. Others might want the improved quality of life that one more day off per week may bring. Remember, the idea is to flourish and thrive, not feel buried and stuck. The bottom line: take time to enjoy the fantastic work that you do.

Manage Yourself Before Others

Many estheticians will put aside their own problems to help someone else with theirs. At face value, this may look quite noble. However, it can mean putting yourself at the bottom of the list. When we exhaustively help people strategize and plot a way in or out of a situation, it can be quite a time stealer. We may find that a colleague or friend does not take our advice, anyway. Ultimately, we have our problems at home to address. Whether they are problems at work, home, or in other areas of our life, it is best to work toward resolving our own issues first, and recognize that other people are equipped to handle their own.

Connect with Your Emotions

Have you ever had a parent, boss, or friend suggest that you should not feel a certain way? It is important to recognize that your health may depend upon the way that you feel. Not allowing feelings to surface creates many different types of blocks and unhealthy patterns. It may be that you are unable to discuss or process your feelings with present company, and you may require a visit with a good, objective friend or therapist. Feelings emerge for a reason. The way that we perceive a specific situation or incident may hold valuable information. Feelings provide a key to resolving a pattern, and more importantly, may be crucial to discovering the continual path to our growth.

YOUR HEALTH: SPIRIT, BODY, AND MIND CONNECTION

In 1948, the World Health Organization defined health in official records as follows: "Health is a state of complete physical, mental and social well-being and not merely the absence of disease or infirmity" (official records of the World Health Organization, no. 2, p. 100). This definition proves to be true today. We might also add a spiritual component to physical, mental, and social well-being, such as in mediation or prayer.

psychoneuroimmunology
Study of how the brain transmits signals along the nerves to stimulate the body's immune system.

The current research from the emerging field of **psychoneuroimmunology** (PNI) shows that there are clear and definite connections between the body and the mind. When the components are in balance, the systems cooperate to keep an individual free from disease and illness. For over 40 years, PNI scientists have studied the way that the brain transmits signals along the nerves to stimulate the body's immune system. Imagine immune cells, which create chemical signals called cytokines, sending signals to the brain. The brain then responds by unleashing neuropeptides to influence the immune system to act and protect the body. This communication is being relayed 24/7 to keep us alive.

When we add emotions to the equation, we also see a mind–body connection. In a practical sense, we have all experienced feeling slightly depressed while having the flu, or feeling bad after an argument that we had with a family member or coworker. We recognize the general malaise that these events bring to the psyche (Figure 1–10). This is a clear demonstration of a mind–body connection. When we look at the benefits of having a positive attitude and its ability to strengthen the immune system, we can also see the body's ability to fend off invaders, such as bacteria and viruses. It also leads to better health care: we are more apt to take the necessary steps to take better care of ourselves if we are emotionally sound and balanced.

Factor In Spirit

Spiritual well-being is as vital as the health of the physical or mental parts of our being, and the spirit, mind, and body are interrelated. With the expression of faith, courage, will, strength, hope, and love, we experience our spiritual being. Each of these contributes to the healthy mind and body. As we know, a spiritual connection will vary from person to person. It may mean following one's intuition, praying, attending a formal organized religious service, volunteering, or being in nature. Many of the struggles that we have today appear to be related to a lack of sense of purpose or place in the world. Having a connection to spirit can provide additional support when our happiness becomes slightly dim, as we know can occur (Figure 1–11).

Serving Our Purpose

There are as many beliefs about spirit as there are people in the world. We can add numbers to that exponentially if we add interpretations of spirit into the equation. For our purposes, we will look at that part

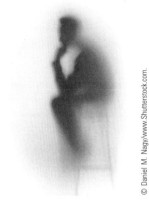

Figure 1–10 The mind–body connection.

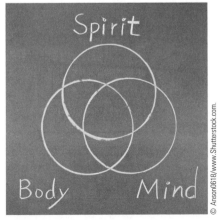

Figure 1–11 The spirit–body–mind connection.

of ourselves that is internal, eternal, and does not change with the whims of current popular culture or a specific trend or viewpoint. We will look at the part of our core being that knows how to be calm, has wisdom, and is connected to a place beyond the worldly issues that we deal with daily. This place is within each of us, and as mentioned, there are many pathways from which to arrive at this place, such as prayer, meditation, a walk on the beach or in the woods, listening to music, feeling grateful, volunteering, and a multitude of other ideas. The main point is that we get to that place of calm, knowing, and have faith that our purpose in life exceeds our current circumstance and that we are here to provide a beacon of light and hope for those around us.

As estheticians, we know this to be at the core of our work with clients, and that the business of our work lives is a vehicle to this most important mission. The more complete we feel in our purpose, the more apt we are to meet the challenges within and without. With our purpose intact, we help people, and we need never forget what we are here to do. It is simple when you think of it this way; the rest of our problems can serve as fuel to inspire us when we are serving our best purpose.

SUMMING IT UP

We need to be clear about our own self-care, as we recommend it to our clients. We must know we matter, because if we cannot care for ourselves, how we will care for others? This notion will prove invaluable in our choosing work environments, projects, employees, employers, vendors, friends, colleagues, and even life partners. Here are five key points regarding self-care for the esthetician or skin therapist:

- We need to take excellent care in all matters that concern our lives, and keep in mind that we will do our best when balanced in *spirit, body, and mind.*
- Stress and stressors are mitigated and manageable when we learn or relearn how to understand our own triggers and to change our perceptions when necessary.
- Worry is useless, negative self-chatter. It is not real. My friend and teacher Brenda Rogers, a life coach and spiritual advisor, states that fear stands for "false evidence appearing real." Do not let fear define or confine you.
- Flourishing is your birthright. We have come to this planet to expand our horizons, to love others in the process, and to serve our purpose with zeal! Expect the best.
- What we do for ourselves, we teach others to do for themselves. Lead by example.

ESTHETICIAN **PROFILE**

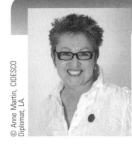

© Anne Martin, CIDESCO Diplomat, LA.

Anne Martin, LA
CIDESCO Diplomat

Licensed Aesthetician and Instructor; Reiki Master; Sole Proprietor, Anne Martin Skin Care Center, Seattle, WA

I was born in Brooklyn, New York, and attended high school in New Jersey. I went to nursing school for six months before moving to Boston, Massachusetts, at age 20. I graduated *magna cum laude* from the University of Massachusetts, majoring in English with a concentration in religious studies and women's studies. I lived on a kibbutz for nearly six months, where my job was milking sheep. I lived in a meditation center for five months and was ordained as a Buddhist nun. I attended Harvard Divinity School for several semesters, concentrating on Buddhist studies and early Christianity, and then attended and graduated from the Elizabeth Grady School of Esthetics. I became a licensed aesthetics instructor in Boston. I taught both theory and practical applications to aesthetic students. I alternated between teaching and salon work.

Training

In 1986, I graduated from the Elizabeth Grady School of Esthetics in Boston, having taken a 900-hour course. I became a licensed instructor within the first year of my studies. I worked in one of the Grady salons and taught theory in the Boston school, where I was also executive coordinator for a time. I studied Reiki in 1988, and received my second degree in the mid 1990s. In 2010, I became a Reiki master practitioner.

In 1990, at age 45, I moved to Seattle. I received a CIDESCO diploma that year and received the first instructor's license offered solely in aesthetics by Washington State. I studied the Dr. Vodder method of manual lymph drainage in both basic and advanced courses and obtained diplomas for both.

Practice Demographic

I specialize in treatments for acne and age management.

The average age of my clients is 40 and above. What I find marvelous is that many of my clients have brought in their children, who have become loyal clients.

Services/Treatments Offered

I offer classic facials and what I call "treatments" (designed for clients with acne). I use the following modalities and techniques: microcurrent LED, galvanic; high frequency; specialty lift-off treatments and masks, vapozone, enzymes, light and superficial peels, extractions, and massage. I offer Reiki, especially to clients who are going through chemotherapy.

Keeping up with advancements is expensive, never-ending, and a completely necessary part of the profession. Selecting those treatments that deliver results, *sustained* results, is my goal. As with many aestheticians, I hear about products or machines from others, I read about them, or the product representatives fills me in. It's a treatment plan, along with visits twice a week for acne, and at-home products that make the most difference in skin care.

Personal Philosophy

I believe that aestheticians work hard to help clients feel better about their skin, which in turn deeply affects how they move through their lives. We bear witness to the lives of others, to events ranging from weddings and births, to a cancer diagnosis and treatment, to divorce, to loss, and to death. We listen to the stories clients tell us, offering empathy and kindness; we deeply understand the suffering acne causes and the fears aging stirs up.

Clients not only look better, but they *feel* better after being with us. Meaning is found in that. I had never known the true value of a facial, and how its simple touch, without judgment, could be so profoundly affecting, before I became an aesthetician and realized the human connection that aesthetics facilitates. Ultimately, it is our own lives as well as those of the clients where a difference is made.

Lecturing feeds my spirit; reaching out to other aestheticians to talk about our work energizes me. Writing does that as well: It is all about the "handshake," the offering of the self.

Additional Contributions to the Industry

I founded the Northwest Aestheticians' Guild (NWAG) in 1994, with the idea of bringing aestheticians together to talk and share and learn. From the beginning, I have had invaluable "couldn't-do-it-without-them" help from a few dedicated colleagues. NWAG offers monthly lectures in Seattle from experts in a wide variety of fields, sponsors day-long classes, and offers a three-day course in the Dr. Vodder method of manual lymphatic drainage.

I began attending the State Advisory Board for Cosmetology, Barbering, Manicuring and Esthetics at its inception in the early 1990s. I was then appointed to the board, and have now served many terms on it. The last several terms, I have served as the chair.

I have spoken on aesthetics at the Face & Body Conference several times (San Francisco, San Jose, and Chicago). SKIN, Inc. has published several of my articles.

With Dr. Mark Lees, I cofounded the Institute of Advanced Clinical Esthetics in 2001 in Seattle, where, along with guest lecturers from around the country, we taught and offered advanced education for licensed aestheticians. Dr. Lees and I also founded the Seattle Skin Care Symposium, where we offer an annual day of education on a variety of topics in advanced education. Over the years, I have offered (and still do) lectures in Seattle and beyond, specializing in massage relating to the acne client, the aging client, empathy in aesthetics, and sales and service.

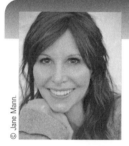

ESTHETICIAN **PROFILE**

Jane Mann, LE
Skin Works, Las Vegas, NV

True Dentistry, Joseph Willardsen, DDS

I was born in Quincy, Illinois, and graduated from the University of Iowa in 1988. I am 45 years old and have been an esthetician in Las Vegas, Nevada, for five years.

My background is in market research and statistics, which is an unemotional approach to products. My mind has been trained to categorize, divide, and look at products with a 360-degree perspective. In my past work, once the data had been processed, I would determine whether the consumers wanted the product, and if so, how to present the product in a way that was attractive for the consumer to buy. This perspective has helped me in the aesthetic field. To a manufacture/marketing company, the beauty industry is based on hope. As badly as women want to be beautiful, estheticians want to deliver beautiful skin to their clients. We all have questions, such as, How do you determine which machines work, which are better? The answer is "knowledge." I became an esthetician because I love problem solving. Whether it is math or fine lines, with the proper data you can solve both problems.

I also entered the esthetics field as a second career because of the flexibility of hours, as well as the opportunity to create my own opportunities.

Along the way, I have had some wonderful opportunities and experiences working with physicians in areas of my interests. I wanted to learn more about acupuncture points in the face and how we might use them with microcurrent therapy. With that in mind, I worked with Dr. Starwynn, dipl. Ac. OMD. Before that, I worked with Dr. Rebecca Fitzgerald, dermatologist and learned about how the face ages from a physician's perspective and belief system. From dermatologist Dr. Jason Michaels, I learned where he places Botox® and how I can use that information when applying microcurrent. Dr. Chan, taught me about temporomandibular joint (TMJ/TMD) dysfunction, which is the musculoskeletal dysfunction of the head and neck, and occlusal disorders. I have also studied craniomandibular orthopedics combined with a neuromuscular approach to therapy.

Training

My education, beyond esthetics school, has been 100 percent self-motivated. I have taken the initiative to look up mentors in areas that I want to specialize in, and dedicated the time to learning with them. In my specific case, I have always been fascinated by microcurrent therapy. It combines my science and research background with beauty. I also love that it is a frontier that has not been explored completely or understood by many estheticians. As my knowledge base has grown, more doors have opened for me.

At one point in my career, I had rented a room in a dental office that specialized in neuromuscular dentistry. I learned that microcurrent therapy helps relieve the tenderness and tightness associated with TMD (temporomandibular joint disorder). TMD is a condition where the temporomandibular joint (TMJ) becomes inflamed primarily due to the grinding of one's teeth. This occurs to the point that the teeth wear down, forcing the bite to close in a way that is not comfortable for the joint in the jaw. I also specialize in acne treatments.

Practice Demographic

My practice demographic is primarily women, ages 30 to 72, typically Fitzpatrick 1 to 5. Many of my clients are concerned about aging and looking for a more natural approach to aid in their process.

Services/Treatments Offered

I offer microcurrent therapy, mild exfoliation, and acne treatments and regimes. I choose microcurrent therapy because it is supported by scientific facts. As more and more research is conducted, I am in awe of the possibilities of this therapy. In fact, I think 95 percent of my clientele gets some type of microcurrent treatment (unless there are contraindications) in a facial. In conjunction with that, I create a skin rejuvenation plan that consists of products geared especially for their skin type and condition.

Services Offered

Microdermabrasion

Microcurrent

Intensive peels and micro peels

IPL

LED

Specialized acne treatments

Personal Philosophy

I love what I do, and that keeps me on a constant track to learn more and stay on top of current trends, research, and breakthroughs. I am very open-minded and not afraid to create something that has not been done before. I have always felt that opportunity is where you create it. I once approached a highly respected cosmetic dentist in my area, and he rented me a room so that I could provide clients with skin care treatments. I was very fortunate because he shared my vision and was also open-minded. That does not mean that people still don't wrinkle their noses and say "I have never heard of an aesthetician in a dental office." However, I am glad, because regardless if I am in a dental office or a retail location, clients still have skin concerns and want to look nice. It is a perfect fit.

Additional Contributions to the Industry

I am NCEA certified. I am developing a class on a nonmanufacture-specific perspective on microcurrent technologies and techniques. With the collaboration of Dr. Willardsen, I am also developing a treatment protocol to meet the needs of TMD clients using microcurrent therapy. I donate time every third Saturday of the month to provide facials and makeup through the Dress for Success program for women on a limited income.

Education:
The Foundation
of Esthetics

> "The difference between an esthetician who 'does facials' and an esthetician who 'practices skin care' is that esthetician's level of education."
>
> *−Mark Lees, PhD, MS, CIDESCO Diplomat*

Chapter 2

Chapter Capture

After completing this chapter, you will be able to:

- Look at esthetics as a second, third, or fourth career.
- Understand the concepts of learning styles and multiple intelligences.
- Appreciate that the brain can continue to learn at any age.
- Recognize that distractions and information overload are impediments to learning.
- Find solutions for building brain capacity.
- Understand adult learning and its requirements.
- Recognize the globalization of esthetic education as well as understand esthetic organizations and their role in education.

LEARN, RELEARN, AND REVIEW BASIC ACADEMIC EDUCATION

The more comprehensive and interdisciplinary our primary, secondary, and postsecondary education is, the more apt we are to make the necessary connections in life. These connections and building blocks will allow us to continue to learn, prosper, and feel rewarded and satisfied with our work as estheticians. Formal and academic educational experiences bring to the individual skills for lifelong learning and the necessary foundation to assimilate information. This then becomes applied knowledge.

Academic disciplines such as the sciences provide multiple opportunities to develop as estheticians. A background in chemistry is beneficial for product knowledge, understanding ingredients, and performing peels; knowledge of anatomy/physiology is important in the understanding and use of technology, massage, and general esthetic applications; and an understanding of skin physiology supports learning about product delivery systems and product penetration. Furthermore, an understanding of nutrition helps in assessing

GUEST SPOT

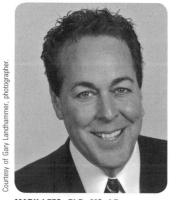

Courtesy of Gary Landhammer, photographer.

MARK LEES, PhD, MS, LE, CIDESCO Diplomat

With all the advancements in skin science, technology, and esthetic treatment, it is imperative that estheticians receive as much science-based education as they can. Not only is the profession becoming more technically advanced, but the skin care consumer is becoming more educated about skin care. If an esthetician is not well read or up on the latest esthetic techniques and skin science, he or she will not continue to succeed in the profession. Well-educated consumers want well-educated professionals.

I would love to see the day when esthetics becomes a full college program requiring background courses in biological sciences and chemistry as well as business and communication skills. There is no doubt in my mind that estheticians who have college degrees in addition to sound professional skin care training are more successful.

skin health, and a background in electronics and electricity in general helps one learn about new devices, which are now mainstream in continuing education for estheticians and necessary for practice growth.

It is a new world for estheticians. In the early days of esthetics training, we may have browsed though sections in a textbook, practiced our massage techniques, and learned the basics of what we now call infection control in order to pass the state board exam. Today, we work in a variety of environments that range from being hands-on as an esthetician in the treatment room, to working as a developmental director for an esthetic journal. Many of us are involved in the research and development of devices, products, and ingredients along with systems and esthetic programs (Figure 2–1). We need to know how to take a concept all the way to the marketplace and how it will function in actual practice. We collaborate with chemists, research scientists, engineers, writers, editors, MDs, PhDs, and EdDs; many estheticians have these designations after their names as well, or will in the future.

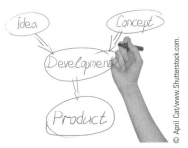

Figure 2–1 Estheticians in product development.

In considering esthetic education from a broad perspective, it becomes important to look at learning as a continual process that runs throughout one's career, whether it is preparatory classes for beginning esthetic students or for seasoned veteran esthetic professionals. It often surprises educators that professionals will pass up classes that they deem below their level because they have been practicing for 25 years. They want something "new," despite not knowing much about anatomy and physiology or the fundamentals of cosmetic chemistry. This becomes challenging later, when clients know as much as estheticians because of the Internet, their own academic studies, online seminars they have attended on skin care and plastic surgery, and classes and webinars they have taken. This happens to all of us at some point, hence the need for a routine assessment of our knowledge.

Take an Esthetics Class

It is always useful to take basic classes for review, whether they are online or in an actual classroom. Basic information is presented differently today; it is reorganized in such a way that we often find we missed something in the first place, years ago. A long-term licensed esthetician attended one class recently and found that she had been applying a device incorrectly for 20 years! Her clients had not been fully benefitting from the treatment; had she not taken a basic technology course, she would not have discovered her error.

Both new and experienced estheticians benefit from combining learning efforts,. In the classroom, educators appreciate both the enthusiasm of the new esthetician and the experience and knowledge of the veteran esthetician.

Brush Up on the Basics

It is a good idea to take an academic class in English, writing, or math, on occasion, just to retool and freshen up on some fundamentals (Figure 2–2). There are wonderful classes at technology institutions and community colleges that can bring us up to speed in these areas if it has been a while since we were in school. Many estheticians are interested in moving into new career pathways and expanding their presence in the industry. Every day, we hear from practitioners who are unsuccessfully trying to find new jobs in the esthetic profession (to move up, so to speak). They often become discouraged. But if they did due diligence in these areas of their education to update and improve their skill sets, they would be in demand. **Globalization**, which is considered a worldwide movement toward integrating cultures, communication, business, and trading, brings a variety of opportunities for estheticians and provides more education. Globalization will ultimately help our industry in the areas of professionalism, respect, and value in business and communications, and further set the stage for anyone who is serious about advancing his or her career.

globalization
a worldwide movement toward integrating cultures, communication, business, and trading.

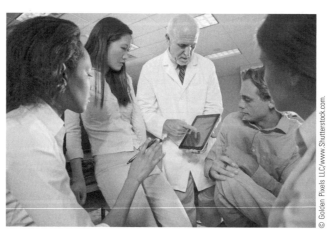

Figure 2–2 Brush up on your basic academics.

© Golden Pixels LLC/www.Shutterstock.com.

Case Study

An esthetician became so disgusted with her job in a salon—she was tired of the petty politics, favoritism shown by her employer, and family dynamics that existed—that she decided to sign up for a class. She hoped this would help her move on in her career. She registered for a course in human resources at her local community college in order to gain a foundation in business and to increase her knowledge of how to deal with personnel issues. She did not know exactly what she would learn in the class, but at a minimum, it would provide a distraction so that she could survive at her current location until she found something new. Her intuition directed her to follow this path. She went to class two evenings a week for two months. Many nights she did not want to go; she worked tirelessly at her job during the day and continued to feel dejected and frustrated about her work situation.

As the weeks went by, she began to learn more about the legalities of personnel issues and began to apply her new knowledge to her job. She learned that there were in fact areas of opportunity at her current location. She also recognized a few safety violations. She became more of an observer, however, and thought hard about her next position rather than trying to fix her current situation. It was her career that she was interested in helping. Once she completed her course, she decided to take a class in marketing and business planning, which she found very interesting. She also began attending online classes about peels, esthetic technologies, and product ingredients. Within three months, a colleague, who was a manager of an outpatient clinic, approached her to interview for the manager position in a new skin care center. The medical team was delighted with her, and she was hired. Within six months, she was seeing patients, managing the skin care center, learning the business from the inside out, and involved in long-range planning and development for the clinic.

Had she not taken these classes, she would still be unhappy in her old job at the salon and looking for somewhere else to go. This was a great outcome, and within the realm of possibility for anyone willing to grow in order to make a positive change in his or her work life (Figure 2–3).

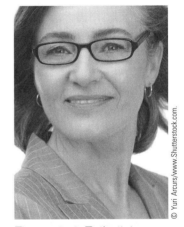

Figure 2–3 Estheticians as clinic managers.

 # ESTHETICS AS A SECOND, THIRD, OR FOURTH CAREER

As discussed in many esthetic articles, a great number of individuals are entering the field as a second, third, or even fourth career. Many are looking for the opportunity to follow their passion, which drives most skin care professionals. Due to downsizing, economical resets globally, and the necessity to reorganize priorities, many newcomers feel that they finally have a chance to do work that they will love to do. This group, who are entering the field in their 30s, 40s, 50s, or 60s, clearly demonstrates that education and learning continue throughout life. Many come to the field of esthetics not only with a passion for it, but with a science or business background. Out of the gate and with many years of experience behind them, they plan to open their own business. This can put more pressure on educators to expand their knowledge base, as these new students are astute and have been successful in other careers. They demand our best.

Older, experienced students may be in an esthetics course to become licensed practitioners and to acquire the skill necessary to serve as a skin therapist; however, their plans may be centered more around lifelong learning rather than being a treatment room esthetician. Many are planning to start their own businesses and are less concerned with trying to plug into a spa, salon, or medical office. Some are licensed massage therapists, cosmetologists, and manicurists and want to add esthetics to broaden their professional options. Others want to teach esthetics or work in research and development or as beauty editors; some plan on working in lifestyle centers as managers of spas and salons that will accommodate the millions of baby boomers who are now beginning to retire (and who will continue to retire for the few decades).

This bodes well for our profession. When life-experienced new estheticians begin to make their debut, it raises the bar for all of us— even though they too will have their challenges (Figure 2–4).

Challenges for Older Students Who Are Learning New Technologies

In this age of technology, we practitioners must be willing to expand our present knowledge in order to be successful. For older students, it can be challenging to learn in the newer IT age. Older students require more in-depth information to make the necessary, systematic connections that will give them a sense of proficiency and ultimate mastery of material. In some cases, older learners fall short of the agility and confidence that it takes to learn new technology. They need to be brought along accordingly by respectful esthetic instructors who possess a healthy understanding of learning styles and depth and breadth of theories and practical applications.

Challenges for Younger Students

Younger students face unique issues plaguing their generation. They have grown up with technology, so they have a clear and decided advantage when learning new applications. However, there is some

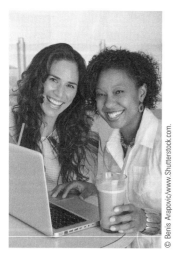

Figure 2–4 Take on esthetics as a second or third career.

© Benis Arapovic/www.Shutterstock.com.

cause for concern in esthetic education, as younger students' learning has been in shorter bites, with some information highlighted in bullet points that can be quickly scanned. Students may then lack a complete understanding of how a theory or practical application actually works. This makes it difficult for them to problem solve, think critically, and in some cases to stay with a task, as they can become easily distracted in favor of the next great idea generated by a group. Social networking is another strong distraction (Figure 2–5).

Whether we are over or under 40, the underlying truth is that we must continue to learn. The more we know about a subject, the more connections we make and the greater our need for more knowledge. Pre- and postgraduation esthetic classes today are filled with individuals of all ages, learning styles, and challenges. This poses special issues for esthetic educators as well as for the student, whether it is a well-seasoned licensed esthetician or a new student just starting out. Much of the accountability and responsibility falls on us, the learner, as we need to know how we learn and to position ourselves to be successful in a variety of learning environments.

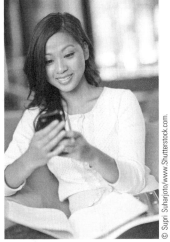

Figure 2–5 Many younger generations can be distracted by social networking.

LEARNING STYLES AND THE MULTIPLE INTELLIGENCES

Recognizing learning styles—both our own and those of others—becomes important to the esthetician at all levels, whether in the treatment room dealing with a client, or in the esthetic classroom. Understanding how people learn relates to how they receive information and how they communicate. People tend to receive information based on their learning style and within their own intelligence inclinations. Each individual may have more than one learning style, but one or two may predominate when the person is learning something new or taking in information.

In 1983, **Howard Gardner, PhD**, psychologist, and professor of education at Harvard University, developed a theory called **multiple intelligences (MI)**. Gardner's theory suggests that there are eight different pathways to learning, which may incorporate a more comprehensive approach to teaching: 1) **linguistic intelligence**, an ability with words or language; 2) **logical-mathematical intelligence**, reasoning capabilities and scientific thinking and investigation; 3) **spatial intelligence**, an ability to visualize through the mind's eye; 4) **bodily-kinesthetic intelligence**, control of one's bodily motions and the capacity to handle objects skillfully; 5) **musical intelligence**,

Gardner, Howard, PhD
Harvard professor who developed the theory of multiple intelligences.

multiple intelligences
A theory created by renowned psychologist Howard Gardner, PhD, that delineates eight different types of intelligence that people possess.

linguistic intelligence
Facility with words and language.

logical-mathematical intelligence
Exceptional ability with numbers and logic.

malleable
Brain's ability to adjust according to new information and situations in the environment.

spatial intelligence
Ability to arrange objects in space or to visualize a process before it takes place.

bodily-kinesthetic intelligence
Excellence in physical movement; an individual who demonstrates this intelligence needs a "hands-on" approach to learning.

musical intelligence
Above-average ability in music; someone who responds to rhythm and sound.

interpersonal intelligence
Talent for dealing with people; higher than usual amount of compassion and emotional depth.

intrapersonal intelligence
Great self-knowledge and self-awareness.

naturalistic intelligence
Strong ability to interact with the natural world.

a natural ability with rhythm, sounds, and music; 6) **interpersonal intelligence**, an ability to understand others; 7) **intrapersonal intelligence**, an understanding of the self; and 8) **naturalistic intelligence**, relating information to one's natural surroundings. Many of us struggle with material that is presented in a statistical or mathematical format (logical-mathematical) for example, and may find blocks or obstructions to assimilating that information. Using the theory of MI, one might take that same information and create a graphic (for visual learners), or write a story about what is being presented (for linguistic learners). This may allow learners to connect with the material quickly and expand upon it as well.

Gardner's theory of eight primary intelligences is defined as follows:

- **Linguistic intelligence**: excellence in the use of words. Writers, teachers, and politicians tend to have linguistic intelligence. Such individuals like to express themselves in writing and favor the use of words in communication (as opposed to gesturing, for example). This individual will want to write and use words while learning. Maya Angelou and Jane Austin are two examples of people with linguistic intelligence.
- **Logical-mathematical intelligence**: exceptional ability with numbers and logic. One is comfortable using statistics, graphs, numbers, and a logical sequence of events to apply learning, understanding, and expression. Physicians, accountants, and engineers have logical-mathematical intelligence. Albert Einstein and Bill Gates are two examples of people with logical-mathematical intelligence.
- **Spatial intelligence**: visually oriented individuals with the ability to move objects in space (as in their mind), or able to visualize something before it is realized. This individual will want to visualize something while learning. Artists, designers, and architects possess spatial intelligence. Michelangelo and Rembrandt possessed spatial intelligence.
- **Bodily-kinesthetic intelligence**: excellence in physical movement. A kinesthetic learner needs a "hands-on" approach to learning (this is true of most estheticians). Women's soccer player Abby Wambach and New York Yankees pitcher Mariano Rivera are two superb examples of people with bodily-kinesthetic intelligence.
- **Musical intelligence**: a high level of musical intelligence. This inclination toward musical intelligence present itself when individuals learn and express themselves through rhythm and sound. Mozart and Ella Fitzgerald were endowed with musical intelligence.

- **Interpersonal intelligence**: demonstrates strength in dealing with people and emotional maturity. This is also known as emotional intelligence. Individuals with this type of intelligence are understanding and compassionate, and express those qualities in their learning and communication styles. Oprah Winfrey and Deepak Chopra possess emotional intelligence.
- **Intrapersonal intelligence**: great self-knowledge and self-awareness. These individuals will also exhibit self-confidence. "Know thyself" is their motto. Gandhi, Buddha, and Abraham Lincoln are all examples of people who possessed intrapersonal intelligence.
- **Naturalist intelligence**: strong ability to interact with the natural world. These people communicate with and work in nature. Charles Darwin, Jane Goodall, and Steve Irwin are examples of naturalists who possess naturalist intelligence.

Gardner's theory has been implemented in varied educational settings in order to maximize learning potential. Most of the information communicated by our culture today appeals to the linguistic and logical-mathematical intelligences. The Internet has improved access for many learners by presenting images, graphics, and multiple forms of media to teach various topics. Many who have struggled in the past with dry explanations or minimal instruction sheets (government documents, business forms, and other tools that have been difficult to follow come to mind) are now able to learn and understand through pictures and videos and audio options.

Knowing what our particular learning styles and intelligences are can be used as a tool to determine our strengths. This knowledge can be beneficial to estheticians in business, in communications, at home, and, most of all, in self-discovery. It can also help in team building to understand the strengths and natural tendencies of colleagues and coworkers. When we understand the gifts and talents that we bring to the workplace, it can serve as a bridge to creating a more cohesive working environment.

THE BRAIN AND LEARNING AT ANY AGE

In understanding learning styles and multiple intelligences, it is not too big of a leap to look deeper into the learning process to see how the brain learns. What scientists know about learning from studies of **brain plasticity** (also known as neuroplasticity) is that our brains are wired to learn. If they were not, we would not be able to learn new skills, have new thoughts, or even to learn how to use a smartphone.

brain plasticity
The idea that the human brain is wired to learn; also known as neuroplasticity.

In *Cognitive Neuroscience*, 3rd ed., by Marie Banich and Rebecca Compton (Cengage Learning, 2011), brain plasticity is defined as the brain's ability to reorganize itself by forming new nerve cells (neurons) and creating connections throughout life (Figure 2–6). The nerve cells can adjust according to new information and situations in our environment through the brain's flexibility.

Everything we do and think shapes our brain. Psychiatrist and neuroscientist Norman Doidge, the author of *The Brain That Changes Itself*, states that the notion of brain plasticity is of great interest to students and educators of all types. There is a great deal of research showing that our brains want to learn and that we can develop a greater capacity for learning by growing neurons and brain cells, forming new synaptic connections. Just as our muscles like to move, our brain likes to learn. The brain operates on a "use it or lose it" model; neurons fire quickly and in turn want to fire even faster. They then begin to build brain capacity. Doidge further states that it is important to increase the RAM and memory in our own brains rather than only focusing on our computers as an outside source of RAM and memory. It is often enticing to rely on our computers, smartphones, iPads, PowerPoint presentations, and other outside devices to serve as a backup for our memory. Neuroscientists believe that it is best for us to use and train our brains and memory to expand our neural networking, which will help us retain memory later in life.

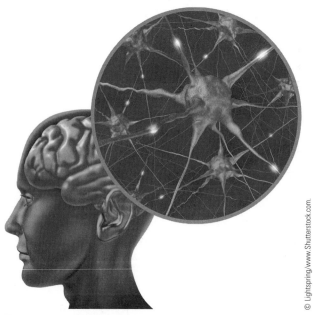

© Lightspring/www.Shutterstock.com.

Figure 2–6 Brain and neuron.

DISTRACTIONS AND INFORMATION OVERLOAD TODAY

We often feel like our brain is in gridlock, or we have trouble turning off the incessant thoughts despite our best efforts to calm and quiet them, even for just a few moments. We see this in our clients: they give us a vacant stare when we begin to explain something or may give an instant redirect to another topic altogether.

People face so many distractions between e-mails, text messaging, computer work, spreadsheets, Web sites—the list is endless. Today, with information being given in small chunks at a time, we have become accustomed to looking at symbols and short spurts of information (Figure 2–7). Our brains are being bombarded continually with trivial pieces of information that are often driving the marketplace; we are directed to purchase but do not really understand the information in a comprehensive way. After a full day of being overwhelmed by imagery, we may feel fatigued.

Sadly, the brain is often being trained to give up our current thought and move on to the next distraction. As esthetic instructors, salon, spa, and clinic managers, we see this in the questions that students or employees may ask during a lecture or a meeting. Often a query will come out of seemingly nowhere, and then we all race to serve that distraction in the moment. It is insidious, as educators and managers become caught up in the new question and strive to provide an answer. There was a time when we used to say, "You are getting ahead of us here, let's stay on track and we will visit this later" rather than jumping off of the current discussion or plan.

As students, employees, or coworkers, we may find it difficult to keep up with our instructors or team leaders in lectures and meetings because our brains are unused to staying on topic for any length of time. We have become accustomed to constant change and the introduction of new information, which may not have anything to do with the topic at hand. For instructors and students, for managers and employees, distraction is the current culture; it is creating difficulty for real learning and the acquisition of knowledge.

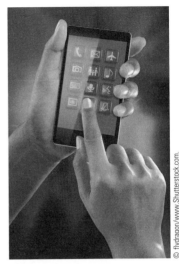

Figure 2–7 Today's adult receives information in short bursts.

 # SOLUTIONS FOR BUILDING BRAIN CAPACITY

When the brain is treated properly, it is freed up to absorb information and to learn. Building brain capacity, is best done by providing focused, educational programs that have depth, and a clear direction. Doidge describes that when we are able to strengthen and expand our brain's capacity, we gain access to skills and thus feel liberated.

It is important that educators, students, and trainers of any type vary their lesson plans and learning endeavors to include more challenging aspects of educational experiences rather than quick-study models and action points. This will build a stronger network in the brain. This type of teaching and learning may appear to take more time; however, in such a deliberate approach, we learn more thoroughly, assimilate (understand) information more readily, and better understand the building blocks of a specific technology, communication, or a science discipline.

There is a solid argument for being able to resist many of the distractions of the current culture by providing our brain with a solid learning experience that reduces distraction. In some cases, this may be as simple as turning off cell phones, e-mail, and other interruptions in the learning environment; staying on task for small periods of time; and then expanding that time in increments.

Blending Art and Science

Great instructors blend art and science, such as Garnis Armbruster-Ollivierre, CIDESCO Diplomat and long-term vocational-certified educator in esthetics and cosmetology. Armbruster-Ollivierre holds a bachelor's degree in psychology and has enjoyed developing multisensory learning pedagogies. Garnis writes her thoughts on learning:

GUEST SPOT

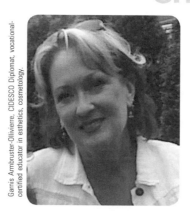

Garnis Armbruster-Ollivierre, CIDESCO Diplomat, vocational-certified educator in esthetics, cosmetology.

**GARNIS ARMBRUSTER-
OLLIVIERRE, BA, LE, CIDESCO**

Intelligence, as in multiple intelligences, has nothing to do with whether a student is academically smart. Our notions about intelligence can powerfully influence our self-concept and beliefs about the abilities and potential of our students and ourselves. Our emotional past experiences have a lot to do with our success in learning. Over time, theorists have sought to break intelligences down into subdivisions or categories, each with its own attributes and psychological reality.

There are four general categories of intelligence.

1. Gardner's theory of multiple intelligences
2. Sternberg's successful intelligence
3. Perkin's reflective intelligence
4. Resnick's effort-based intelligence

Gardner's concept of multiple intelligences consists of eight general types: linguistic, logical-mathematical, musical, spatial, bodily-kinesthetic, interpersonal, intrapersonal, and naturalist intelligence. Such intelligences recognize our diverse attitudes and aptitudes, and let's not forget, emotional history. Defining each one of these domains may be realized by creating a specific type of assessment such as writing or artwork, as opposed to standardized testing. Let's also address environment, sound, light, temperature, scent, and design of the classroom. These considerations are essential in an all-inclusive classroom and potentially student marketability. The instructor sets the stage.

The human brain can only absorb approximately 20 to 30 minutes of a particular topic of instruction at a time. Changing the content of instruction every half hour will utilize both hemispheres of the brain. This method, known as "distribution of practice," will keep the students interested.

In this time of "instant gratification" and sensationalism provided by new devices and state-of-the-art communications, the student is truly dependent on this connection and ultimate distraction, as mentioned previously. There is no room in the classroom for this type of distraction.

In the past, I have assigned projects to students that engage their interaction and creativity. One of the learning modalities in aesthetics in particular is anatomy and physiology. I gave students "free reign" to choose an art medium to demonstrate their knowledge of the bones, muscles, and nerves of the human skull and face. They were to design and label all of the listed criteria. Students were allowed to use Styrofoam head blocks, paint, puzzles, and stained glass, among other materials. Students were asked to label the insertion and origin of the muscles as to properly apply a beneficial massage technique.

Did the lesson take longer? Yes, but none of the students left class looking in the textbook to determine where the buccinators are. Yes, in time, that information will fade away if not used. So once the student is in the clinical segment of his or her education, it is imperative to continue to use the clinical terminology.

I have had a delightful and exciting career helping students realize their potential and guiding them into a whole new aspect of their lives with a sense of accomplishment.

Armbruster-Ollivierre makes a wonderful case for her interest in helping students realize their potential and gain entry into their future with confidence.

The Salon Professional Academy

Katherine Morgason, an extraordinary esthetics educator for The Salon Professional Academy in Tacoma, Washington, has a course called *The Skin Histology Project* (Figure 2–9). The students use a variety of mediums to present and demonstrate skin histology, which delineates the layers of the skin in a profile format. In Morgason's class, students also experience public speaking early on in the program, which facilitates learning objectives and broadens their options in the marketplace.

Activity

Open your own creative pathways by taking an art class in glass blowing, watercolor or oil painting, or even sculpting. Make a skin profile for one of your projects, starting with the layers of the skin. Put as much detail in the work as you can, and use color! Share what you know and create passion about it every day by putting the magnificent art piece in your waiting room or lobby. This is an exciting experience even if you decide not to put it on display. It is a fun process that involves both sides of the brain. If you do decide to exhibit your work, your clients or patients will love it.

fyi

If you are a long-term professional and would like to expand your horizons and develop an additional revenue stream, put your "brave on" and give public speaking a go. Great speakers can make excellent money. It is a necessary skill to develop. The classroom is a great place to start, whether you are an undergraduate or graduate esthetician.

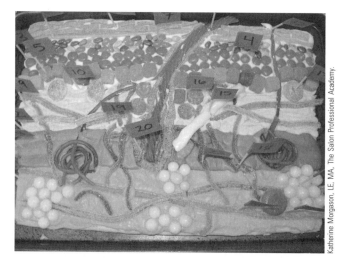

Katherine Morgason, LE, MA, The Salon Professional Academy.

Figure 2–9 Tiffany Craig, student at The Salon Professional Academy, Tacoma, WA, creates a depiction of skin layers using edible products.

As we know, estheticians are often excellent public speakers and invited as keynote speakers in a variety of settings and industries.

Business Courses in Esthetics for Both Students and Professionals

In another case, an instructor had students develop a business plan for their own practice. They developed the name for their business, mission/vision statements, researched products they would retail, created a menu of services, and financial documents such as profit and loss reports, cash flow, and balance sheets. Students had an understanding of what it would take to start up a business when their esthetic course was completed, and they learned what it would take to be an excellent employee by going through the exercise.

This is also a great class for an existing salon or spa owner or employee to take to keep on track and to grow a business. Many spa and salon owners do not take the time to do this, and never know how close they are to realizing their goals. It is good business to have a business plan. (See Chapter 7 on business planning.)

There are many examples of great learning experiences all over the world today, and it is necessary for us to put them into practice for our clients, our employees, our students, our educators, our children, and ourselves. Adult learning has its own precepts, and it is important to set the stage to continue to learn and grow.

ENVIRONMENT FOR ESTHETICIANS AS ADULT LEARNERS

There are some basic requirements to foster an environment for learning to take place, for both learners and instructors. Adult learners have some specific learning needs, as we have a variety of real-life experiences to draw from along with other learning experiences. We can become impatient if we assess that the learning environment is not conducive to meeting our needs, and even more so if the environment is not beneficial to our objectives, which is often about applying information for career gains.

Adult learning has its own mixed bag of opportunities. Adults often think about learning in terms of gaining knowledge to facilitate professional growth, or to acquire a new skill. There is a real and well-documented reason for this approach to learning. **Dr. Malcolm Knowles**, known as "the father of adult education," developed a theory, called **andragogy**, that is a set of assumptions about how adults learn. The focus of Knowles's theory allows teachers, instructors, and facilitators to create lessons, which are part of a relevant learning environment for adult learners/students. In his theory, Knowles shares that adults need to know *why* they should learn something. As children, we are told *what* and often *how* we are to learn; this works with varying degrees of success.

Part of being an effective instructor involves understanding how adults learn best. Compared to children and teens, adults have special needs and requirements as learners. Adult learning is a relatively new area of study, and not without its challenges. As adult learners, we need to understand how we learn as individuals, and be accountable to that by choosing our learning environments. It may also be suggested that we exercise some flexibility and acquire a degree of agility in order to learn in today's educational environments (Figure 2–10).

Here are some ideas on how both esthetic adult learners and educators can benefit from Dr. Knowles's research into adult learning characteristics:

- Adults are **autonomous** and self-directed, thus need to be free to direct their selves. Our teachers must actively involve us as participants in the learning process and serve as facilitators rather than an all-knowing force, feeding us information. We do not respond well to a top-down approach, such as the "teacher knows best" model.

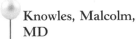

Knowles, Malcolm, MD
Known as "the father of adult education."

andragogy
Theory developed by Malcolm Knowles, PhD, that focuses on relevant learning and teaching methods for adults.

autonomous
Independent in origin action or function; self-governing.

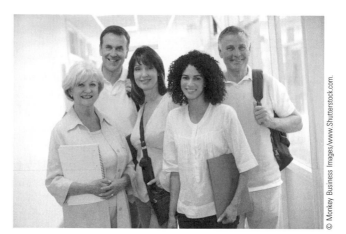

Figure 2–10 A group of adult learners.

Specifically, educators must understand our perspectives about what topics to cover and let us work on projects that reflect our interests. Educators should allow participants to assume responsibility for presentations and group leadership. Instructors need to be sure to act as facilitators, guiding us to our own knowledge rather than supplying us with facts. Finally, teachers must show us how the class will help us reach our goals.

- As adults, we have accumulated a foundation of life experiences and knowledge that may include work-related activities, family responsibilities, and previous education. Educators need to connect learning to our knowledge/experience base. To help us do so, they should draw out the participants' experience and knowledge, which is relevant to the topic. They must relate theories and concepts to us and recognize the value of experience in learning. While this can be alienating to some younger students, as they may not have the experiences to draw from, they need to be open to learning from others' experiences. Older students need to be patient with both younger instructors and younger students.

- Adults are goal-oriented. Upon enrolling in a program, we usually know what we want to achieve by taking the class. Adults appreciate an esthetic educational program that is organized and has clearly defined elements. Instructors must show us how this class will help us attain our goals. This classification of goals and course objectives must be done early in the class, webinar, seminar, or course.

- Adults are *relevancy oriented*. We must see a reason for learning something. Learning has to be applicable to our work or other responsibilities to be of value to us. Therefore, instructors must identify objectives for adult participants before the course begins. This means that theories and concepts must relate to a setting familiar to us. The key to achieving this is to have we adult learners choose projects that reflect our own interests.

- Adults are practical, focusing on the aspects of a lesson most useful to them in their work. They may not be interested in knowledge for its own sake. Instructors must tell participants explicitly how the lesson will be useful to them in the spa, salon, clinic, or other workplace environment.

- As do all learners, adults need to be shown *respect*. Instructors must acknowledge the wealth of experiences that adult participants bring to the classroom. Adults need to be treated as equals in experience and knowledge, and allowed to voice their opinions freely in class, provided they are relevant to the topic. Adult learners must also realize that long drawn-out personal stories can derail the best educational programs. It is important to choose any input to the class wisely.

 ## GLOBALIZATION OF ESTHETIC EDUCATION

As many esthetic professionals today communicate with friends from various countries, or have moved from one country to another, we see a great deal of diversity in the levels of education. Esthetic programs in the United Kingdom, Germany, France, Canada, South Africa, China, Australia, New Zealand, and Belgium all favor comprehensive educational programs for the skin care professional. Topics tend to be more alike than different, and programs run consistently from six months to three years; however, the depth of study may vary greatly. In some countries such as the United Kingdom and Germany, esthetics programs can begin at the secondary education level, preparing esthetic students to continue their advanced education while being able to work once they graduate. Here are some of the basic educational subjects offered in various countries:

- In the United Kingdom, a skin therapist or beauty therapist has three years of study. This includes academic studies, such as cosmetic chemistry, human biology, anatomy and physiology, physics, electricity, public speaking, business management, and art and design, along with hairdressing and nails. The beauty therapist portion of the course includes skin physiology, disorders and diseases, exercise, posture, diet and nutrition, skin treatments with and without devices, ingredients, and general skin health practices.

- In New Zealand, some schools have optional programs lasting six months, one year, or one and a half years; they depend upon the track one chooses, such as spa, beauty therapist (also called beautician), or body therapist. These courses range from anatomy and physiology to massage to skin care and treatments, such as hygiene, cleansing, analysis, masks, electrical machines, makeup, eyelash and brow treatments, manicures, pedicures, and waxing.

- South Africa refers to estheticians as beauty therapists and offers programs ranging from six months to two years. Some beauty therapists will train for three years in advanced therapies. The longer programs consist of dermatology, anatomy and physiology, massage, nutrition, hygiene makeup, waxing, manicure and pedicure, electrolysis and epilation, exercise, first aid, nail extensions, and electrical body treatments. Other educational offerings in basic training, which may incorporate some academic studies, are psychology, business administration, aromatherapy, permanent makeup, laser theory, pathology, reflexology, spa therapies, lymphatic drainage, and pathology.

- In Canada, esthetic programs range from six months to one year for basic programs. Within the programs, the subjects include basic facials, bacteriology, nutrition, anatomy and physiology, manicure and pedicure, skin disorders and disease, chemistry, pharmacology, waxing, lash and brow tint, body treatments, marketing, physics, electricity, and spa management.

- Australia esthetic programs begin with a one-year curriculum that provides a diploma of beauty therapy. It typically involves manicure/pedicure, body treatments, financial/business classes, skin biology, anatomy and physiology, electricity, nutrition, cosmetic chemistry, developing treatment plans, product knowledge, makeup, lash and brow tint, applied facial and body applications, hair removal/epilation, bleaching, communication, retailing, and safe working practices (infection control).

- In China, educational program can vary greatly, and programs can last from three weeks to six months. Subjects vary as well and may range from academic classes to professional programs, which may involve makeup, eyebrow tattooing, eyelash curling, manicure/pedicure, personal hygiene, skin structure and function, dermatology, electricity and facial devices, massage, peeling facial and body treatments, and product knowledge.

- In Germany, esthetic and cosmetology training requires theoretical training in anatomy, physiology, dermatology, chemistry, physics, and nutrition. Practical training includes manicures, pedicures, skin analysis, massages, and color theory. The range of hours is from 1,000 to 1,500 hours total of training.
- In France, esthetic training includes training in makeup, fragrance, sales, face and body care, and cosmetics. There are many specialization options in programs for esthetic professionals, such as esthetics in gerontology, nutrition, and dermatology. The programs range between one and three years, depending upon the program and the specialization.

Global Online Learning

Web-based learning enables estheticians to take classes on topics at any point in their day, and in just about any location. We can study chemistry, physiology and anatomy, business practices, infection control, client services, product knowledge, cultural differences, and a variety of subjects. We can literally hear about an issue in one moment, and register for a class on it within the next.

Estheticians, nurses, physicians assistants, physicians, and dental hygienists need to take lab classes and perform practical applications; however, there is much theory and even some demonstrations of procedures that can be learned through good online classes. When you think back about how the brain learns, remember that each time we create a foundation for acquiring knowledge, we are providing another building block for the learning to take place.

Online Esthetic Classes

Online esthetic classes support various learning styles, use multiple intelligences models, and often provide classes in multiple languages. If a practitioner is following a live demonstration, he or she can participate in hands-on learning or a **kinesthetic** experience through an online class. This medium is great for "hands-on" learners if they set themselves up properly before the class begins. Many estheticians will have a model, products, devices, and other materials prepared and will follow along with the educator, making it "live" for themselves. Online esthetic instructors will answer questions during or after the presentation (Figure 2–11).

Bandwidth issues and computer limitations aside, if we are willing to take the steps required to update our technology, we can provide online classes for our staff members, students, and colleagues regularly,

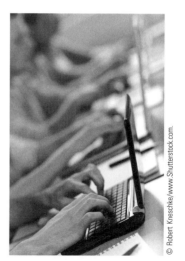

Figure 2–11 Update classroom technology to promote Web-based learning for students and staff.

kinesthetic
Tendency to respond positively to physical movement.

anywhere in the world. Online learning in the way of Web casts, webinars, and seminars is part of our current learning culture.

Electronic Applications (Apps)

As you know, the market has delivered wonderful applications to put on our cell phones in a variety of topics, including cosmetic chemistry, ingredients, anatomy/physiology, business operations with forms, service menu options, medical terminology, skin disorders and diseases, spa design applications, and many more to come (and in a variety of languages). Pay special attention to the new applications from skin care and textbook publication companies. In the near future, you will see electronic applications for a variety of treatments and services, along with those for test taking for continuing education and basic esthetic studies.

ESTHETIC ORGANIZATIONS, ASSOCIATIONS, AND EDUCATION

Esthetic organizations and associations have been vital to the heartbeat of esthetics education throughout the many decades worldwide. They have provided the impetus for growth and change, education, standardization, professionalism, and ethics. For today's estheticians and skin therapists who are interested in furthering or rounding out their education, here are some organizations that have provided excellence in education, advocacy, and guidance for decades.

WEB RESOURCE

www.beautyschools.org

American Association of Cosmetology Schools (AACS)

AACS was founded in 1924 as a nonprofit educational association to bring together all parts of the cosmetology industry—meaning students, teachers, suppliers, and educators—to further the education at all levels of the cosmetology art and sciences as a discipline. It also represents the interest of cosmetology and its constituents before the U.S. Department of Education, Congress, and state legislatures.

AACS focuses on updating its membership with new teaching methods, current industry information, and changes in legislation that can affect the industry. It serves as lobbyists and representatives in protecting the interests of cosmetology schools in Washington, DC. AACS sponsors and holds meetings, conferences, and conventions throughout the year, which are geared toward education and providing networking opportunities. AACS also has an educational arm, Cosmetology

Educators of America (CEA); its activities are planned and implemented by a volunteer team of beauty and wellness school professionals and industry partners supported by AACS staff.

Aesthetics International Association (AIA)

Founded in 1972, the AIA's goal is to bring esthetic professionals together to network, share knowledge, and establish a presence in the industry. AIA has consistently worked toward raising the standards of education and public awareness of the esthetics industry, and has been instrumental in influencing esthetic licensing as a separate entity in the United States.

AIA offers continuing education, a school affiliate program, and a skin care professional networking program in which professionals may share information. AIA also publishes *Dermascope*, a professional skin care magazine dedicated to providing support to the busy professional.

WEB RESOURCE

www.aestheticsassociation.com

Associated Skin Care Professionals (ASCP)

Headquartered in Golden, Colorado, ASCP was created in January 2007 by the founders of a professional association for massage therapists, an organization with a 20-year track record serving wellness professionals. During the company's growth, an increasing number of massage therapists obtained additional licensing as estheticians, so membership was extended to skin care practitioners in 1997.

WEB RESOURCE

www.ascpskincare.com

ASCP provides a membership association that connects skin care professionals, provides online education, and offers consumers a valuable online skin care referral service, which provides a resource explaining different treatments and their benefits. Members can purchase professional liability insurance coverage while connecting to the profession through business support, continuing education, and an advocacy voice with legislators and the media. ASCP has a presence at trade shows, actively supports skin care schools, and networks regularly on behalf of the profession in regulatory and practice matters.

Professional Beauty Association (PBA)

The Professional Beauty Association's purpose is to advance the professional beauty industry by providing its members with business tools, government tools, government advocacy, educations, networking, events and more to ensure business and career success with integrity. PBA is the largest organization of salon professionals with members representing salons and spas, distributors, manufacturers and beauty professionals with the addition of the National Cosmetology Association (NCA).

National Coalition of Estheticians, Manufacturers/ Distributors & Associations (NCEA)

NCEA was founded by Susanne Warfield in 2000 to support the skin care professional by working to increase the hours of training necessary to be successful in the skin care industry. Other goals for NCEA have included creating a standard for an esthetician job task, which has been realized; to increase the standards through the state regulatory boards in maintaining consumer safety, to obtain license reciprocity from state to state, and to develop international recognition.

Additionally, NCEA works toward standardizing continuing education on a national basis (in the United States) and serves to train esthetic educators and instructors through National Education for Teacher Training (NETT).

WEB RESOURCE

www.ncea.tv

Comité International d'Esthétique et de Cosmétologie (CIDESCO)

CIDESCO, Comité International d'Esthétique et de Cosmétologie, was founded in Brussels in 1946 by Belgian Georges Dumont and Frenchman Jacques Poirsons. The goals of the founding fathers were to bring members together, to exchange ideas, and to share knowledge. Additionally they wanted to connect with doctors, surgeons, and dermatologist and cosmetic chemists and to work with others in the esthetic and cosmetology industry to demonstrate that their work was of serious value. The final and most noted goal, which has manifested over time, was to establish a structure of educational esthetic programs and form schools that complied with the precepts as outlined by CIDESCO. There are over 200 CIDESCO schools today in 33 countries, and no doubt there will be more to come in the future. CIDESCO's head office is located in Zurich, Switzerland.

CIDESCO Diplomats undergo a rigorous training experience, which involves 1,200 hours of training that is both theoretical and practical in a CIDESCO registered school. A CIDESCO Diploma takes one anywhere in the world, as skin care professionals are familiar with the standards set by the organization and it is well documented that a CIDESCO Diplomat is well trained.

WEB RESOURCE

www.cidesco.com

International Therapy Examination Council (ITEC)

ITEC is an international examination board with centers in 38 countries that has been in existence since 1947. The headquarters is based in London, and the qualifications are accredited by the UK government.

WEB RESOURCE

www.itecworld.co.uk

There are four levels of study for the beauty therapist, which range from basic facial techniques to body therapies to advanced skin care therapies, such as laser hair removal and skin rejuvenation. There are opportunities to obtain certification and diplomas in over 52 categories. One must seek an ITEC college to obtain the necessary training and examination.

 ## SUMMING IT UP

In working as an esthetician, it is necessary to routinely increase our knowledge of the skin and its responses to what we are applying to it, which requires education in techniques, applications, treatments, and analysis.

As we know, there is literally a class for every type of product and treatment on the market. Courses are beginning to include case studies, in which estheticians share their findings with other professionals and thus learn more about what does and does not work in skin care issues. Many of us have spent a large part of our time in trial and error, which is certainly one method. However, to be able to gain knowledge from reputable educators, physicians, estheticians, esthetic organizations and associations, and manufacturers in the global marketplace certainly improves our chances of obtaining the best options for our practices and our clients. The support and the level of education in educational settings and online have never been better and will continue to improve going forward. Online classes will continue to gain interest, as they allow estheticians and other industry professionals access to courses and material that have not been available in the past.

Education gives a lifelong tool that when applied is the key to freedom, independence, and prosperity. Estheticians and beauty professionals, in general, have had and will continue to experience opportunities that are not found in most professions.

ESTHETICIAN **PROFILE**

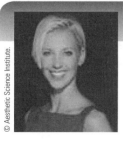

© Aesthetic Science Institute.

Michelle D'Allaird Brenner, LE
CIDESCO Diplomat

Aesthetic Science Institute, Latham, NY; School Owner

I am Michelle D'Allaird, a licensed cosmetologist, esthetician, CIDESCO Diplomat, school owner, author, speaker, and consultant. I first entered the world of beauty in cosmetology school in 1987.

I had big dreams of owning my own hair salon, but quickly realized that not only did I not like doing hair, but I was not very good at it!

I loved skin and nails, and decided to open my own little skin care business next to a friend who had a hair salon.

Knowing very little about the skin, I was determined to read every book and to study and learn what I could about the skin. I certainly had not learned this in cosmetology school, and esthetics licensing was not yet in existence in New York State.

After two years, I was offered a position as the director of esthetics for a franchise of skin care centers on the East Coast. My job was to develop a two-week training program and hire and train all of their new estheticians. This was the fear of a lifetime! I now had to train estheticians who had come out of 600 hours of esthetics school and actually had a license, when all I had was cosmetology school and my own hard work.

It was those six years that inspired my passion for the skin, for teaching, and for raising the bar of our profession from the bottom up. I believe that continuing education is critical. However, you cannot build a house on a weak foundation, and the core esthetics curriculum is that foundation.

I opened the Aesthetic Science Institute in 1993. Today, I travel the country and the world educating and speaking about the skin and product ingredients. I have graduated over 600 estheticians who are part of the amazing profession of skin care, and I continue to grow and further my experiences through writing, curriculum development, and working with top skin care chemists, scientists, and researchers across the globe.

Training

Colonna Beauty School, Albany, NY

CIDESCO certification exam in Independence, Missouri

Dr. Vodder Lymphatic Drainage—International Dermal Institute

Reiki practitioner—Reiki Room, Saratoga Springs, NY

Medical esthetician/laser technician—Aesthetic Science Institute

I attend a minimum of two continuing education classes every year as well as teach over 10 advanced classes per year.

Practice/School Demographic

- 98 percent female
- Ages 17–72
- Average age is 30
- Most students are stay-at-home mothers returning to work, career changers, and individuals searching for something to do during retirement
- 14 students in a class, maximum limit
- Full-time and part-time classes that run year-round
- Offer courses in esthetics, medical esthetics, laser, waxing, and nail specialty
- Full continuing education programs for licensed professionals

School Spa Services/Treatments Offered

Full clinic open to the public *only* after students have completed at least 175 hours

- Basic facials
- Enzyme/alpha-beta/lactic/glycolic facials
- Microdermabrasion
- Salt scrubs
- Cellulite wraps
- Chocolate body wraps
- Full face, body, bikini, and Brazilian waxing
- Microdermabrasion
- Full electricity used in every facial (unless there is a contraindication)

Personal Philosophy

I am thrilled and honored that every day I have the ability to provide others with the knowledge, skills, and tools to create their own futures and success. My goal is to inspire, motivate, and create passion in future professionals in my field while in turn being inspired and motivated by each student who brings something different to my life.

My drive for success and belief in myself and my profession has allowed me to sustain my business growth and success. Quitting is not an option, it is simply an opportunity to look at a situation from a different point of view.

Additional Contributions to the Industry

This area brings me continuous pride!

- Developed one of the first medical esthetics and laser curriculum approved by the NY State Department of Education
- Lead author of *Milady Standard Makeup* textbook
- Regular contributing author for *Les Nouvelles Esthétique* and *Dermascope* magazine
- Host and speaker for esthetics conferences across the United States
- Master skin health educator and consultant for artistry
- International speaker and educator in over 17 countries
- Educational director of Aesthetics International Association
- Member of ASCP and esthetics school board member
- Member of AACS
- Part of the most amazing profession of beauty, health, and youth that exists—a professional esthetician
- Active member of NY State Esthetics Licensing Advisory Committee and Laser Advisory Committee

I thank my lucky stars every day for the people in my life who have supported me, for the professionals who believed in growing the reputation of the industry, and for my commitment to never settling. When you reach for the moon, you may fall short, but at least you will be a star.

ESTHETICIAN **PROFILE**

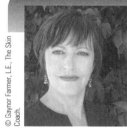

© Gaynor Farmer, L.E., The Skin Coach.

Gaynor Farmer, LE
CIBTAC

Senior Instructor, Eve Taylor Aromatherapy and Skin Care, Peterborough, England.

I am from England, and my initial attraction to esthetics industry, as for many other estheticians whom I have met over the years, was to become a makeup artist. I wrote to the BBC in London at the age of 14 to inquire what the qualifications were to pursue this career. One route was rather academic, requiring the study of history, English literature, and art at an advanced level. I was happy to study art, but English and history bored me, so I chose dressmaking. This was much more suited to my creative side, even though it wouldn't further my career. The other route was a three-year hairdressing and beauty therapy certificate. I opted for the latter. This was 1982. I lived in Birmingham, the second largest city in England, which boasted two universities and several colleges. However, none of the colleges offered the course I was looking for at the time, so I had to travel out of the city for my training.

Training

I attended Solihull College of Technology for three years. For the first year, I studied mainly hairdressing; the second year was split between hairdressing and beauty therapy (skin care), with subjects such as cosmetic chemistry, human biology, anatomy and physiology, physics, electricity, public speaking, business management, and art and design. The third year was beauty therapy with a focus on electrical modalities for face and body.

I was awarded a diploma from the Confederation of International Beauty Therapists and Cosmetologists (CIBTAC) and City & Guilds certificate in beauty therapy. This proved that I was qualified to do my work, but more importantly, my education taught me professional ethics, which have guided my decisions for the past 28 years. I then went back to college to earn a teaching certificate to assist with my visa applications, as I wanted to travel. In 2001, I trained at the International Dermal Institute in Los Angeles.

Once licensed, I worked in a beauty salon located inside women's gym. Then I decided I wanted to work for myself, so I became a mobile beauty therapist. I traveled to women's homes providing facials, waxing, electrolysis, manicures, pedicures, lash tinting, makeup, and body massage within the northeast area of Birmingham, England. I then opened a salon with a good friend who was also a mobile therapist. I then moved a little further afield and began working on cruise ships traveling all over the world. The experience was phenomenal for expanding my awareness and appreciation of other cultures. I cruised for six years; five with a British-based company called Allders International.

In 2001, I moved to the United States, and went to train and subsequently to work for Dermalogica and the International Dermal Institute (IDI) in Los Angeles. I became a trainer and opened the flagship store in Santa Monica, CA. I then moved to the Central Coast region of California, where I operated a training/consulting business, The Skin Coach. I also offered classes at Alexander's Aesthetics in Burlingame, CA, and worked for Bio-Therapeutic, Inc., as an independent educator training estheticians on their newly purchased devices. I am now the Senior Instructor for Eve Taylor Aromatherapy and Skin Care in Peterborough, England.

Services Offered

As the Senior Instructor of Eve Taylor and Aromatherapy and Skin I serve in the following areas:

- Creating new curriculum, specifically skin related, to expand on the tried and tested methods taught by Eve for the past 40 years

- Work closely with R & D department to expand the skin care line to ensure we meet the needs of our customer demands
- Travel nationally and internationally to teach our methods, protocols and product knowledge to distributors and their customers
- Compile training manuals/brochures to supplement new products
- Assist with new website development
- Create curriculum in developing markets such as China and India

Personal Philosophy

My personal philosophy is to stay current with new trends via education, trade magazines, journals, and exhibitions and to remain flexible and open to new possibilities. I often find that things do not always turn out how we expect them to, and I have learned that if we are too rigid in our thoughts and expectations we may miss a golden opportunity.

I also believe that it is important to love what you do. There are so many things that I love about my work. First, I love variety. One day I may be writing an article, another day teaching an esthetician a new massage technique to reduce puffiness around the eyes, and yet another teaching a class full of eager esthetic students how to use a device. Secondly, I love to learn. My work allows me to continually study and learn new techniques, ingredients, technology so that I can pass this information onto my fellow estheticians and students. Sustainability is important in esthetics as it is a dynamic marketplace.

Contributions to the Industry

I love to help people through teaching and sharing my knowledge. When we are of service to others, we are fulfilling our purpose of contribution. Eve Taylor, a wonderful mentor and friend states, "Knowledge is useless unless we share it with others."

Infection Prevention Guidelines for Estheticians: The CDC, OSHA, and HIPAA

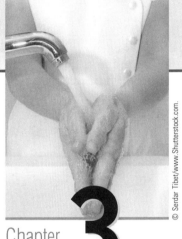

© Serdar Tibet/www.Shutterstock.com.

> "With my strong background in health care, I focused on taking the traditional beauty/therapy role to the next level with a strong focus on skin health … I learned to always look behind the surface for a complete overview of the body's functioning, which has helped my team and me to treat and correct many skin conditions."
>
> −Louise Gray, RN, Beauty Therapist, Educator, Founder and Owner of Louise Gray Skin Care centers, New Zealand

Chapter **3**

Chapter Capture

After completing this chapter, you will be able to:

- Practice basic safety guidelines.
- Understand the CDC and its mission.
- Comply with OSHA standards.
- Understand bloodborne pathogens.
- Understand the causes of diseases.
- Understand the decontamination methods.
- Understand how to break the chain of infection.
- Understand safety, confidentiality, and HIPAA.

BASIC SAFETY GUIDELINES

Basic safety guidelines for esthetic professionals are the same in all working environments anywhere in the world. Various countries have their own standards and government entities that dictate the rules, regulations, and laws governing infection control practices. Not only must we comply with these regulations, but in general, we need to know how to keep ourselves, our clients, and the public safe by using safe practices at all times in and out of the workplace. Once you know how potentially **pathogenic** (harmful, disease causing) microorganisms are transmitted, it is important to share that information with family members, friends, coworkers, and others with whom you come in contact. It is our responsibility as licensed professionals to share the knowledge of infection control that will keep infections from spreading. It is very simple: practice standard precautions.

As we recall from our basic esthetic training, standard precautions are a set of guidelines devised by the Centers for Disease Control that require us to treat all body fluids as if they were infectious and all tissue as if it were hazardous. Frequent hand-washing, proper infection control, the wearing of gloves, and the use of appropriate body protection devices during treatments, services, and cleanup are essential to following these regulations. We will look at two agencies that have brought forth regulations and prevention methods that have made the workplace safer.

pathogenic

Harmful microorganisms that can cause disease or infection in humans when they invade the body.

CENTERS FOR DISEASE CONTROL AND PREVENTION

In 1946, the Centers for Disease Control and Prevention (CDC) was created in Atlanta, Georgia. The CDC was founded as the Malaria Control in War Areas (MCWA), which focused on fighting malaria through killing mosquitoes during World War II.

The CDC is the premier U.S. agency involved in health promotion, disease, prevention, and preparedness; it is a global leader in public health. It works in public health efforts to prevent and control infectious and chronic diseases, injuries, workplace hazards, disabilities, and environmental health threats.

The CDC is recognized globally for conducting research and investigations and for its action-oriented approach. The CDC applies research and findings to improve people's daily lives and responds to health emergencies. The CDC works with states and other partners to provide a system of health surveillance to monitor and prevent disease outbreaks (including bioterrorism), implement disease prevention strategies, and maintain national health statistics. The CDC also guards against international disease transmission, with personnel stationed in more than 25 foreign countries, monitoring for transmittable pathogens throughout the world.

THE OCCUPATIONAL SAFETY AND HEALTH ADMINISTRATION

The Occupational Safety and Health Act of 1970, the Chemical Right to Know Law of 1983, and the Bloodborne Pathogens Standard of 1992 created the agency known as OSHA (Occupational Safety and Health Administration). OSHA was specifically designed to protect employees at work in any industry by identifying and establishing certain risks that put workers and customers in danger. By addressing the hazards in the workplace for salons, spas, skin care centers, and clinics, OSHA serves as a governing board to which all must comply for the health and safety of employees and our patrons.

The Bloodborne Pathogens Standard was created in response to the additional exposure to diseases such as hepatitis B, hepatitis C, and human immunodeficiency (HIV) viruses as faced by health care professionals. States must use federal OSHA standards or develop a state plan that is least as strict as OSHA (which is a federal agency).

If you are practicing in a country without these standards, you have a tremendous opportunity to help that community. By slowing and stopping the transmission of infection in your own practice, you may save lives. It is also necessary to share information if we fail to meet the expected standards of a profession; this may open estheticians and beauty industry professionals to civil liability and subsequent charges of negligence.

BLOODBORNE PATHOGENS STANDARD

The Bloodborne Pathogen Standard, as created by OSHA, was developed to minimize the transmission of HIV and hepatitis viral infections in health care workers, specifically those workers who can be reasonably anticipated to come in contact with blood and other body fluids considered to be other potentially infectious material (OPIM).

Case Study

An esthetician reported having stuck herself with a lancet, post-extraction. She had forgotten that she was to drop the used lancet into the sharps container. When she attempted to move the lancet, it penetrated the skin on her index finger. She instantly realized that she could be at risk for a bloodborne pathogen to enter her bloodstream from microorganisms left on the lancet from the extraction she had performed on her client.

She immediately cleaned the area, applied a bandage, and went to her supervisor to report the incident. Next, she met with an occupational health specialist for testing. She was offered a post-exposure prophylaxis (PEP) with doses of hepatitis B immune globulin (HBIG), which provided approximately 75 percent protection from transmission. She decided that it was better to take all of the extra precautions available. The client or source individual's blood was tested, and did not present with a pathogen. The esthetician received further counseling from the occupation heath specialist and returned to work to a follow-up session on bloodborne pathogen transmission from her immediate supervisor and the clinic administrator. She filled out an OSHA Form 200 at that time. She was made aware of the record of the exposure and that the document is to be kept for 30 years.

She realizes today that she was fortunate that there were no further complications to her situation and that she should not have set the lancet down, but should have placed it immediately in the sharps container.

Estheticians who work in spas, salons, skin care centers, and medical offices and who perform facials with extractions, work with post-operative patients, and apply microdermabrasion treatments face an increased likelihood of exposure to bloodborne pathogens. The Bloodborne Pathogens Standard is designed to look at all aspects of exposure as real and potential. It follows a logical path from prevention of transmission, to dealing with exposure incidents, to employing follow-up measures if one has been exposed, to legal record keeping.

It is important to have plenty of sharps containers within reach for disposal of sharps of any type at the moment you are finished using it. Do not walk with a lancet or other sharp to another location, or have sharps containers within reach of children visiting the salon, spa, or medical facility.

Here are the key elements of the Bloodborne Pathogens Standard:

1. Universal and standard precautions: Standardized systems have been created to treat all body fluids as if they were infectious and to assume that all tissue is hazardous. Frequent hand washing, the wearing of gloves, the use of appropriate body protection devices during services, treatments, and cleanup and disinfecting are essentials to following the standard.

2. Engineering controls and work practice controls: Protection devices must be provided by the employer. This includes antiseptic soap, splashguards, masks, safety glasses, eye flush stations, sharps disposal containers for lancets, gloves, and appropriate labels for biohazardous materials (Figure 3–1).

3. Personal protective equipment: There are precautions in addition to engineering and work practice controls. They consist of lab coats, uniforms, safety glasses, masks, gloves, and laundering and cleaning supplies, which are also supplied by the employer.

4. Cleanliness of the work areas: The employer is to ensure a work environment that is clean and safe. All surfaces must be decontaminated after procedures using a hospital disinfectant. In addition, gloves must be worn in all treatments and procedures and at any time during a potential exposure to OPIM. All surfaces must be cleaned and then disinfected with an Environmental Protection Agency (EPA) registered disinfectant.

5. Hepatitis B vaccine: This must be made available to employees within 10 days of beginning to work in a job where there is reasonably anticipated risk to exposure of bloodborne pathogens. The vaccine is given in three doses over a six-month period. As estheticians, we are considered a Group One Classification, as we are exposed to body fluids while performing services and treatments. Refusing to have the vaccine is not advisable. If one decides not to receive the hepatitis B vaccine, the employee signs a waiver that is then put into the employee's file. The individual may have the vaccine at a later date if it is requested. Those who are pregnant, nursing, or sensitive to yeast or its components should not take the vaccine.

6. Follow-up after exposure: The employer must make a documented confidential medical evaluation detailing:
   a. The circumstances surrounding the event
   b. The route of exposure (how it happened)
   c. The identification of the person who was the source of the exposure
   d. Immediate washing of the exposed area with soap and running water, or flushing in the case of eye exposure
   e. The exposed employee must be tested for HBV, HCV, and HIV (and must provide consent)
   f. A request for the source individual's blood to be tested for HBV, HCV, and HIV is made; the esthetician's employer covers the cost of the test

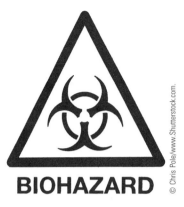

BIOHAZARD

Figure 3–1 The standard biohazard symbol.

© Chris Pole/www.Shutterstock.com.

WEB RESOURCES

You can find an EPA-approved list of disinfectants by going to the EPA's Web site at www.epa.gov and searching for "EPA-registered disinfectants."

g. The employee is offered prophylaxis or HB vaccine follow-ing a confidentiality guarantee

h. The employee is counseled regarding precautions to take to avoid transmission

i. An OSHA 200 Form is filled out

j. Medical record of employee exposure is to be kept for 30 years; full confidentiality is guaranteed

Environmental Protection Agency

The EPA registers all types of disinfectants sold and used in the United States. Disinfectants are products that destroy all bacteria, fungi, and viruses (but not spores) on nonporous surfaces. The two types that are used in salons, spas, medical offices, and medi-spas are hospital disinfectants and tuberculocidal disinfectants.

Hospital disinfectants are effective for disinfecting blood and body fluids after cleaning the items or area. They can be used on any non-porous surface in the salon, spa, or clinic. (Nonporous means that an item is made or constructed of a material that has no pores or open-ings and cannot absorb liquids.) Hospital disinfectants control the spread of disease. Tuberculocidal disinfectants are proven to kill the disease-causing bacteria that are transmitted through coughing or sneezing. These bacteria are capable of forming spores, so they are difficult to kill.

Tuberculocidal disinfectants are one kind of hospital disinfectant. The fact that tuberculocidal disinfectants are more powerful does not mean that you should automatically reach for them. Some of these pro-ducts can be harmful to salon, spa, and esthetic tools and equipment, and these products require special methods of disposal. Check the rules in your state to be sure that the product you choose complies with state requirements.

It is against federal law to use any disinfecting product contrary to its labeling. Before a manufacturer can sell a product for disinfecting surfaces, tools, implements, or equipment, it must obtain an EPA-registration number that certifies that the disinfectant may be used in the manner prescribed by the manufacturer's label. Misusing a product for disinfecting may cancel its efficacy for disinfecting. This also means that if you do not follow the label instructions for mixing, contact time, and the type of surface the disinfecting product can be used on, you are not complying with federal law. If there is a lawsuit, you can be held responsible.

REVIEW OF TERMS FOR THE CAUSES OF DISEASE

As we learned in our basic esthetic courses, there are many disease-causing microorganisms, which range from bacteria, viruses, fungi, and parasites; they all have different characteristics and modes of replication. Our job is to reduce our exposure to them by preventing their transmission to ourselves, our coworkers, and our clients. Here are some of the basic terms that serve as a reminder to use and practice infection control (Table 3–1).

Table 3–1 The Causes of Disease

Term	Definition
Bacteria	One-celled microorganisms having both plant and animal characteristics. Some are harmful and some are harmless. A single bacterium may replicate 16,000,000 times in 12 hours.
Direct Transmission	Transmission of blood or body fluids through touching (including shaking hands, sexual intercourse, and kissing where body fluids are exchanged).
Indirect Transmission	Transmission of blood or body fluids through contact with an intermediate contaminated object such as a razor, extractor, nipper, or an environmental surface.
Infection	Invasion of body tissues by disease-causing pathogens.
Germs	Nonscientific synonym for disease-producing organisms.
Microorganism	Any organism of microscopic to submicroscopic size.
Parasites	Organisms that grow, feed, and shelter on or in another organism (referred to as the host), while contributing nothing to the survival of that organism. Parasites must have a host to survive.
Toxins	Various poisonous substances produced by some microorganisms (bacteria and viruses).
Virus	A parasitic submicroscopic particle that infects and resides in cells of biological organisms. A virus cannot reproduce outside a living cell.

PATHOGENIC BACTERIA

Bacteria have three distinct shapes that help to identify them. Pathogenic bacteria are classified as described below.

- *Cocci* are round-shaped bacteria that appear singly (alone) or in groups.
- *Staphylococci* are pus-forming bacteria that grow in clusters like bunches of grapes. They cause abscesses, pustules, and boils. Some types of *staphylococci* (or staph, as many call it) may not cause infections in healthy humans.
- *Streptococci* are pus-forming bacteria arranged in curved lines resembling a string of beads. They cause infections such as strep throat and blood poisoning.
- *Diplococci* are spherical bacteria that grow in pairs and cause diseases such as pneumonia.
- *Bacilli* are short, rod-shaped bacteria. They are the most common bacteria and produce diseases such as tetanus (lockjaw), typhoid fever, tuberculosis, and diphtheria.
- *Spirilla* are spiral or corkscrew-shaped bacteria. They are subdivided into subgroups, such as *Treponema pallidum*, which causes syphilis, a sexually transmitted disease (STD), and *Borrelia burgdorferi*, which causes Lyme disease.

Bacterial Growth and Reproduction

Bacteria generally consist of an outer cell wall that contains liquid called protoplasm. Bacterial cells manufacture their own food through what they absorb from the surrounding environment. They give off waste products, grow, and reproduce. The life cycle of bacteria consists of two distinct phases: the active stage and the inactive or spore-forming stage.

Active Stage

During the active stage, and when conditions are favorable, bacteria grow and reproduce. Bacteria multiply best in warm, dark, damp, or dirty places. When they reach their largest size, they divide into two new cells. This division is called binary fission. The cells that are formed are called daughter cells and are produced every 20 to 60 minutes, depending on the bacteria. The infectious pathogen *Staphylococcus aureus* undergoes cell division every 27 to 30 minutes. When conditions become unfavorable and difficult for them to thrive, bacteria either die or become inactive.

Inactive or Spore-Forming Stage

Certain bacteria, such as the anthrax and tetanus bacilli, coat themselves with wax-like outer shells. These bacteria are able to withstand long periods of famine, dryness, and unsuitable temperatures. In this stage, spores can be blown about and are not harmed by disinfectants, heat, or cold. When favorable conditions are restored, the spores change into the active form and begin to grow and reproduce.

Bacterial Infections

There can be no bacterial infection without the presence of pathogenic bacteria. Therefore, if pathogenic bacteria are eliminated, clients cannot become infected. You may have a client who has tissue inflammation, a condition in which the body reacts to injury, irritation, or infection. *Staphylococci* are among the most common bacteria that affect humans and are normally carried by about a third of the population. Staph bacteria can be picked up on doorknobs, countertops, and other surfaces; however, in salons, spas, medical facilities, and medi-spas they are more frequently spread through skin-to-skin contact (such as shaking hands) or through the use of contaminated tools or implements. Although lawsuits are rare considering the number of services performed in a salon or spa or medi-spa, every year many facilities are sued for allegedly causing staph infections.

Staph is responsible for food poisoning and a wide range of diseases, including toxic shock syndrome. Some types of infectious staph bacteria are highly resistant to conventional treatments such as antibiotics. An example is the staph infection called Methicillin-resistant *Staphylococcus aureus* (MRSA). Historically, MRSA occurred most frequently among persons with weakened immune systems or those who had undergone medical procedures in hospital or medical facilities (here, it is called **hospital-associated Methicillin-resistant *Staphylococcus aureus* [HA-MRSA]**). As MRSA has spread, and is more common today, it is found in communities in the general population (and called **community-associated Methicillin-resistant *Staphylococcus aureus* [CA-MRSA]**).

Clients who appear completely healthy may bring this organism into the salon, spa, or skin care center, where it can infect others. MRSA initially appears as a skin infection, such as pustules, rashes, and boils, that can be difficult to cure. Without proper treatment, the infection becomes systemic and can have devastating consequences that can result in death. Because of these highly resistant bacterial strains, it is important to clean and then disinfect all tools and implements used in the salon or spa; do not perform services if the client shows visible signs of abrasion or infection.

hospital associated Methicillin-resistant *Staphylococcus aureus* (HA-MRSA)
Type of staph infection that is highly contagious, resistant to antibiotics, and originates in a hospital setting.

community-associated Methicillin-resistant *Staphylococcus aureus* (CA-MRSA)
Type of staph infection that is highly contagious, resistant to antibiotics, and found in the community.

VIRUSES

A virus is a parasitic submicroscopic particle that infects and resides in the cells of a biological organism. A virus cannot live outside of a living cell. Some viruses cause common colds and other respiratory and gastrointestinal (digestive tract) infections. Other viruses that plague humans are measles, mumps, chicken pox, smallpox, rabies, yellow fever, hepatitis, polio, influenza, and HIV, which causes AIDS.

CAUTION!

All salon, spa, and medical facility practitioners should receive the hepatitis B vaccine. Health authorities recommend that service provid-ers in industries with direct contact with the public—including estheticians, nail techs, cosmetologists, teachers, florists, and bank tellers—ask their doctor about receiving this vaccine.

One difference between viruses and bacteria is that a virus can live and reproduce only by taking over other cells and becoming part of them, while bacteria can live and reproduce on their own. Bacterial infections can usually be treated with specific antibiotics, but antibiotics have no affect on viruses.

Through immunization or vaccination, our immune system becomes equipped to fight an infectious agent. A vaccination protects the individual from communicable diseases by introducing a customized type of substance, which is similar to the infectious agent; then our body's own immune system can rally to overcome the real infectious agent.

Hepatitis

Hepatitis is a bloodborne virus that causes disease and can damage the liver. In general, it is difficult to contract this disease; however, hepatitis is easier to contract than HIV because it can be present in all body fluids of those who are infected. Unlike HIV, hepatitis can live on a surface outside the body for long periods of time. For this reason, it is vital that all surfaces with which a client comes into contact are thoroughly cleaned and disinfected.

There are three types of hepatitis that are of concern in the salon, spa, or medical facility: hepatitis A, hepatitis B, and hepatitis C. Hepatitis B is the most difficult to kill on a surface, so check the label of the disinfectant you use to be sure that the product is effective against hepatitis B. Hepatitis B and C are spread from person to person through blood and, less often, other body fluids, such as semen and vaginal secretions.

HIV/AIDS

Human immunodeficiency virus (HIV) causes acquired immune deficiency syndrome (AIDS), which is a disease that breaks down the body's immune system. HIV is spread from person to person through blood and, less often, other body fluids, such as semen and vaginal secretions. A person can be infected with HIV for many years without having symptoms, but testing can determine whether a person is infected within six months after exposure to the virus. People who are HIV-positive may never have been tested and do not know they have the potential to infect other people.

CAUTION!

HIV and hepatitis can be spread by the following methods:

- Blood and body fluids, secretions, excretions (except perspiration)
- Contact with mucus membranes and nonintact skin (cuts, abrasions, open lesions)
- Open mouth, full-contact kissing, in which mucus and body fluids such as semen are exchanged
- Sharing toothbrushes and razors
- Personal sexual devices

HIV and hepatitis are not spread by the following methods:

- Toilet seats
- Holding hands
- Sharing food
- Sharing kitchen utensils
- Sharing phones, remotes, pens, electronic devices
- Hugging, holding, caressing
- Perspiration

fyi

Pathogenic bacteria, viruses, or fungi can enter the body through:

- Broken, inflamed skin, such as a cut, scratch, or rash
- The mouth (contaminated water, food, or fingers)
- The nose (inhaling different types of dust or droplets from a cough or sneeze)
- The eyes or ears
- Unprotected sex

The body prevents and controls infections with:

- Healthy, unbroken, intact skin, which is the body's first line of defense
- Body secretions, such as perspiration and digestive juices
- White blood cells that destroy bacteria
- Antibodies produced by the immune system

CAUTION!

If you accidentally cut a client, the tool will be contaminated. You cannot continue to use the implement without cleaning and then disinfecting it. Continuing to use a contaminated implement without cleaning and disinfecting it puts you and others in the salon, spa, or medical facility at risk of infection. Follow the OSHA Bloodborne Pathogen Standard precautions and protocols; treat client and implements accordingly.

The HIV virus is spread mainly through the sharing of needles by intravenous (IV) drug users and by unprotected sexual contact. Less commonly, HIV is spread through accidents with needles in health care settings. The virus is less likely to enter the bloodstream through cuts and sores. It is not spread by holding hands, hugging, sharing food, or using household items such as the telephone or toilet seats. There are no documented cases that indicate that HIV can be spread by food handlers, insects, or casual contact during hair, skin, nail, and standard pedicure salon services.

 FUNGI

Fungi are microscopic plant parasites that include molds, mildews, and yeasts. They can produce contagious diseases, such as ringworm. Mildew, another fungus, affects plants or grows on inanimate objects but does not cause human infections in the salon, spa, or skin care center. Depending upon the type, fungi grow in single cells or in colonies. Also called vegetable parasites, fungi obtain nourishment from dead organic matter or from living organisms. Most fungi are nonpathogenic and make up many of the body's normal flora. Fungal infections usually affect the skin, as they live off of *keratin*, a protein that makes up the skin. The most basic cause of fungal infections are **dermatophytes**, the fungi that cause skin, nail, and hair infections.

Common types of fungal infections are ***tinea pedis***, or athlete's foot; ***tinea corporis***, or ringworm; and ***onychomycosis***, a nail infection. *Tinea barbae*, also known as barber's itch, is a superficial fungal infection that commonly affects the skin. It is primarily limited to the bearded areas of the face and neck or around the scalp. This infection occurs almost exclusively in older adolescent and adult males. A person with *tinea barbae* may have deep, inflamed or noninflamed patches of skin on the face or the nape of the neck.

Other types of fungal infections are those brought about by yeast. These include ***tinea versicolor***, also known as sun spots, which are characterized by white or varicolored patches on the skin and are often found on arms and legs. ***Intertrigo*** is another type of fungal infection found in the body folds of the skin in areas such as the underarms and in the groin. Thrush is a fungal infection found in the mouth and vaginal areas. Both intertrigo and thrush are caused by ***candida albicans***, a yeast that thrives in dark, moisture-rich environments.

Both bacterial and fungal infections will spread to other people unless all implements, surfaces, towels, and everything that touches the client is properly cleaned and disinfected before reuse, or is thrown away after use. It is always important to assume that all clients may have infections (standard precautions) and to use proper infection control measures at all times.

PARASITES

Parasites are organisms that grow, feed, and shelter on or in another organism (referred to as a host), while contributing nothing to the survival of that organism. Parasites must have a host to survive. Parasites can live on or inside of humans and animals. They can also be found in food, on plants and trees, and in water. Humans can acquire internal parasites by eating fish or meat that has not been properly cooked. External parasites that affect humans on or in the skin include ticks, fleas, and mites.

Head lice are a type of parasite responsible for contagious diseases and conditions. One condition caused by an infestation of head lice is called ***pediculosis capitis*** (Figure 3–2). Scabies is also a contagious skin disease and is caused by the itch mite, which burrows under the skin. Contagious diseases and conditions caused by parasites should only be treated by a doctor. Contaminated countertops, tools, and equipment should be thoroughly cleaned and then disinfected with an EPA-

dermatophytes
Fungi that cause skin, nail, and hair infections.

tinea pedis
Medical term for fungal infections of the feet; red, itchy rash of the skin on the bottom of the feet and/or in between the toes that is usually found between the fourth and fifth toes.

tinea corporis
Fungus commonly known as ringworm.

onychomycosis
Type of nail infection.

tinea barbae
Also known as barber's itch; a superficial fungal infection that commonly affects the skin and is primarily limited to the bearded areas of the face and neck or around the scalp.

tinea versicolor
White patches where production of melanin has been compromised.

Intertrigo
Type of fungal infection found in the body folds of the skin in areas such as the underarms and in the groin.

candida albicans
Yeast that thrives in dark, moisture-rich environments.

pediculosis capitis
Infestation of the hair and scalp of head lice.

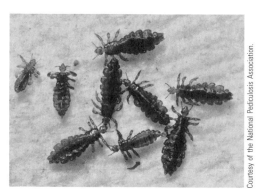

Courtesy of the National Pediculosis Association.

Figure 3–2 Head lice.

registered disinfectant for the time recommended by the manufacturer or with a bleach solution for 10 minutes.

Bed Bugs

Bed bugs are a type of parasite scientifically known as *climex lectularius* or *cimicidae*. They are approximately 6 mm as adults, red-brown in color, and are more of a nuisance than a true health threat in normal circumstances. A secondary infection such as a bacterial infection may occur if one has multiple bed bug bites, which may require medical intervention and treatment with antibiotics. In most cases, the bites will resolve or an OTC topical antibiotic may be all that is required.

We are seeing more bed bugs today, with traveling and moving around the globe made so easily. They can crawl into luggage, tote bags, and clothing, yet prefer mattresses, sofas, and linens—making our homes a perfect breeding ground. Bed bugs are found in hotel rooms, on cruise ships, in dorms, and in a variety of suitable breeding grounds. If an infestation is discovered in your place of business, you must take immediate steps toward pest control. There are Web sites that offer great suggestions and information about bed bugs.

WEB SITE REVIEW

http://www.howto-getridofbedbugs. com

http://www.bedbugbitesusa.com/

climex lectularius
Parasite commonly known as a bed bug.

cimicidae
Parasite commonly known as a bed bug.

DID YOU KNOW ❓

The bed bug feeds on human and animal blood, and has a clever, two-pronged, tubular-structured approach to feeding. It works primarily at night to source a host. It injects a person or animal with its saliva through one tube, which serves as an anesthetic, and simultaneously through its other tube draws blood from the host, who does not feel the bite. The bites look like mosquito bites, and are often mistaken for them.

With clients traveling, and the globalization of our industry, it is necessary to take our knowledge of infection control, including practicing standard precautions at all times, and to certain to share the information with other practitioners, regardless of licensure. Proper decontamination methods can prevent the spread of disease caused by exposure to potentially infectious materials on an item's surface. Decontamination will also prevent exposure to blood and visible debris or residue such as dust, hair, and skin.

 # DECONTAMINATION

There are new guidelines for the levels of decontamination, which is the removal of blood or OPIM on an item's surface and the removal of visible debris or residue such as dust, hair, and skin. There are two methods of decontamination:

- Decontamination method 1: Cleaning and then disinfecting with an appropriate EPA-registered disinfectant.
- Decontamination method 2: Cleaning and then sterilizing.

Historically, state regulatory agencies believed there was a lower risk of infection in salons, spas, and skin care centers than in medical facilities, where sterilizing is commonplace. However, two states— Texas and Iowa—now require a step up in sterilization and require salons that have nail departments to use autoclaves. We may see this adopted by other states.

At a minimum, salons, spas, and skin care centers will use decontamination method 1: cleaning and then disinfecting. Estheticians working in medical facilities will use a combination of both decontamination methods 1 and 2. Many states have upgraded their infection control standards in salons and spas that perform nail services to decontamination method 2: cleaning and sterilizing. When done properly, decontamination method 2 results in the destruction of all microbes through steam, heat, and pressure in an autoclave.

Decontamination Method 1

Decontamination method 1 has two steps: cleaning and disinfecting. Remember that when you clean, you must remove all visible dirt and debris from tools, implements, and equipment by washing with a liquid soap or detergent and warm water and by using a clean and disinfected brush to scrub any grooved or hinged portions of the item. Follow your state regulations for cleaning an item and to determine what constitutes cleaning in your state, as there are some variances. Follow the regulations closely to remain in compliance.

A surface is properly cleaned when the number of contaminants on it is greatly reduced. In turn, this reduces the risk of infection. The vast majority of contaminants and pathogens can be removed from the surfaces of tools and implements through proper cleaning. If left on the implement surfaces, the protective covering of oils may prevent a disinfectant's capability to kill them. This is why cleaning is an important part of disinfecting tools and equipment. A surface must be properly cleaned before it can be properly disinfected. Clean surfaces can still harbor small amounts of pathogens, but the presence of fewer pathogens means that infections are less likely to be spread. Proper cleaning of hands requires rubbing hands together and using liquid soap, warm running water, a nail brush, and a clean towel. Do not underestimate the importance of proper cleaning and hand washing. They are the most powerful and important ways to prevent the spread of infection.

There are three ways to clean your tools or implements:

1. Washing with soap or detergent and warm water, and then scrubbing them with a clean and properly disinfected scrub brush.
2. Using an ultrasonic unit. Check to make sure that your ultrasonic product is capable of cleaning an item. If it is an enzymatic product, you may need to clean the implement first. Follow the manufacturer's recommendation.
3. Using a cleaning solvent (e.g., on metal bits for electric files).

The second step of decontamination method 1 is disinfection. Remember that disinfection is the process that eliminates most, but not necessarily all, microorganisms on nonliving surfaces. This process is not effective against bacterial spores. In the salon or spa setting, disinfection is extremely effective in controlling microorganisms on surfaces such as comedone extractors, microdermabrasion tips, and other tools and equipment. Any disinfectant used in the salon or spa should carry an EPA-registration number and the label should clearly state the specific organisms the solution is effective in killing when used according to the label instructions.

Remember that disinfectants are products that destroy all bacteria, fungi, and viruses (but not spores) on nonporous surfaces. Disinfectants are not for use on human skin, hair, or nails. Never use disinfectants as hand cleaners, since this can cause skin irritation and allergy. Disinfectants are pesticides and can be harmful if absorbed through the skin. If you mix a disinfectant in a container that is not labeled by the manufacturer, you must label the container properly with the contents and the date it was mixed. All concentrated disinfectants must be diluted exactly as instructed by the manufacturer on the container's label.

While disinfecting, it is important to heed the amount of contact time that a manufacturer recommends to destroy all potential pathogens such as bacteria, virus, and fungi. Manufacturers have proven to the EPA that their product does in fact destroy these microorganisms at specific levels, and once the solution has become contaminated, it must be replaced with fresh disinfectant.

Decontamination Method 2

Decontamination method 2 also has two steps: cleaning and sterilizing. The word *sterilize* is often used incorrectly. Sterilization is the process that completely destroys all microbial life, including spores.

The most effective methods of sterilization use high-pressure steam equipment called an autoclave. Simply exposing instruments to steam is not enough. To be effective against disease-causing pathogens, the steam must be pressurized in an autoclave so that the steam penetrates the spore coats of the spore-forming bacteria. Dry-heat forms of sterilization are less efficient and require longer times at higher temperatures. Dry-heat sterilization is not recommended for use in salons or spas.

It is important to understand how to use an autoclave correctly. For example, dirty implements cannot be properly sterilized without first being properly cleaned. Autoclaves need regular maintenance and testing to ensure they are in good working order. The color-indicator strips that are used on autoclave bags can provide false readings, so they should never be used solely to determine whether instruments have been sterilized. These strips are only an indication, not verification, that the autoclave is working.

The CDC requires that autoclaves be tested weekly to ensure that they are properly sterilizing implements. The accepted method is called a spore test. Sealed packages containing test organisms are subjected to a typical sterilization cycle and then sent to a contract laboratory that specializes in autoclave performance testing. You can find laboratories to

---

CAUTION!

Improper mixing of disinfectants—to be weaker or more concentrated than the manufacturer's instructions, for example—can dramatically reduce their effectiveness. Always add the disinfectant concentrate to the water when mixing and follow the manufacturer's instructions for proper dilution. Safety glasses and gloves should be worn to avoid accidental contact with eyes and skin.

As with all disinfecting materials, it is necessary to follow the manufacturer's recommendations for product and device use. A failure to do so may result in injury, incomplete decontamination results, or a loss of warranty by some manufacturers.

The benefits of sterilization are:

- Sterilization is the most reliable means of infection control.
- Sterilized tools and implements in sealed bags assure clients that you are using fresh instruments during the service. The bag should be opened just before the service to show clients that the tools and implements have been sterilized and that the salon or spa owners and staff care about the safety of their clients.

perform this type of test by simply doing an Internet search for autoclave spore testing. Other regular maintenance is also required to ensure that the autoclave reaches the correct temperature and pressure. Keep in mind that an autoclave that does not reach the intended temperature for killing microorganisms may create a warm, moist place where pathogenic organisms can grow and thrive.

Safety Tips for Disinfectants

Do:

- Keep a Material Safety Data Sheet (MSDS) on hand for the disinfectant(s) you use.
- Wear gloves and safety glasses when mixing disinfectants.
- Avoid skin and eye contact.
- Add disinfectant to water when diluting (rather than adding water to a disinfectant) to prevent foaming, which can result in an incorrect mixing ratio.
- Use tongs, gloves, or a draining basket to remove implements from disinfectants.
- Keep disinfectants out of reach of children.
- Carefully measure and use disinfectant products according to label instructions.
- Follow the manufacturer's instructions for mixing, using, and disposing of disinfectants.
- Carefully follow the manufacturer's directions for when to replace the disinfectant solution in order to ensure the healthiest conditions for you and your client. Replace the disinfectant solution every day—and more often if the solution becomes soiled or contaminated.

accelerated hydrogen peroxide (AHP)
Disinfectant based on stabilized hydrogen peroxide that needs to be changed only every 14 days. It is nontoxic to the skin and the environment.

DID YOU KNOW ?

The EPA has recently approved a new disinfectant for use in salons, spas, and medical facilities called **accelerated hydrogen peroxide (AHP)**. Available in a spray, immersion form, and wipes, this disinfectant is based on stabilized hydrogen peroxide and needs to be changed only every 14 days. It is nontoxic to the skin and the environment. There are test strips available to check the effectiveness during the 14-day period. One AHP formula is available for disinfecting pedicure tubs. As it is a new product, it is a good idea to have the EPA registry information readily available for inspector visits. As always, read the labels of all types of disinfectants closely. Choose the one that is most appropriate for its intended use and the safest for you and your clients.

Do Not:

- Let disinfectants come in contact with your skin. If you do get disinfectants on your skin, immediately wash the area with liquid soap and warm water. Then rinse the area and dry the area thoroughly.
- Place any disinfectant or other product in a marked container. All containers must be labeled.

 BREAKING THE CHAIN OF INFECTION

The spread of infection is described as a chain with six links connected in a circle (Figure 3–3). Each link has its own name and a function that it serves to keep the infection going. If we break any one link, we can stop the transmission of the infection. In Table 3–2, we explore what each link does and how it creates a medium for the transmission of infection.

Keep a Logbook

Salons, spas, skin care centers, and medi-spas should always follow manufacturers' recommended schedules for cleaning and disinfecting tools and implements and sinks and basins. It is necessary to schedule regular service visits for equipment and replace parts when needed. Although your state may not require you to keep a logbook of all equipment usage, cleaning, disinfecting, testing, and maintenance, it is advisable to keep one. Showing your logbook to clients provides them with peace of mind and confidence in your ability to protect them from infection and disease.

 MATERIAL SAFETY DATA SHEET

Federal and state laws require that manufacturers supply a MSDS for all products sold and used (Figure 3–4). The MSDS contains information compiled by the manufacturer about product safety, including the names of hazardous ingredients, safe handling and use procedures, precautions to reduce the risk of accidental harm or overexposure, and flammability warnings. The MSDS also provides useful disposal guidelines and medical and first aid information. When necessary, the MSDS can be sent to a medical facility so that a doctor can better assess and treat the patient. OSHA and state regulatory agencies require that MSDS documents are to be kept available in the salon, spa, or medical office for all products. OSHA and state board inspectors can issue fines for salons, spas, medical offices, or medi-spas for not having MSDS documents available during regular business hours.

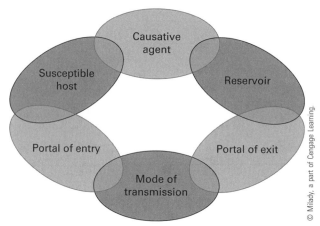

Figure 3–3 The chain of infection.

© Milady, a part of Cengage Learning.

Table 3–2 Breaking the Chain of Infection

Name of Link in Chain	What Is It?	How Do I Break the Chain of Infection?
Infectious agent	Bacteria, virus, fungi, parasite	Hand washing, disinfecting implements and objects in the workplace and home, vaccinations, eating well
Reservoir	A person, plant, animal, or object in which an infectious agent can live; often wet or damp areas.	Cleaning, disinfecting work stations, esthetic rooms, staying well, handling food properly
Portal of exit	The way the infectious agent leaves the reservoir out into the environment such as nose, mouth, body fluids	Covering mouth when coughing and sneezing, handling waste products safely, covering scratches, abrasions and cuts
Mode of transmission	Any mechanism in which infectious material can spread from a reservoir to a person, whether directly or indirectly, such as in unwashed hands, mucus, or airborne particles	Hand washing, wearing gloves, cleaning and disinfecting high-touch areas, maintaining and using standard precautions at all times
Portal of entry	A break in the skin, or eyes, nose, or mouth, where the infectious material can gain entry into the person	Using personal protection devices, goggles, gloves, masks, covering wounds when working, not drinking or eating in service or treatment areas, not touching face or mouth if hands are not clean
Susceptible host	A person vulnerable to the infectious material, or one lacking the necessary resistance to the pathogen	Maintaining good health, vaccinations, maintaining good skin health, not smoking or drinking excessively

© Milady, a part of Cengage Learning.

Material Safety Data Sheet (MSDS)

Section I

Product Name or Number	Emergency Telephone No.
Manufacturer's Name	Manufacturer's D-U-N-5 No.
Address (Number, Street, City, State, Zip)	
Hazardous Materials Description and Proper Shipping Name (49.CFR 172.101)	Hazardous Class (49.CFR 172.101)
Chemical Family	Formula

Section II — Ingredients (list all ingredients)   CASE REGISTRY NO.   %

Section III — Physical Data

Boiling Point (F) (C)	Specific Gravity (H_2O = 1)	
Vapor Pressure (mm Hg) ———	Percent Volatile by Volume (%)	
(psl) ———		
Vapor Density (Air = 1)	Evaporation Rate (= 1)	
Solubility in Water	pH =	
Appearance and Odor	Is material: Liquid Solid Gas Paste Powder	

Section IV — Fire & Explosion Hazard Data

Flash Point (method used)	Flammable Limits	LEL	UEL
( )			
( )			
Extinguishing Media			
Special Fire Fighting Procedures			
Unusual Fire and Explosion Hazards			

Figure 3–4 An MSDS document.

SAFETY TIPS FOR THE SALON, SPA, SKIN
CARE CENTER, OR MEDICAL SETTING

1. Clean your space systematically and routinely. This is an area where we cannot be too compulsive. Use approved cleaning solutions and EPA-registered disinfectants after each direct contact, service, treatment, or procedure. Clean and disinfect all bottles, caps, sinks, and surfaces and follow with disinfecting practices. Follow with autoclave use where appropriate.

2. Follow the correct hand-washing regulations and practices. Frequent hand washing is the first preventative measure to control the transmission of microorganisms, therefore disease. A standard hand washing protocol is:

   i. Use a dry paper towel to turn on the faucet (sinks are considered contaminated).

   ii. Wet hands with warm water (not hot), use a liquid soap, and lather for two minutes. (Hot water can dry the skin and create small open pathways, or **fissures**, for pathogens to enter the body.)

   iii. Use a brush to clean under nails.

   iv. Rinse thoroughly, without touching the faucet.

   v. Use paper towels to dry hands and then discard them. Use another paper towel to turn off the faucet, and then another to open the bathroom door.

   vi. When hand washing is unavailable, the CDC recommends using an alcohol-based hand sanitizer that contains at least 60 percent alcohol, which can quickly reduce the number or germs on hands in some situations. The CDC recommends using hand sanitizers as follows:

   - Apply the product to the palm of one hand.
   - Rub your hands together.
   - Rub the products over all surfaces of your hands and fingers until your hands are dry.

3. Wear gloves for all services, treatments, and procedures where you can reasonably anticipate coming in contact with OPIM. Wear them for cleaning and mixing solutions. Remove gloves immediately after use to avoid contaminating other surfaces. Then perform a hand washing.

4. Follow standard precautions for disposing of all OPIM.

   i. Put all used sharps into a sharps container.

   ii. Put all cotton swabs, used gloves, and other used materials into an approved red biohazard bag, which is collected and

fissures
Cracks in the skin that penetrate the dermis; examples include severely cracked and/or chapped hands or lips.

disposed of according to protocol for biohazardous materials.

5. Read and follow MSDS. Create your own MSDS notebook for easy reference by including all the sheets that you have for the products that you retail in one section and those that you use in practice in another.

6. Create a room-cleaning and disinfecting checklist. This should be up to date in case you are audited by inspectors of any type (state inspections, OSHA, clinic administrator). Your checklist will show frequency of cleaning and disinfecting of the esthetic rooms on a daily, weekly, monthly, and quarterly basis, including sinks, equipment, floors, product bottles, vents, walls, beds, chairs, ceilings, trash and biohazard units, and all other items in the room (Figure 3–5).

7. Be prepared for inspections. The esthetic professional never knows when he or she may be visited by state and government inspectors, therefore, it is good to be prepared. OSHA inspections can take place without notice and cannot be rescheduled.

   If you do have an inspection, you can expect the inspector to present his or her credentials and ask to speak to the owner, manager, or administrator of your facility. The inspector will describe the scope of the visit and discuss the procedures that are to be followed. Your OSHA records, charts, cleaning lists, and esthetic rooms will be inspected, and a general walk-through will be conducted. The inspector may speak to employees. If there are any violations, they will be served to the owner, manager, or the administrator. Make certain to have the OSHA regulations posted where all employees can view them.

   The reasons for their visit are typically in order as follows:

   a. There is an immediate danger to employees.
   b. There has been a fatality or accident (in which three or more employees were injured).
   c. A complaint has been filed.
   d. The occasion is random (and was perhaps assigned by computer).

   If you are visited by an OSHA inspector:
   - Do not panic.
   - Do not volunteer information.
   - Answer questions truthfully.
   - Document the inspector's name, badge number, the time and date of the visit, and the areas inspected.

ROOM-CLEANING FORM

Month of: _____

DAILY FREQUENCY:
1. Scrub and clean sinks and faucets _____ (INT)
2. Floors mopped and cleaned _____ (INT)
3. Trash and red HAZMAT cans cleaned, wiped down and relined _____ (INT)
4. Spillage on walls or doors to be whipped down _____ (INT)
5. Facial bed, microdermabrasion equipment, bowls, countertops to be cleaned after each client/patient _____ (INT)
6. Facial scope _____ (INT)

WEEKLY FREQUENCY:
1. Clean all air conditioning or heating grills/vents _____ (INT)
2. Clean walls of esthetic room _____ (INT)
3. Clean H$_2$O steamer and other facial equipment hardware _____ (INT)

QUARTERLY:
1. Clean room ceiling _____ (INT)

*Some of these duties may be performed by a professional cleaning service.
*OSHA will expect that you have an updated form readily available.

Figure 3–5 A room-cleaning checklist.

 SAFETY AND CONFIDENTIALITY

Another area of public safety falls in the realm of confidentiality. Regardless of where we work, we must keep all matters concerning records of clients, customers, and employees confidential. The Department of Health and Human Services (HHS) developed federal privacy standards called the Health Insurance Portability Accountability Act (HIPAA) of 1996 in order to protect patients in medical settings with respect to their health information, and regarding health plans, physician notes and records, and general patient information and how that information is used.

The same goes for estheticians in any setting. As estheticians and salon, spa, and skin care professionals, it is vitally important from a legal standpoint to protect clients' information from being exposed to other staff members, other clients, and the public. This means that we do not share the details of a client's visit in a consultation, in a service, at home, or anywhere else with anyone other than that client. There have been incidences in which information has been shared publically about clients and customers, which resulted in litigation. This lowers the standards for our profession. Do not ever post information online or on social networking sites. This is unprofessional, and one may end up having to defend oneself in a court of law for having passed on sensitive information about a client. Every time you share private information about a client, consider: "How would this sound if I had to defend myself in court?" It is always advisable to keep all information about a client confidential.

 ## SUMMING IT UP

Infection control needs to be the number one focus of the practicing esthetician. As we look at new and improved ways to keep our clients, coworkers, and the public safe, it is necessary to continually research new methods of decontamination and stay up on the latest information as provided by OSHA and the CDC. As we move forward, we will undoubtedly face more areas of exposure and need to adjust our protocols accordingly. It is also advisable to continue to train new members of our profession on the importance of breaking the chain of infection.

ESTHETICIAN **PROFILE**

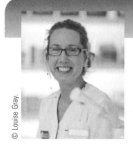

Louise Gray, RN
Beauty Therapist

Owner, Louise Gray Skin Care Centers, Mission Bay, Auckland, and Ponsonby, New Zealand

I am a registered general nurse and worked extensively in intensive care. With this type of nursing, you realize how the body works as a whole and that you cannot compartmentalize things. I often saw how my patient's facial skin reacted to various medications and how stress from illness/disease or trauma is portrayed on the skin. I loved my role, especially working with people, and had never intended to leave, but in the end, I wanted and needed to move on. I still wanted to involve myself with patients/people on a health level, so I began my beauty therapy training in 1995. Dividing my time as a nurse and skin care/beauty therapist, I came to realize that I had a real passion for skin health. I loved helping others with skin problems, and enjoyed true success.

With my strong background in health care, I took the traditional beauty therapy role to the next level in skin health by founding Every-Body Skin and Body Care in 1998. We focus on looking behind the surface for a complete overview of the body's functioning to treat and correct many skin conditions. My centers have won the premier beauty therapy of New Zealand award, "Beauty Therapist of the Year NZ," in 2003; the Dermalogica Therapist of the Year in 2009; and Dermalogica Skin Care Centre of the Year in 2011. I believe these awards are a tribute to my true desire to treat the largest organ of the body with respect and knowledge.

Training

1976–1979	Registered general and obstetric nurse training
1988	Postgraduate intensive care therapy course
1995–1996	Student beauty therapist, Joyce Blok Institute; received thesis prize
1997	Joyce Blok Institute/electrolysis tutor
2003	New Zealand Beauty Therapy Awards, "Best Therapist"
2002–2005	Dermalogica Platinum Clinic
2006–2008	Dermalogica Premier Platinum Clinic
2008–2011	Dermalogica Award, "Skin Centre of Excellence"
2009–2011	Dermalogica Award, "Commitment to Education"
2011	Dermalogica Skin Care Centre of the Year

Practice Demographic

Our client base is primarily in the 30- to 60-year-old age bracket; we focus mostly on age management, skin rebalancing due to hormonal disturbances, and hyperpigmentation.

We also have great success with treating many other skin conditions, from sensitive/sensitized skins to imbalanced skins to irritated skins, including dermatitis and eczema.

Services/Treatments Offered

Our tried-and-tested skin bar achieves an 80-percent-retail to 20-percent-service ratio and gives clients the ability to use the product themselves on their skin in a setting that mimics what they will be doing at home. Using Micro-Zone services, we take treatments out of the treatment room—we offer 20–minute, targeted treatments that provide maximum results in the minimal amount of time.

We also offer a full beauty therapy service menu with a core facial treatment; this is a 60-minute treatment with no description, as it is customized for the client.

Consumer research shows that the number of consumers who receive regular beauty therapy and spa treatments globally is in decline; only 5 percent of consumers in the U.S., Canada, UK, and Australia partake of this service. However, the consumption of professional skin care products has doubled in the last eight years. Clients have become self-selectors and want facilities where they can make informed decisions guided by professionals. Time has become a precious commodity with working families, seven-day trading, financial pressure, and complex lifestyles. Consumers today are now extremely results driven, and demand, "Prove to me that it is worth it! I don't have time or money to waste!"

Personal Philosophy

I believe that Louise Gray Skin Care clinics are more than just skin care centers: they have shown success in changing people's emotional outlook and the employees have also enjoyed success.

Education, I believe, is the main driving factor that has made the clinics so successful. Louise Gray Professional Skin Care therapists follow a training program that ensures they are educated to the highest industry standard; their skills go beyond product knowledge and techniques to include in-depth skin histology, client care, and business skills. We therapists need to become masters in the art of understanding people. We all have different personalities, so we need to be able to assist them in the best way possible.

Additional Contributions to the Industry

Continuing with my strong passion for education, I have been an educator for the Joyce Blok Institute, focusing on electrolysis, and with Dermal International NZ, focusing on its core classes. I always believe in giving back to the community in which we work, as our community is what supports us the most. I regularly support local businesses, schools, and community-based projects by offering service gifts, speaking at local schools on skin health, and providing support and encouragement for clients who have completed an amazing physical feat.

ESTHETICIAN **PROFILE**

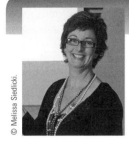

© Melissa Siedlicki.

Melissa Siedlicki, LE
CIDESCO Diplomat

Medical Esthetics Instructor, Clover Park Technical College, Tacoma, WA, USA

I was born and raised in Tacoma, Washington. I became an esthetician because I have a fascination with the skin; it amazed me then and still does today. I went to esthetics school in 1987 at Clover Park (Vocational) Technical College. At that time, the program was a combination license–manicuring and esthetics for a total of 500 hours. Esthetics was new in Washington, and the majority of my early business was nails, silk tips, and acrylics. Applying artificial nails was not my favorite thing to do, but I became fast and was good at it. I slowly turned my steady nail clientele into skin care clients.

I obtained my CIDESCO international diploma in 2003. I have obtained certification in laser practices and safety through Rocky Mountain Laser College, and will soon be certified in cosmetic chemistry through UCLA extension courses offered by Rebecca James Gadberry.

Training

As an educator, I am always learning. I have trained with the following companies and educators:

- International Dermal Institute
- Peter Pugliese, MD
- Mark Lees, PhD
- Rebecca James Gadberry, UCLA
- Janna Ronert, Image Skin Care
- PCA
- Bio-Therapeutic
- Rocky Mountain Laser College (laser hair reduction, IPL, pigment reduction, and skin tightening)
- Dr. Vodder manual lymphatic drainage
- Jane Iredale

Practice/School Demographic

Clover Park Technical College is a state college. Our students come from all walks of life. While the primary student demographic is female, we have had over the past few years some male students as well. The youngest student I have had was 17 in the running start program; the oldest student was 67.

When I started teaching at CPTC, I taught what is now referred to as "basic esthetics," which included facials, waxing, makeup, body wraps, anatomy and physiology, diseases, disorders, safety, and sanitation. In 2003, I saw a need for advanced training, real, in-depth training. A lot of situations were arising from a lack of adequate training in chemical peels, rapid exfoliations, and even microdermabrasion and "not-so-simple" laser applications. A solid educational foundation is the key to students' doing well in class, in students' practices, and in increasing safety in the marketplace.

School Spa Services Offered (Also Incorporated into Courses)

At Clover Park Technical College, we have a program called "esthetic sciences." This course incorporates two separate programs: the basic licensing course (600 hours as currently required by Washington State), and "medical esthetics," which is an additional 600 hours of advanced technologies. Since I developed this program, I have seen articles published that support the need for students to obtain these skills in order to work as medical estheticians. Our licensing program incorporates a working clinic, in which the public can come in and receive services at a reduced fee, including facials, waxing, Vichy room treatments, and makeup applications. The courses and services are as follows:

- Manual lymph drainage
- Microdermabrasion: three different styles of machine (aluminum-oxide crystals, diamond-encrusted tips, and nylon/plastic or silk tips), so students have a well-rounded education in any microdermabrasion machine modality

- Three different peel lines (PCA Skin, Neostrata, and Image) with their complimentary skin care products, mostly focusing on repair and wound or inflammation
- Jane Iredale mineral makeup (our focus is on camouflage post)
- LED therapies
- Bio-dermology cellulite treatments; students not only learn how to apply these technologies but receive a lecture series on each modality
- In-depth laser physics and theory course
- Hands-on laser training
- Advanced cosmetic chemistry

Personal Philosophy and Rewards

It warms my heart to see students "get it" with the smiles and excitement they exhibit when they have learned something new. I really get excited for them. They know when they come to me with a question, however, that I am not just going to answer it for them. I walk them through it, and ask them to tell me why they chose *that peel*, or why they want to use a *specific technology*, for example. I empower them to be independent thinkers and play out each scenario, from a peel to a laser treatment. The key to success and in sustaining oneself in this industry is to love what you do, to gain as much continuing education as possible, and to reinvest in yourself regularly.

Additional Contributions to the Industry

I have four Washington State licenses: esthetician, cosmetologist, manicurist, and instructor. I hold a CIDESCO international diploma. I develop curriculum and am an instructor for the advanced medical esthetics program at CPTC. I have presented to the Washington State Department of Licensing at cosmetology and esthetic meetings in favor of increasing hours for esthetician programs. I am an advisory member for the NW Aestheticians Guild and teach classes at the Guild on laser and light therapies.

Enzyme, Chemical, and Layering Peels

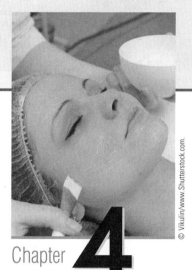

"A chemical peel can be one of the most powerful, versatile, and efficacious treatments available to the aesthetician. With a wide variety of applications that can produce dramatic results, the chemical peel merits strong consideration as the treatment of choice."

—Amy Classen, Clinical Aesthetician-Hecht Aesthetic Center, Bellingham, Washington

Chapter **4**

Chapter Capture

After completing this chapter, you will be able to:

- Analyze the skin you are peeling.
- Implement the skin analysis classification tools.
- Understand the pH of peeling products.
- Identify the variables in chemical peeling.
- Perform an enzyme peel.
- Perform a chemical peel.

UNDERSTANDING THE SKIN YOU ARE PEELING

In many cases, peels are the best application for skin rejuvenation, and preparation is critical to the successful outcome of any peel. Peels are economical for the esthetician and easy to apply. However, they are anything but easy if one has limited experience or does not follow protocols. It is important to stay within your scope of practice. A salon peel is vastly different from a medical grade peel, and the recovery time and experience from a chemical peel is in direct relationship to the level of peel you are using and the skin type you are peeling. A client's **Fitzpatrick skin type** is also of primary concern with respect to the type of peeling agent that you select. The higher the Fitzpatrick type, the more risk there is for pigment changes and scarring.

As we have learned, chemical peels are designed to increase exfoliation by applying skin-type- and condition-specific peeling products to the skin, which stimulates cell renewal by releasing old cells from the stratum corneum. In peels that penetrate deeper into the papillary dermis, or into the dermis, creating a wound response creates stimulation of the **fibroblasts**. This upregulates collagen and elastin production, increases the thickness of the dermis and makes the skin look firm, less wrinkled, and fuller. Deeper peels are always performed by a physician or other qualified medical personnel.

Fitzpatrick skin type
Scale used to measure the skin type's ability to tolerate sun exposure.

fibroblasts
Cells that are responsible for making connective tissue such as collagen.

The Analysis

The analysis conducted during the consultation becomes the primary method to determine whether you will use a chemical peel, which one you will use, and whether your treatment will include technology. We have found that some technologies that offer product penetration such as microcurrent and galvanic therapies can make peeling solutions more unpredictable and are therefore not recommended for use during the peeling phase of stronger, deeper peels. It is best to always follow the manufacturer's recommendations and attend their certification courses.

> **CAUTION!**
>
> In most states, esthetician licensure allows us to perform superficial peels. Make certain to know and understand the rules and regulation regarding peels in your state. Unless you are working in a medical facility and are under the direction of a physician, do not perform peels that are beyond your licensure: in doing so, you may risk the skin health of your clients and possibly your license to practice.

GUEST SPOT

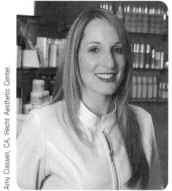

Amy Classen, CA, Hecht Aesthetic Center.

AMY CLASSEN, CLINICAL AESTHETICIAN

Amy Classen, a clinical aesthetician from the Hecht Aesthetic Center in Bellingham, Washington, shares information on chemical peeling:

As with other forms of treatment, chemical peels will bring about changes to the tone and texture of skin as well as reducing surface lines and wrinkles. However, one advantage of a peel is that a customized mixture of acids can offer the versatility of treating multiple conditions at once. The application of a progressive series of chemical peels can also lead to dramatic results without the trauma or downtime that can come from a deeper laser treatment.

The peels I use are superficial, simply meaning that they only treat the topmost layers of the skin. This means the client can leave my office with very little to no downtime.

Types of Chemical Peels

The types of chemical peels I find most effective are modified and enhanced Jessner's and blended TCA (trichloroacetic acid) peels. The exfoliating agents I use are a blend of lactic acid, salicylic acid, and an array of natural skin lighteners, such as **Kojic** and citric acids. I can use these acids to treat a variety of issues. For example, I will treat an acne client who has post-inflammatory hyperpigmentation (PIH) with a **tyrosinase inhibitor** such as Kojic acid and then with salicylic acid for smoothing and reducing impactions and as an anti-inflammatory agent.

Preparing the Client

Preparing the client begins with the consultation. The first step is to determine the issue and the goal of the client. It is important to set realistic expectations about what the chemical peel can accomplish. I always give clients a very informative, step-by-step explanation of the process of the chemical peel as well as the pre- and post-care. My client will know everything that will happen and everything that could happen. Educating the client is critical to ensure that there are no surprises, that the client knows what to expect, and that he or she will get the most out of the treatment. How a client takes care of the skin post-treatment is as important as the peel itself. Some peels require that the client follow rules regarding sun exposure in the weeks or days following treatment, for example, that would actually aggravate the skin's condition.

Medical History and Documenting Observations

It is also essential to get a full medical history of your client prior to applying a peel to determine whether he or she has any contraindications, such as recent isotretinoin use or herpetic (herpes) outbreaks. If a client has a history of herpes, refer the client to his or her physician for

Kojic acid
Type of tyrosinase inhibitor used to stabilize and reduce melanin production.

tyrosinase inhibitor
A product or ingredient that inhibits the melanin producing enzyme tyrosinase.

fyi

There are many sophisticated tools on the market today that provide interesting skin analysis profiles. They are great marketing tools and have a variety of accessories. However, these devices may or may not help us decide which peel preparations to use, as many of them are very expensive. They are also often relegated for use in a pretreatment sales presentation by a nonpractitioner for the client or patient. Every esthetician preparing to provide chemical peels must be able to make assessments based on the skin type and condition that he or she is treating, with experience with the product that will be applied.

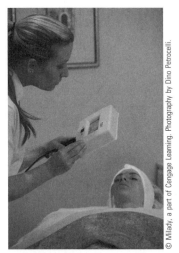

Figure 4–1 Using a Wood's lamp for analysis.

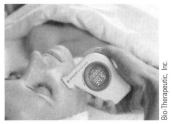

Figure 4–2 A moisture reading tool.

 home care compliance
Clients or patients using products at home in a manner consistent with a plan created by an esthetician and physician.

reepithelialized
Formation of new epidermis and dermis over an area of injury in which epithelial cells from the wound margin and the pilosebaceous units migrate to repair damage.

an evaluation and prescription for antiviral medication. Any health issues or deviations on the client intake form should be well researched prior to beginning a peeling series.

Along with analysis tools and classifications that we will discuss, a simple Wood's lamp and a moisture reading device are examples of good practice in making accurate observations, documentation, and in setting up a treatment plan (Figure 4–1; Figure 4–2).

Home Care Compliance

Home care compliance is stressed when it comes to the client's ability to care for a peel, whether it be a light enzyme peel, a superficial chemical peel, or one that is more complicated and involves technology. From products and prescriptions used to prepare for a peel to post-peel soothing, calming, and healing applications, it is necessary to watch clients closely in the first few days and weeks before and after the peel. It is important to make certain that they are not pulling on peeling skin; using home devices prematurely; or using retinoic acid, retinol, or AHAs or BHAs in higher concentrations before they are fully **reepithelialized**, or healed.

Many estheticians and skin care providers and their clients have enjoyed exceptional experiences and results with chemical peels. When done well, they are an excellent choice for age management and photo damage.

SKIN TYPES

Whether we are just beginning our work as estheticians or are long-term practitioners, we know that we must have a good understanding of the skin type and condition for which we plan to peel, regardless of the peel formula. There are skin analysis classification tools that we may use to guide our decision making toward successful outcomes. They have been developed by true pioneers in dermatology: dermatologists Thomas B. Fitzpatrick, Richard G. Glogau, Mark G. Rubin, and Alfred M. Kligman. It is to them that we owe our gratitude and success.

Fitzpatrick Skin Types

As we remember from our basic training, one of the first tools to use in skin assessment is the Fitzpatrick Skin Type Scale. It continues to serve as a guide in determining the strength and type of peeling agent we might use. Whether a client is very light and burns easily or has darker skin and more resistance to burning, we have a point of reference to anchor our decisions for a peeling formula (Table 4-1).

Table 4–1 Fitzpatrick Skin Types

Fitzpatrick Skin Type	Characteristics
Skin Type I	Always burns. Has light blue or green eyes, may have **ephelides** (light freckles). Has a pink undertone to the skin. Usually has white, blond, or red hair. May become **erythemic** (present redness) with peels and take time to heal.*
Skin Type II	Always burns, may tan lightly. Has blue or green eyes. Skin is slightly warmer than skin type I. Is a good candidate for peels as he/she will generally not develop pigment problems.
Skin Type III	Sometimes burns, tans easily. May have dark green or brown eyes, and darker hair. May pigment easily. May need to use pre-peel lightening agents, but typically tolerate peels well.
Skin Type IV	Rarely burns, tans easily. Typically has dark eyes and hair. Will pigment easily. Best to do more frequency, lower-level peels. Avoid **postinflammatory hyperpigmentation** (pigment changes created by trauma, injury, and peels or stronger products).
Skin Type V	Rarely burns, tans effortlessly. Dark eyes and hair. At risk for **hypopigmentation** (loss of pigment) and **hyperpigmentation** (increase in pigmentation). Not a candidate for many resurfacing procedures or deep peels. May scar easily and develop **keloids** (raised scars).
Skin Type VI	Does not burn. Dark black eyes and hair. Can pigment, hypogpigment, scar, and develop keloids. Use lower-level exfoliants in both treatment and home care plans. Do not overstimulate **melanocytes** (cell factories that create the pigment melanin) by overuse of vacuuming, abrading (microdermabrasion), or peeling.

© Milady, a part of Cengage Learning.

*Note that some higher-level skin types may burn and be reactive to the sun, chemical peels, and other forms of skin exfoliation. It is always advisable to patch test all skin types with the peeling product you plan to use.

ephelides
Light-colored freckles.

erythema
Redness caused by inflammation.

postinflammatory hyperpigmentation
Dark melanin splotches caused by trauma to the skin that can result from acne pimples and papules.

hypopigmentation
Absence of pigment that results in light or white splotches.

hyperpigmentation
Overproduction of pigment.

keloid
Thick scar resulting from excessive growth of fibrous tissue (collagen).

melanocytes
Cell that produces pigment granules/melanin in the basal layer of the epidermis.

Glogau Photodamage Classification

The **Glogau Photodamage Classification** presents four levels of photodamage, ranging from minimal to extreme. Glogau classification measures wrinkle activity that can be seen on the face, whether the face is in motion or at rest, at four levels. The first level is observing no

Glogau Photodamage Classification
Categorization of wrinkle activity developed by Richard Glogau, MD.

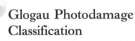

wrinkles while the face is at rest or moving. The second level is observing wrinkles only while the face is moving, such as smiling or laughing. The third level is observing wrinkles while the face is at rest and there is no facial activity. The fourth and final level is when wrinkles are a predominate feature of the face, whether it is at rest or moving. The four levels are as follows (Table 4-2):

keratosis
Abnormally thick buildup of cells.

lentigines
Technical term for freckles; small, yellow-colored to brown-colored spots on skin exposed to sunlight and air.

Table 4–2 Glogau Photodamage Classification

Type	Wrinkle Activity	Characteristics
I	No wrinkles at rest or while moving	Early photoaging • Mild pigment changes • No **keratosis** (dead cellular buildup) • No wrinkles • Upper teens to 30s • Minimal acne scarring
II	Wrinkles only in motion (person is speaking, laughing, frowning)	Early to moderate photoaging • **lentigines** (pigmented lesions historically called liver spots) • Wrinkles forming • Light keratosis • Nasolabial fold forming • 30s to 40s
III	Wrinkles at rest (visible while not moving)	Advanced photoaging • Hyperpigmentation • Telangiectasia • Keratosis
IV	Wrinkles as predominate characteristic	Severe photoaging • Sallow, ashen skin color • Prior skin cancers • Wrinkles are all over face

© Milady, a part of Cengage Learning.

Rubin Photodamage Classification

The Rubin Photodamage Classification is a system that categorizes the level of photodamage based on the depth of visible changes in the skin. This form of analysis allows the practitioner to determine the level of peel that will best treat the condition. This can be used with a combination of other classifications to apply the best peel possible for the client (Figure 4–3).

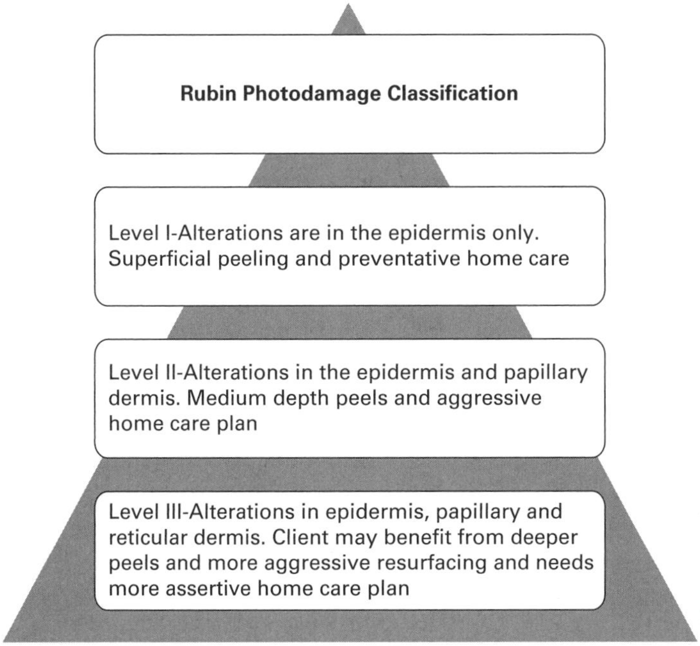

Figure 4–3 Rubin Photodamage Classification.

Kligman Acne Classification

Alfred Kligman, MD, developed an acne classification system for identifying levels of acne from the least to the greatest amount (Table 4-3).

Table 4–3 Kligman Acne Classification

	Characteristics
Grade I	Open and closed comedones with transitory, noninflamed lesions
Grade II	More open and closed comedones, with a few pustules and papules
Grade III	Open and closed comedones; many pustules and papules; may present with cystic lesions, pigment changes, and inflammation; may exhibit erythema; may be painful
Grade IV	Exhibits all of the above stages at more advanced levels and may develop mental and/or psychological issues due to condition

PEELS AND pH

Knowing the pH (potential hydrogen) of a peel product is as important as understanding the skin type you are peeling. Simply put, if a 15 percent glycolic peel has a peel pH level of 1.0, it is going to be much more aggressive than a compound with a 3.8 ph containing the same percentage of glycolic.

Buffered and Nonbuffered Peels

A nonbuffered, nonchemically altered pH peel will be stronger than a buffered peel. If a buffered peel has a pH of 3.8, for example, and the nonbuffered peel has a pH of 1, and both have 30 percent glycolic acid, the nonbuffered peel will be stronger and cause more irritation. For some skin types, such as oily and acneic, this may be advantageous. Buffering a peel allows the active product to stay on the skin longer without irritation and may prove in the end to be a better choice for normal skin types or sensitive reactive skin types.

 # VARIABLES IN PEELING

Standardizing the peeling process will help the esthetician control the peel as much as possible in order to ensure a positive outcome. If the peel preparation, the peeling process, and the post-peel care are consistent, with little deviation, there is a greater chance for success each time. If we are constantly trying a different preparation or peeling product or protocol, it will be difficult to determine which step affected the process, whether positive or negatively.

The variables in peeling are as follows:

- The type of peel
- The percentage of the peeling ingredient
- The pH
- Whether the peel is buffered or nonbuffered
- The amount of layers applied
- The length of time the peel is left on
- The client's skin type and condition
- The pre-peel preparation
- The post-peel care
- Home care compliance

Long-term professionals who have used thousands of peels and peel preparations will state that it is always important to be consistent in all phases of peeling to obtain the best results and to rule out any deviations to the success of a given peel preparation. Consistency is the key to using peels in your practice.

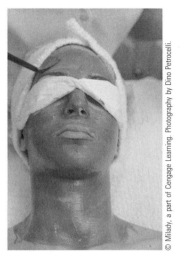

Figure 4–4 An enzyme peel application.

ENZYME PEELS: PAPAYA, PUMPKIN, AND PINEAPPLE

Historically, enzyme peels have been used for sensitive, dry, and dehydrated skin types and conditions and have been excellent for acneic skin, which does not tolerate other types of peeling products. (It is worth noting, however, that certain enzyme peels can be very aggressive.) Clients must be using regular home care products for their skin type and condition as preparation for any type of peel, and to support healing. Make sure they are using environmental protection with an SPF of at least 30. Enzymes may be gentler in many ways than acid-based chemical peels but can be just as unforgiving when used incorrectly. Erythema, hyperpigmentation, and irritation may result from a chemical peel if the client's skin has not been properly prepped, if the client has allergies to the enzyme peel ingredients, or if an inappropriate enzyme peel has been used (Figure 4–4).

The Objective

Your objective in applying an enzyme peel is to perform a superficial exfoliation of the stratum corneum. Enzyme peels will be tolerated by most skin types and conditions. The peel has reached its optimum benefit when the skin has an even, slightly pink tone. If some areas are turning red or if the client is experiencing discomfort, remove the enzyme peel. Conduct patch testing before applying any peels.

The more preparation you do before the peel in home care and patch testing, the better your results will be. This is true for all enzyme and chemical peels.

Indications

Clients who have the following conditions are the best candidates for enzyme peels:

- Dehydration
- Aging
- Fine lines
- Superficial hyperpigmentation

Contraindications

Clients who have the following conditions are not candidates for enzyme peels:

- Isotretinoin use within a year (must obtain a physician's recommendation)
- Herpetic outbreak (cold sores)
- Open wounds (acne lesions or other bleeding lesions)
- Pregnancy and lactation
- Cancer
- Autoimmune disorders
- Sunburn
- Dermatitis
- Eczema

PROCEDURE 4–1: ENZYME PEEL

Supplies List
- Gloves
- Brush
- Water
- Glass bowl
- Timer
- Gauze
- Sponges or towels
- Eye pads
- Informed consent document

Products
- Enzyme peel product
- Cleanser
- Hydrating serum
- Soothing cream (azulene, allantoin)
- Environmental protection product with SPF 30

Protocol
1. The client signs the informed consent document. Prep client with standard protocols, secure his or her hair with a headband, and apply eye protection.

2. With cleansed, gloved hands, apply a thin layer of the product, starting at the forehead.

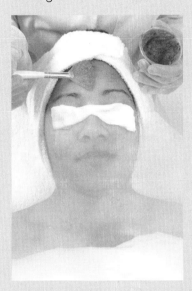

3. While applying peel to the forehead, use steam for activation if required by the product.

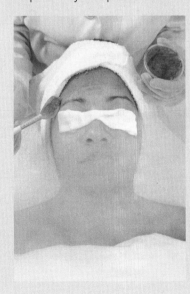

4. Apply enzyme peel to the nasal area, and continue.

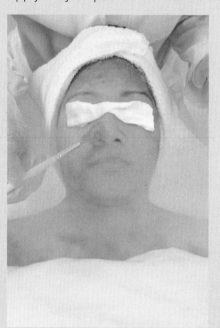

5. Apply the enzyme peel to the cheeks.

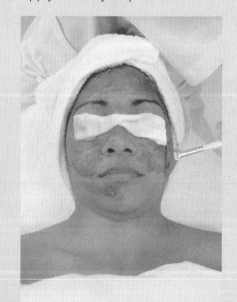

6. Apply the enzyme peel to the chin.

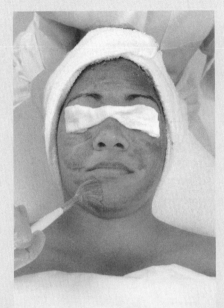

7. Apply the enzyme peel to the entire face.

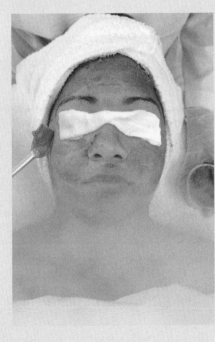

8. Apply the enzyme peel to the neck.

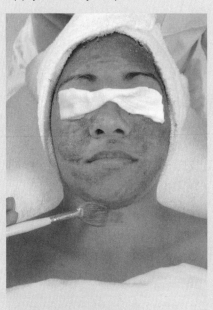

9. Apply the enzyme peel to the décolleté.

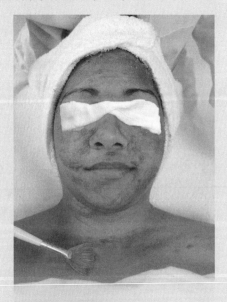

10. Continue to apply enzyme peel to the décolleté until you achieve full coverage.

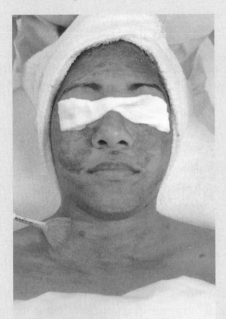

11. Leave on the skin for 10 to 15 minutes or as directed by manufacturer.

12. Remove the enzyme peel with warm towel, soaked sponges, or gauze.

13. Follow up with hydrating serum and cream.

14. Use an environmental protection product with an SPF of at least 30.

15. Cleanse your hands.

16. Send your client home with written instructions on avoiding alpha hydroxy acids (AHAs), beta hydroxy acids (BHAs), retinoic acid, and other aggressive exfoliants for four to five days or as recommended by the manufacturers of enzyme peel product. Include a list of the products the client should use at home and have him or her sign a document stating that he or she will follow the home care protocols.

17. See the client to the retail area. Make product recommendations, sell through, and schedule the client's next appointment. Enzyme peels can be performed every two to three weeks.

18. Disinfect the work area and brushes.

19. Make chart notes.

See Table 4–4 for pre- and post-peel information.

CHEMICAL PEELS

As discussed previously, before you apply any peels, you must conduct a thorough consultation with your client or patient. You must understand the type of skin that you are peeling and ensure that the peel preparation is the correct one for the skin type and condition that you are treating. Make certain the client or patient understands and acknowledges his or her responsibilities in post-peel care.

Lactic Acid Peel

Lactic acid peels are among the lightest of AHA peels and are tolerated by most skin types. A client should use an exfoliant, AHA, or BHA in his or her home care program prior to having a lactic acid peel to increase cell renewal and thus condition the skin for post-peel healing. For those clients in higher Fitzpatrick skin type categories, it is beneficial to add hydroquinone, Kojic acid, or other tyrosinase inhibitors to stabilize and reduce post-peel melanin production. This may avoid postinflammatory hyperpigmentation (PIH). This advice applies to all peels. It is necessary to include skin type and condition hydrators, anti-oxidants, and environmental protection products with both chemical and physical sunscreen ingredients with an SPF of at least 30 in all home care protocols.

The Objective

Your objective in applying a lactic acid peel is to perform a superficial exfoliation of the stratum corneum. The lactic acid peel is one of the lightest AHA peels and tolerated by most skin types and conditions. The peel has reached its optimum benefit when the skin has an even, slightly pink tone. If some areas are turning red faster than the skin overall, then those areas are peeling at a faster rate than the others and must be neutralized with the manufacturer's recommended neutralizing product. It is unlikely that a lactic acid peel will produce white areas, or "frosting," which you might experience with a glycolic peel. However, if the client does respond quickly by showing signs of erythema, it might be necessary to remove the peel earlier than you had anticipated. Remember that patch testing is necessary for all peels (Figure 4–5).

The more preparation you do before the peel in home care and patch testing, the better your results will be. This is true for all peels.

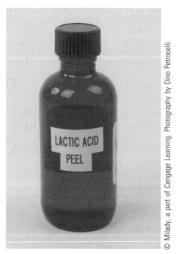

Figure 4–5 A lactic peeling solution.

© Milady, a part of Cengage Learning. Photography by Dino Petrocelli.

Indications

Clients who have the following conditions are the best candidates for a lactic acid peel:

- Dehydration
- Aging
- Fine lines
- Superficial hyperpigmentation

Contraindications

Clients who have the following conditions are poor candidates for a lactic acid peel:

- Isotretinoin use within a year (must obtain physicians recommendation)
- Herpetic outbreak (cold sores)
- Open wounds (acne lesions or other bleeding lesions)
- Pregnancy and lactation
- Cancer
- Autoimmune disorders
- Diabetes
- Sunburn
- Dermatitis
- Eczema
- Bleeding disorders

PROCEDURE 4-2: LACTIC ACID PEEL

Supplies List

- Gloves
- Brush
- Water
- Glass bowl
- Timer
- Gauze
- Eye pads
- Sponges
- Informed consent document

Products
- Peel product
- Stripping solution (oil extracting)
- Cleanser
- Hydrating serum
- Soothing cream (azulene, allantoin)
- Environmental protection product with SPF 30

Protocol
1. The client signs the informed consent document.
2. Prep client with standard protocols, secure his or her hair with a headband, and apply eye protection.
3. With cleansed, gloved hands, apply one to two layers of the lactic acid peel with a brush to a cleansed and degreased skin, beginning at the forehead. Using light, even strokes, work your way down to the cheeks, the sides of the face, and the chin. (Leave the eye, neck, and décolleté areas for last, as these can be more sensitive.)

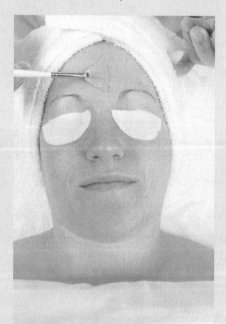

4. Apply the lactic peel to the sides of the face with a brush.

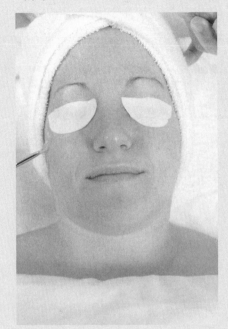

5. Continue to apply the peel down the sides of the face.

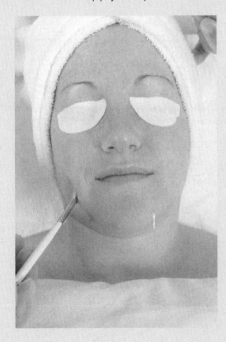

6. Apply the peel to the nasal region.

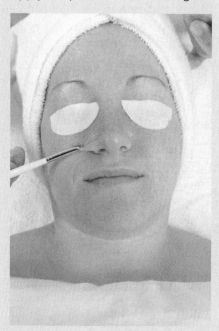

7. Apply to the chin.

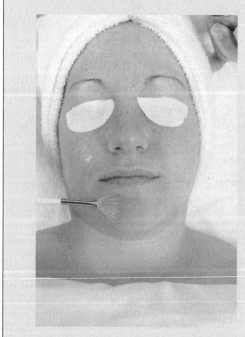

8. Repeat on the other side.

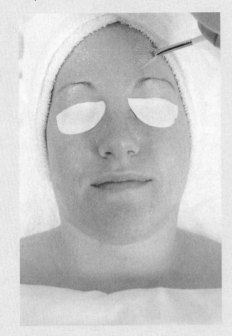

9. Continue to apply to the other side of the face.

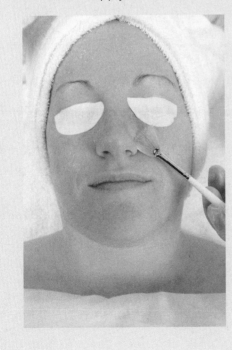

10. Continue to apply the peel to the whole face.

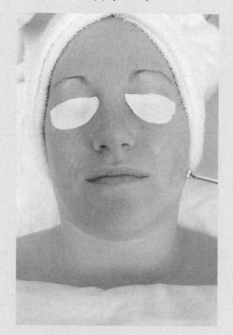

11. Apply the lactic peel to the chin.

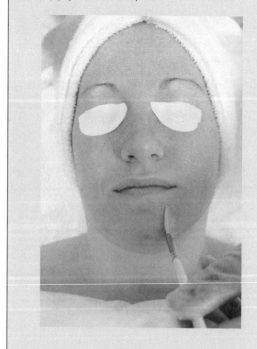

12. Apply the lactic peel to the neck.

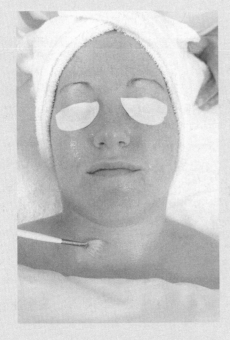

13. Apply the lactic peel to the décolleté.

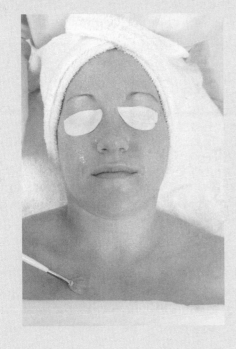

14. Set the timer for the recommended peeling agent. Follow the guidelines as recommended by the manufacturer for time and layering protocols.

15. Monitor changes in the client's skin at all times. If one area becomes redder or develops "hot spots," neutralize those areas at once for a more even peel.

16. Neutralize the peel with the approved neutralizing solution and remove it with gauze or sponges.

17. Apply calming, soothing hydrating serum and moisturizing cream with azulene and/or allantoin.

18. Apply an environmental protection product with SPF of 30.

19. Cleanse your hands.

20. Send your client home with written instructions on avoiding AHAs, BHAs, retinoic acid, and other aggressive exfoliants for two weeks. Include a list of products that your client should use at home and have him or her sign a document stating that he or she will follow the home care protocols. Use the peel manufacturer's recommendation on post-peel home care. At a minimum, this should include a soothing cleanser, a moisturizer, and a sunscreen with an SPF of at least 30.

21. See the client to the retail area. Make product recommendations, sell through, and schedule the client's next appointment. Lactic acid peels can be performed every two to three weeks.

22. Disinfect the work area and brushes.

23. Make chart notes.

See Table 4–4 for pre- and post-peel information.

CAUTION!

Higher-level and nonbuffered peels are to be performed in a medical setting only, with qualified medical training and certification.

Glycolic Peel: Alpha Hydroxy Acid

A client should use an exfoliant, retinoic acid, AHAs, or BHAs in his or her home care program prior to having a glycolic peel to increase cell renewal and thus condition the skin for post-peel healing. For those clients in higher Fitzpatrick skin type categories, it is beneficial to add hydroquinone, Kojic acid, or other tyrosinase inhibitors to stabilize and reduce post-peel melanin production. This may avoid PIH. This applies to all peels. It is necessary to include skin type and condition hydrators, antioxidants, and environmental protection products with both chemical and physical sunscreen ingredients with an SPF of at least 30 in all home care protocols.

The Objective

Your objective in applying a glycolic peel is to perform a superficial exfoliation of the stratum corneum. The peel has reached its optimum benefit when the skin has an even, slightly pink tone. If some areas are turning red faster than the skin overall, then those areas are peeling at a faster rate than the others and must be neutralized with the manufacturer's recommended neutralizing product. If the skin is turning white, or "frosting," remove the peel at once. You are approaching a much deeper peel than a superficial peel, and the client's skin is responding faster than anticipated. If, however, you are working in a physician's office and have been trained to work with a higher concentration of peel solution, follow the direction of your supervising medical personnel. If you are a sole practitioner, you may need to opt for a lighter peel or an enzyme for that skin type. Patch testing is necessary for all peels.

The more preparation you do before the peel in home care and patch testing, the better your results will be. This is true for all peels.

Indications

Clients who have the following conditions are the best candidates for a glycolic peel:

- Dehydration
- Aging
- Fine lines
- Light hyperpigmentation

Contraindications

Clients who have the following conditions are poor candidates for a glycolic peel:

- Isotretinoin use within a year (must obtain physicians recommendation)
- Herpetic outbreak (cold sores)
- Open wounds (acne lesions or other bleeding lesions)
- Pregnancy and lactation
- Cancer

- Autoimmune disorders
- Diabetes
- Sunburn
- Dermatitis
- Eczema
- Bleeding disorders

PROCEDURE 4-3: GLYCOLIC PEEL

Supplies List

- Gloves
- Brush
- Water
- Glass bowl
- Timer
- Gauze
- Eye pads
- Sponges
- Informed consent document

Products

- Peel product
- Stripping solution (oil extracting)
- Cleanser
- Hydrating serum
- Soothing cream (azulene, allantoin)
- Environmental protection product with SPF 30

Protocol

1. The client signs the informed consent document.
2. Prep client with standard protocols, secure his or her hair with a headband, and apply eye protection.
3. With cleansed, gloved hands, apply one to two layers of the glycolic acid peel with a brush to a cleansed and degreased skin, beginning at the forehead. Using light, even strokes, work your way down to the cheeks, the sides of the face, and the chin.

(Leave the eye, neck, and décolleté areas for last, as these can be more sensitive).

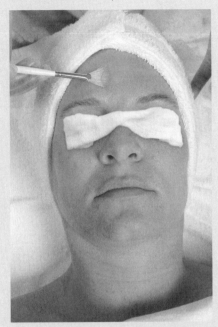

4. Continue to apply the glycolic peel to the forehead.

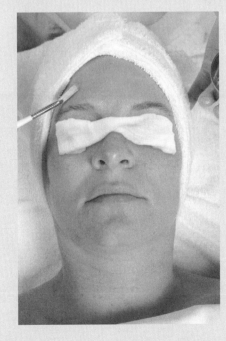

5. Apply the glycolic to the cheeks and down the sides of the face.

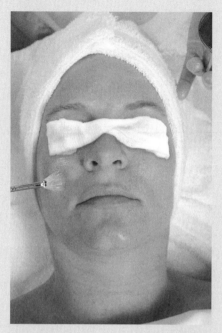

6. Repeat on the other side of the face.

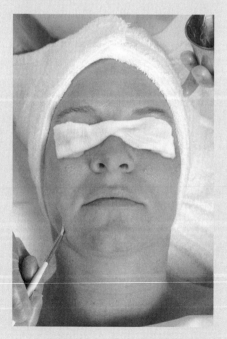

7. Continue to apply glycolic peel down the other side of the face.

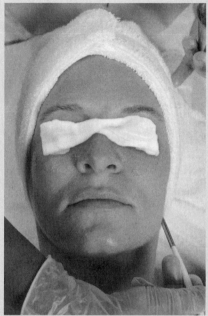

8. Continue to apply the peel to the whole face.

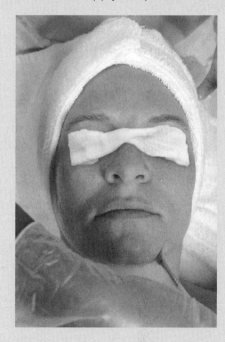

9. Apply the peel to the chin.

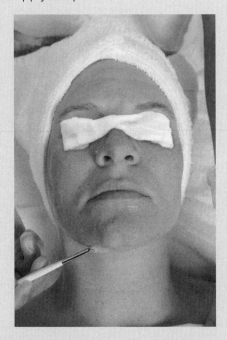

10. Apply the peel to the neck.

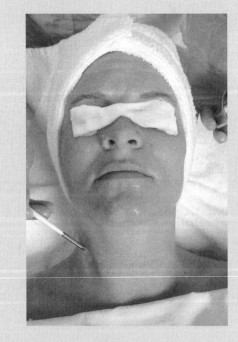

11. Continue to apply the peel to the neck.

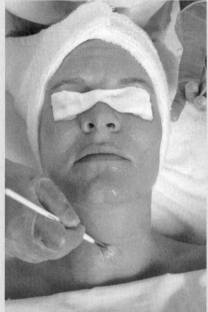

12. Apply the peel to the décolleté.

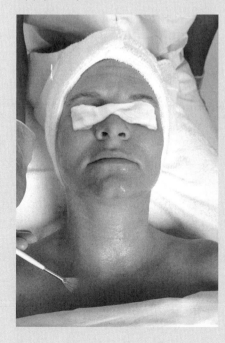

13. Continue to the apply peel to the décolleté.

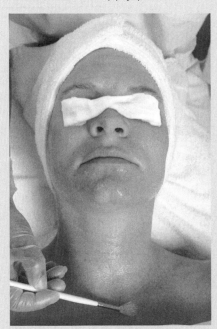

14. Set the timer for the recommended peeling agent. Follow the guidelines as recommended by the manufacturer for time and layering protocols.

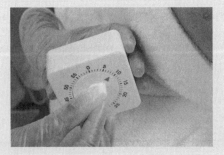

15. Monitor changes in the client's skin at all times. If one area becomes redder or develops "hot spots," neutralize those areas at once for a more even peel. If the skin turns white, the skin is "frosting," and you are moving into a more aggressive peel. Neutralize and remove the peel in this case.

16. Neutralize the peel with the approved neutralizing solution and remove it with gauze or sponges.

17. Apply calming, soothing hydrating serum and moisturizing cream with azulene and/or allantoin.

18. Apply an environmental protection product with an SPF of 30.

19. Cleanse your hands.

20. Send your client home with written instructions on avoiding AHAs, BHAs, retinoic acid, and other aggressive exfoliants for two weeks. Include a list of products that your client should use at home and have him or her sign a document stating that he or she will follow the home care protocols. Have the client follow the manufacturer's recommendations for post-peel home care use. At a minimum, this should include a soothing cleanser, a hydrator, and a sunscreen with an SPF of at least 30.

21. See the client to the retail area. Make product recommendations, sell through, and schedule his or her next appointment. Glycolic peels can be performed every three to four weeks.

22. Disinfect the work area and brushes.

23. Make chart notes.

See Table 4–4 for pre- and post-peel information.

> **CAUTION!**
>
> Higher-level nonbuffered peels are to be performed in a medical setting, with qualified medical training and certification.

Salicylic Acid Peel: Beta Hydroxy Acid Peel

For years, the salicylic acid peel has been the gold standard peel for acne, as it serves as an antibacterial and has anti-inflammatory benefits. This type of peel is excellent for removing open and closed comedones and, unofficially, some of us have found it to have a slight lightening effect on pigmented lesions in lower Fitzpatrick skin types. A client should use an exfoliant, retinoic acid, AHA, or BHA in his or her home care program prior to having a salicylic peel to increase cell renewal and thus condition the skin for post-peel healing. For those clients in higher Fitzpatrick skin type categories, it is beneficial to add hydroquinone, Kojic acid, or other tyrosinase inhibitors to stabilize and reduce post-peel melanin production and help avoid PIH. This applies to all peels. It is necessary to include skin type and condition hydrators, antioxidants and environmental protection products with both chemical and physical sunscreen ingredients with an SPF of at least 30 in all home care protocols (Figure 4–6).

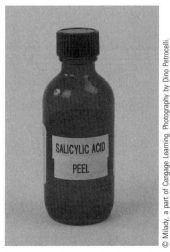

Figure 4–6 A salicylic acid peeling solution.

© Milady, a part of Cengage Learning. Photography by Dino Petrocelli.

The Objective

Your objective in applying a salicylic peel is to reduce oil and acne by performing a superficial exfoliation of the stratum corneum. An oil-soluble peel, a salicylic peel can be gentler than a glycolic peel and is excellent for clearing congested follicles. The peel has reached its optimum benefit when the skin has an even, slightly pink tone. If some areas are turning red faster than the skin overall, then those areas are peeling at a faster rate than the others and must be neutralized with the manufacturer's recommended neutralizing product. Some areas may turn white, or "frost," with a salicylic peel. You may need to remove the peel earlier than you had anticipated if you are approaching a deeper peel in those areas, so watch the skin closely. Some frosting around acne lesions is common, but if the peel has created a general whitening, or frosting, it is best to remove the peel at once. You may need to opt for a lighter peel or for an enzyme for that skin type. Patch testing is necessary for all peels.

The more preparation you do before the peel in home care and patch testing, the better your results will be. This is true for all peels.

Indications

Clients who have the following conditions are the best candidates for a salicylic peel:

- Oily skin
- Acne
- Aging
- Uneven texture
- Superficial hyperpigmentation

Contraindications

Clients who have the following conditions are poor candidates for a salicylic peel:

- Allergy to salicylates (e.g., aspirin and other medicines containing salicylates)
- Isotretinoin use within a year (must obtain physicians recommendation)
- Herpetic outbreak (cold sores)
- Open wounds (acne lesions or other bleeding lesions)

- Pregnancy and lactation
- Cancer
- Autoimmune disorders
- Diabetes
- Bleeding disorders
- Sunburn
- Eczema
- Dermatitis

PROCEDURE 4–4: SALICYLIC ACID PEEL

Supplies List
- Gloves
- Water
- Glass bowl
- Timer
- Gauze (could use brush for application if preferred)
- Eye pads
- Sponges
- Fan (salicylic acid peels tend to generate heat)
- Informed consent document

Products
- Peel product
- Stripping solution (oil reducing/extracting)
- Cleanser
- Hydrating serum
- Soothing cream (azulene, allantoin)
- Environmental protection product with an SPF of 30

Protocol
1. Client signs the informed consent document.
2. Prep the client with standard protocols, secure his or her hair with a headband, and apply eye protection.
3. With cleansed, gloved hands, apply one to two layers of the salicylic acid peel with gauze to a cleansed and degreased skin, beginning at the forehead. Using light, even strokes, work your way down to the cheeks, the sides of the face, and the chin.

(Leave the eye, neck, and décolleté areas for last, as these can be more sensitive.)

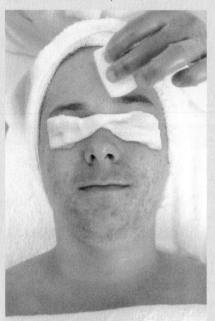

4. Continue down the side of the face.

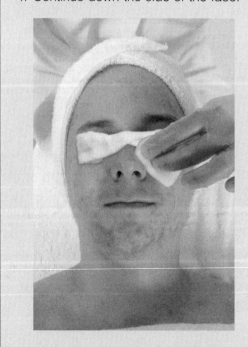

5. Apply to the chin.

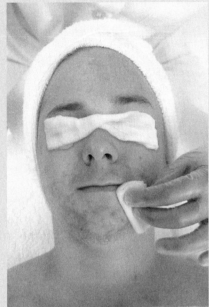

6. Continue to apply to the chin.

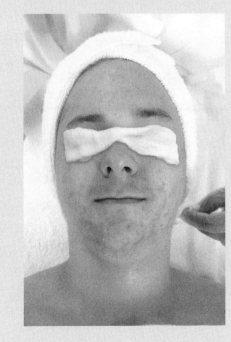

7. Apply peel on the other side of the face.

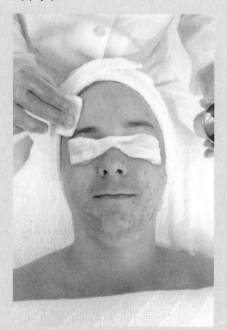

8. Continue to apply to all areas of the other side of the face.

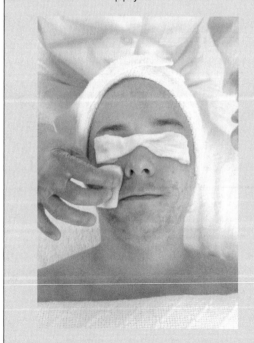

9. Turn on the fan and wait two minutes between layers.

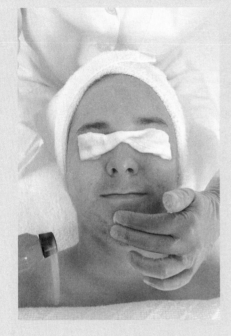

10. Note any "frosting" on the client.

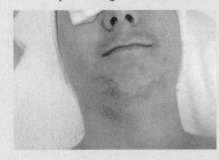

11. Apply a second layer.

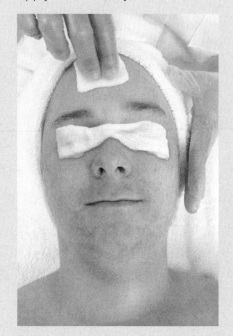

12. Continue with the second layer.

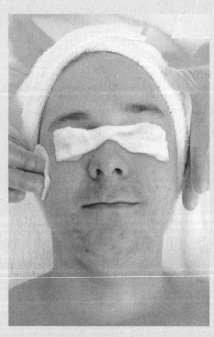

13. Continue applying the second layer.

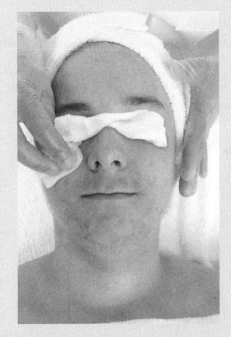

14. Continue applying the second layer to the full face.

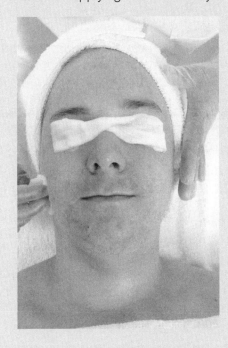

15. Complete the second layer.

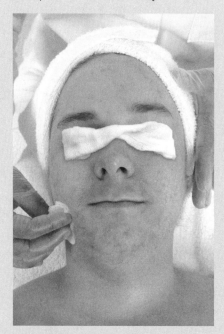

16. If recommended by the manufacturer, set a timer for the recommended peeling agent. For clients with oilier, thicker skin, a third application may be indicated.

17. Monitor the changes in the client's skin at all times. If one area becomes redder or develops "hot spots," neutralize those areas at once for a more even peel. If the skin turns white, the skin is "frosting," and you are moving into a more aggressive peel. Neutralize and remove the peel in this case.

18. Neutralize the peel with the approved neutralizing solution and remove it with gauze or sponges.

19. Apply a calming, soothing, anti-inflammatory product and a hydrator with azulene and/or allantoin.

20. Apply an environmental protection product with an SPF of 30.

21. Cleanse your hands.

22. Send the client home with written instructions on avoiding AHAs, BHAs, retinoic acid, and other aggressive exfoliants for two weeks. Include a list of products that your client should use at home and have him or her sign a document stating that he or she will follow the home care protocols. The client will need a soothing cleanser, a light hydrating serum, and a sunscreen with an

SPF of at least 30. Have the client follow the manufacturer's product recommendations.

23. See the client to the retail area. Make product recommendations, sell through, and schedule his or her next appointment. Salicylic acid peels can be done every two weeks depending upon skin type and the level of acne that you are treating.
24. Disinfect work area and brushes.
25. Make chart notes.

See Table 4–4 for pre- and post-peel information.

Jessner's Solution Peel

A Jessner's solution peel is excellent for many indications. It is useful for acne, age management, and the general improvement of skin topography. The original peel was developed by dermatologist Max Jessner and included 14 percent of these preparations: salicylic acid, lactic acid, and resorcinol (phenol-based). Some Jessner's solution peels have been modified and include glycolic acid; they may also offer a lower percentage of the key peeling ingredients. A client should use an exfoliant, retinoic acid, AHAs, or BHAs in their home care program prior to having a Jessner's solution peel to increase cell renewal and condition the skin for post-peel healing. For those clients in higher Fitzpatrick skin type categories, it is beneficial to add hydroquinone, Kojic acid, or other tyrosinase inhibitors to stabilize and reduce post-peel melanin production. This will help avoid PIH. This applies to all peels. It is necessary to include skin type and condition hydrators, antioxidants, and environmental protection products with both chemical and physical sunscreen ingredients with an SPF of at least 30 in all home care protocols.

The Objective

Your objective in applying a Jessner's solution peel is to reduce oil and acne, increase suppleness, and improve texture by performing a superficial exfoliation of the stratum corneum. This peel can penetrate deeper than the stratum corneum, so it is best to have some experience with peels on a variety of skin types prior to performing a Jessner's solution peel.

A Jessner's solution peel is performed in layers, and the upper layers of the epidermis may show signs of frosting. This is normal. Estheticians must understand the level of peel that they are trying to achieve and proceed cautiously with one or two layers, at the most. Some Jessner's peels may not be neutralized, but diluted with water instead. Others are left on the skin and worn out of the clinic. Modified versions may have other protocols, so it is necessary to follow the manufacturer's recommendations for all peels. Patch testing is necessary for all peels.

CAUTION!

Higher-level and nonbuffered peels are to be performed in a medical setting only, with qualified medical training and certification.

CAUTION!

Each peel manufacturer has protocols that need to be followed implicitly. Some companies will have neutralizers and others may not. Some may require that you apply a peel in layers and time each layer and others may not. If you change peel products, make certain that you use the new peel protocol. Some peels have higher or lower pH values, and may be buffered or nonbuffered. All of these factors will affect the outcome of the peel. It is important that you know the peel you are using and the skin you are peeling. Follow the pre- and post-peel instructions and teach your clients to do the same.

The more preparation you do before the peel in home care and patch testing, the better your results will be. This is true for all peels.

Indications

Clients who have the following conditions are the best candidates for a Jessner's solution peel:

- Oily skin
- Acne
- Aging
- Uneven texture
- Superficial hyperpigmentation

Contraindications

Clients who have the following conditions are poor candidates for a Jessner's solution peel:

- Allergy to salicylates (e.g., aspirin and other medicines containing salicylates)
- Isotretinoin use within a year (must obtain physicians recommendation)
- Herpetic outbreak (cold sores)
- Open wounds (acne lesions or other bleeding lesions)
- Pregnancy and lactation
- Cancer
- Autoimmune disorders
- Diabetes
- Bleeding disorders
- Sunburn
- Eczema
- Dermatitis

PROCEDURE 4–5: JESSNER'S SOLUTION PEEL

Supplies List
- Gloves
- Water
- Glass bowl
- Timer
- Gauze (can use brush for application if preferred)
- Eye pads
- Sponges

- Fan (Jessner's solution peels tend to generate heat)
- Informed consent document

Products

- Peel product
- Stripping solution (oil reducing/extracting)
- Cleanser
- Hydrating serum
- Soothing cream (azulene, allantoin)
- Environmental protection product with an SPF of 30

Protocol

1. Client signs the informed consent document.
2. Prep the client with standard protocols, secure his or her hair with a headband, and apply eye protection.
3. With cleansed, gloved hands, apply one to two layers of the Jessner's solution peel with gauze to a cleansed and degreased skin, beginning at the forehead. Using light, even strokes, work your way down to the cheeks, the sides of the face, and the chin. (Leave the eye, neck, and décolleté areas for last, as these can be more sensitive.)

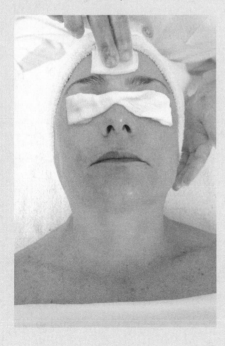

4. Apply the peel down the side of the face.

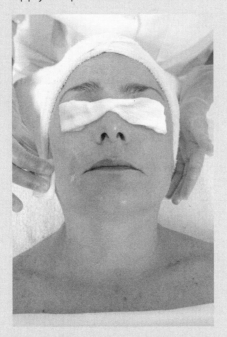

5. Continue down the side of the face.

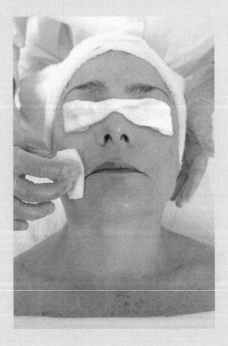

6. Apply Jessner's peel to the upper lip.

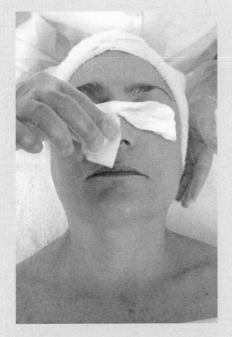

7. Repeat the application to the other side of the face.

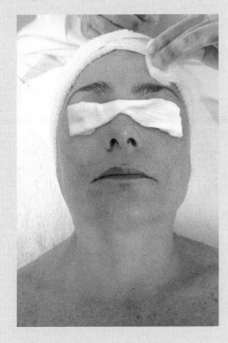

8. Continue down the side of the face.

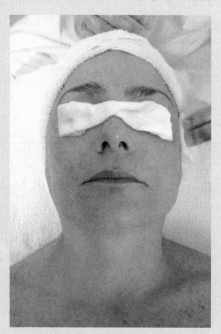

9. Continue down the side of the face.

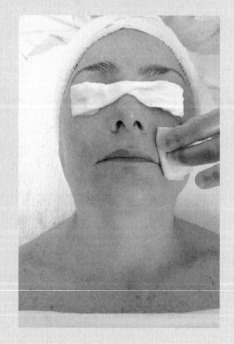

10. Continue down the side of the face.

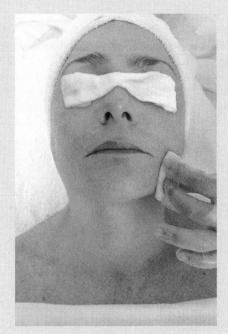

11. Apply the peel to the chin.

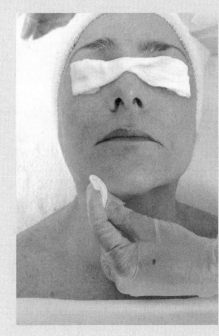

12. Applying the peel to the neck.

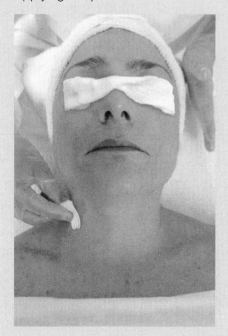

13. Apply the peel to the neck.

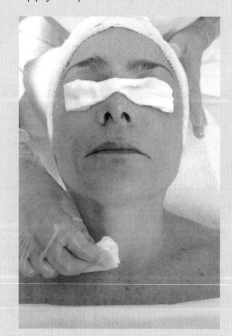

14. Apply the peel to the décolleté.

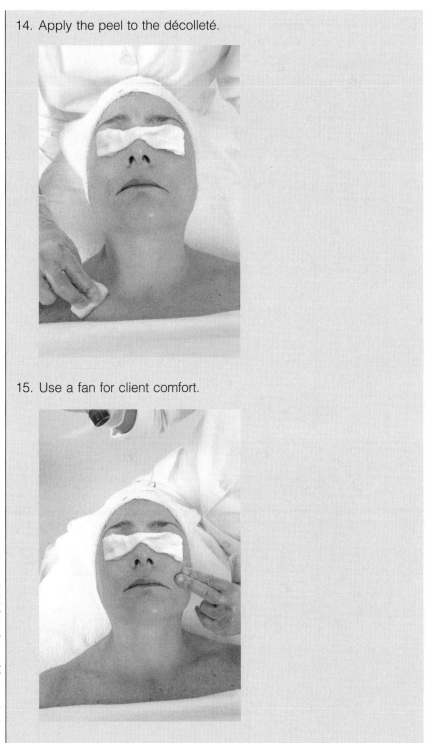

15. Use a fan for client comfort.

16. Set a timer for the manufacturer's recommended time; apply a second layer if desired.

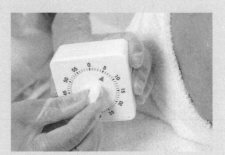

17. Neutralize, if directed by the manufacturer.

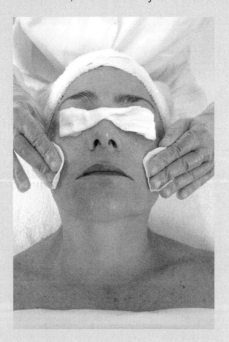

18. Continue to neutralize if directed by the manufacturer.

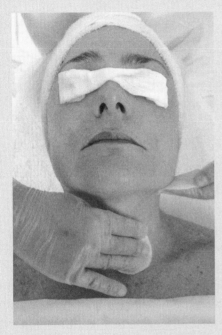

19. Set a timer for the recommended peeling agent. Follow the guidelines as recommended by the manufacturer for time and layering protocols. For clients with oilier, thicker skin, a second or third application may be indicated.

20. Monitor changes in the client's skin at all times. If one area becomes redder or develops "hot spots," neutralize or dilute those areas at once for a more even peel. If the skin turns white, the skin is "frosting," you are moving into a more aggressive peel. Neutralize and remove the peel in this case.

21. Neutralize the peel (if recommended by manufacturer) or dilute it with water, using gauze or sponges.

22. Apply a calming, soothing, anti-inflammatory product and a hydrator with azulene and/or allantoin.

23. Apply an environmental protection product with an SPF of 30.

24. Cleanse your hands.

25. Send the client home with written instructions on avoiding AHAs, BHAs, retinoic acid, and other aggressive exfoliants for two weeks. Include a list of the products that the client should use at home and have him or her sign a document stating that he or she will follow the home care protocols. Have the

CAUTION!

Higher-level and nonbuffered peels are to be performed in a medical setting only, with qualified medical training and certification.

client follow the manufacturer's recommended post-peel products. At a minimum, these should include a soothing cleanser with azulene or allantoin, a hydrating moisturizer with hyaluronic acid, and a sunscreen with an SPF of at least 30.

26. See the client to the retail area. Make product recommendations, sell through, and schedule his or her next appointment. Jessner's solution peels can be done every month depending upon the skin type, condition, and/or the level of acne that you are treating.

27. Disinfect the work area and brushes.

28. Make chart notes.

See Table 4–4 for pre- and post-peel information.

Trichloroacetic Acid

A trichloroacetic acid (TCA) peel is excellent for many indications. It is useful for acne, age management, a general improvement of texture, hyperpigmentation, and in some cases produces a tightening effect. TCA peels come in a variety of strengths, so it is important to make sure that you are licensed to perform the chosen level of the formulation. Some states allow estheticians to perform 8 to 10 percent TCA peeling solutions; others do not allow estheticians to perform TCA peels at all. Additionally, some regulations state that you may perform them under a physician's supervision. Make certain that you are in compliance.

TCA peels that are above 10 percent—such as the Obagi Blue Peel developed by dermatologist Zein Obagi—are for use only under the direction of a qualified physician. The risk of scarring and hyperpigmentation with TCA peels is higher. This is a huge liability for estheticians. You can put your clients and patients at risk if you attempt to apply these peels without the training and direction by a qualified medical practitioner.

Pre-peel Home Care

A client should use an exfoliant, retinoic acid, AHAs, or BHAs in their home care program prior to having a TCA peel to increase cell renewal and condition the skin for post-peel healing. For those clients in higher Fitzpatrick skin type categories, it is beneficial to add hydroquinone,

Kojic acid, or other tyrosinase inhibitors to stabilize and reduce post-peel melanin production. This will help avoid PIH. This applies to all peels. Include a list of products that your client should use at home and have him or her sign a document stating that he or she will follow the home care protocols. Include skin type and condition hydrators, antioxidants, and environmental protection products with both chemical and physical sunscreen ingredients with an SPF of at least 30 in all home care protocols.

The Objective

Your objective in applying a TCA peel is to smoothen skin texture, brighten and lighten the skin, and peel off layers of photodamaged skin.

A TCA peel may be performed in layers. The upper layers of the epidermis may show signs of whitening, or "frosting." This is normal. However, estheticians must understand the level of peel that they are trying to achieve. Proceed cautiously, with one or two layers at the most. Modified versions may have other protocols, so you need to follow the manufacturer's recommendations for all peels. Patch testing is necessary for all peels (Figure 4–7). Most TCA peels are left on the skin and are not neutralized. The more preparation you do before the peel in home care and patch testing, the better your results will be. This is true for all peels.

Indications

Clients who have the following conditions are the best candidates for a TCA peel:

- Aging, photo-damaged skin
- Hyperpigmentation
- Acne and acne scarring
- Uneven skin texture
- Elastosis

Contraindications

Clients who have the following conditions are poor candidates for a TCA peel:

- Isotretinoin use within a year (must obtain physicians recommendation)
- Herpetic outbreak (cold sores)

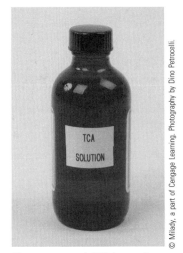

Figure 4–7 A TCA peeling solution.

© Milady, a part of Cengage Learning. Photography by Dino Petrocelli.

- Open wounds (acne lesions or other bleeding lesions)
- Pregnancy and lactation
- Cancer
- Autoimmune disorders
- Diabetes
- Bleeding disorders
- Sunburn
- Eczema
- Dermatitis
- Hypertrophic scarring

PROCEDURE 4-6: TCA (TRICHLOROACETIC) PEEL

Supplies List
- Gloves
- Water
- Glass bowl
- Timer
- Gauze
- Eye pads
- Fan (TCA peels generate heat)
- Informed consent document

Products
- TCA (8 to 10%) peel product
- Stripping solution (oil reducing/extracting)
- Cleanser
- Hydrating serum
- Soothing cream (azulene, allantoin)
- Environmental protection product with an SPF of 30

Protocol
1. Client signs the informed consent document.
2. Prep the client with standard protocols, secure hair with a headband, and apply eye protection.
3. With cleansed, gloved hands, apply one to two layers of the TCA peel with gauze to a cleansed and degreased skin, beginning at the forehead. Using light, even strokes, work your way down to

the cheeks, sides of the face, and chin. (Leave the eye, neck, and décolleté areas for last, as these can be more sensitive.)

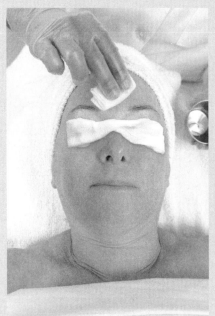

4. Continue on the side of the face.

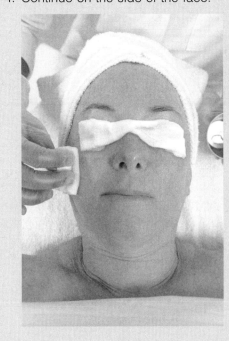

5. Continue on the side of the face.

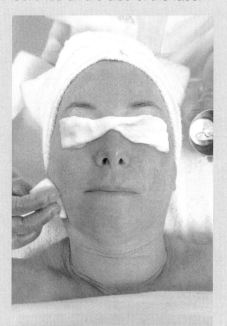

6. Apply to the nasal region.

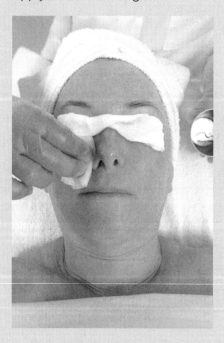

7. Apply the TCA peel to the chin.

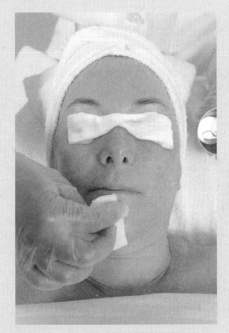

8. Repeat on the other side.

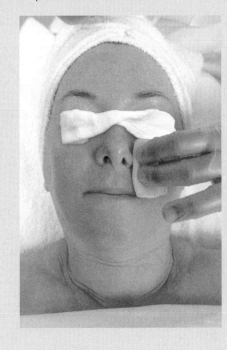

9. Continue on the other side.

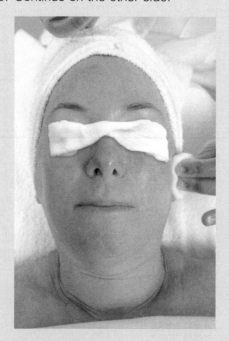

10. Continue applying the TCA peel.

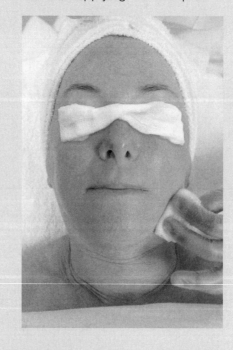

11. Apply to the neck.

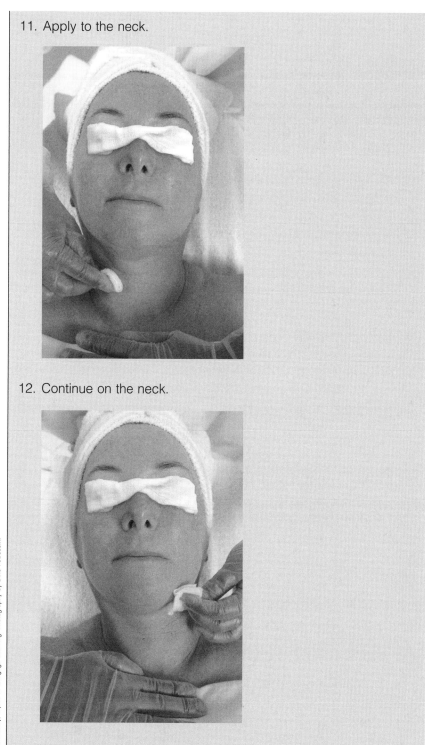

12. Continue on the neck.

13. Follow the guidelines as recommended by the manufacturers for time and layering protocols. For clients with oilier, thicker skin, a second or third application may be indicated.

14. Monitor changes in the client's skin at all times. If one area becomes redder, develops "hot spots," and begins to frost (whiten), make certain that you wait two to three minutes between each layer to achieve an even peel.

15. Apply cold compresses (4" × 4" pads dipped in cool water work well for this).

16. Apply a calming, soothing, anti-inflammatory product, a hydrator with azulene and/or allantoin, or post-peel balm, as recommended by the manufacturer.

17. Apply an environmental protection product with an SPF of 30.

18. Cleanse your hands.

19. Send the client home with written instructions on avoiding AHAs, BHAs, retinoic acid, and other aggressive exfoliants for two weeks. Include a list of the products that your client should use at home and have him or her sign a document stating that he or she will follow the home care protocols. Have the client follow the manufacturer's product recommendations: soothing and calming products for the first 8 to 10 days.

20. See the client to the retail area. Make product recommendations, sell through, and schedule his or her next appointment. Very low-level TCA peels can be done every month depending upon the strength of the peeling solution, the skin type, and the indications that you are treating. Make certain that the client has the approved protocol for home care, including post-peel care instructions and a product kit. Tell the client not to use anything else on his or her skin for the duration of the peeling process. Also remind the client not to pull or peel the skin as it begins to peel off. This activity can and will create a scar.

21. Disinfect the work area.

22. Make chart notes.

See Table 4–4 for pre- and post-peel information.

CAUTION!

Higher-level and nonbuffered peels are to be performed in a medical setting only, with qualified medical training and certification.

PEEL SELECTION

In brief, experience will be your best guide. Having the appropriate training on each peel preparation is paramount to a successful outcome. Each manufacturer offers classes on peeling, and it is advisable for you to receive as much training and certification as possible. As you know (or will come to know), each manufacturer has its own recommendations on protocols for neutralizing a product (or not), the amount of time a peel should be left on the skin (which can be related to whether a peel is buffered or nonbuffered), and home care products and applications. There is a full spectrum of reasons that you will follow their direction for applying their peels.

Knowing the skin type that you are peeling and using the analysis tools as provided by the Fitzpatrick Skin Type Scale, Glogau's Photodamage Classification, Rubin's Photodamage Classification, and Kligman's Acne Chart will give you a basis from which to formulate your plan. If your objective is age management while treating a client with photodamage, and the client fits the indication and contraindication profiles, you will use a peel with more constituents, such as a Jessner's peel. Conversely, if your client has a few acne lesions and no photodamage but struggles with extra oil and hydration, you will want to use a preparation that is not only a **keratolytic** (exfoliation process), but has antibacterial properties, such as a salicylic acid peel.

Case Scenario I

Client I is in her early 20s. She has Fitzpatrick skin type II, Glogau type 1, Kligman's grade II acne, and has some **PIH** (postinflammatory hyperpigmentation) from her acne. She is a college student and notices acne flare-ups when she becomes very stressed out during finals. She is on a good home care program; she uses a **BHA** (beta hydroxy acid) cleanser, a hydrating serum with licochalcone (licorice extract) for lightening and oil balancing, and an ultrasonic peeling device twice week. This has kept her skin clear. However, she still wants the benefit of a chemical peel to smooth out her older acne scarring.

Beta hydroxy acid peel
Exfoliating organic acid; salicylic acid; milder than some alpha hydroxy acids; excellent for oily skin.

Peel Recommendation

In this case, we would start with a weekly series of salicylic acid peels to reduce oil and for smoothing. While we are applying the peel series, we would have her stop using her ultrasonic device, and gradually work toward a Jessner's solution peel monthly for pigment control and additional smoothing. She may be a candidate for microdermabrasion and later skin resurfacing if she continues to scar.

Case Scenario II

Client II is in her 40s, and her skin is dull, dry, and dehydrated. She has Fitzpatrick skin type III, Glogau Photodamage Classification III,

Rubin Photodamage Classification II, and has melasma from two pregnancies. She feels that her skin is not as tight as it was and has noticed that lines around her eyes and mouth are worsening. Her home care consists of a glycolic acid cleanser, a hydrating toner, a serum with hyaluronic acid, and cream with peptides for cell renewal and collagen production. She uses SPF 30 daily and gives herself a collagen and brightening masque weekly to help with the dryness, dehydration, and pigmentation problems.

Peel Recommendation

Client II would benefit from a series of three light TCA peels for lightening, tightening, stimulation, and wrinkle smoothing. She should use an SPF of the highest level to avoid more pigmentation, as she is prone to producing extra melanin. She must watch her UV exposure.

Introducing Routine Skin Care Back into the Postpeel Plan

Each peeling agent is unique, and reactivity to the peels can be as well. You will introduce AHAs, BHAs, retinoic acid, and other active products back into the client's home care program once he or she has fully peeled and the barrier is intact. This can range from five or six days to a month depending upon the depth, pH level, buffered or nonbuffered type of peel, and the client's skin type and condition. Some clients may need to remain on a gentle cleanser, hydrator, and emollient longer than expected before going back to more aggressive exfoliants and active products.

 LAYERING PEELS

Layering peel products and solutions can be very effective depending upon your experience, the client's skin type and condition, and his or her willingness to follow protocols. As we know, a beautiful peel can be ruined by a noncompliant client who decides to ignore environmental protection requirements, the need for hydration, and the adequate healing time of a peel before applying a caustic product or another aggressive service.

Peels that are combined or layered with excellent results have been lactic and glycolic, glycolic and salicylic, glycolic and TCA, salicylic and TCA. You must have had the appropriate training when combining peeling preparations, and you must be certified to use them.

For higher concentrations of peeling solutions, it is vital that you only perform the peels under the supervision of qualified medical personnel.

Layering Lactic Acid and Glycolic Peels

As with all peels, home care compliance care is vital to receiving excellent results with layered peels. The client receiving a peel layered with lactic and glycolic should be well selected: this is a good preparation for the client; the client has sensitive skin that has tolerated both of these peels separately; and the client wants a boost to his or her regular peel program. The layered approach may be alternated with single peels: you may apply a layered peel in one visit, and then a single peel in the next. This is an excellent choice for sensitive, dry, dehydrated skin types, which have been well prepared with home care containing AHA/BHA ingredients in their products. The client should also have been using hydrating serums, creams, and environmental protection with an SPF of 30.

The Objective

Your objective in applying a layered lactic acid and glycolic peel is to perform a superficial exfoliation of the stratum corneum. The lactic acid peel is one of the lightest AHA peels, which has one of the largest molecular structures (glycolic has the smallest, and can penetrate deeper). The lactic peel layer will help remove some of the spent cellular debris and prepare the skin for the glycolic acid layer. You must perform a layered peel with just one to two layers for each layer until you are acquainted with the skin you are peeling and have experience with your peeling solutions.

The peel has reached its optimum benefit when the skin has an even, slightly pink tone. If some areas are turning red faster than the skin overall, then they are peeling at a faster rate than the others and must be neutralized with the manufacturer's recommended neutralizing product. It is unlikely that a lactic acid peel will produce white areas or "frosting" (it may result from glycolic peel, however). If the client does respond quickly by showing signs of erythema, you might need to remove the peel earlier than you had anticipated. Patch testing is necessary for all peels. Make certain to test both peel preparations in the patch test.

The more preparation you do before the peel in home care and patch testing, the better your results will be. This is true for all peels.

Follow all indications, contraindications, preparation, and protocols for the lactic and glycolic acid peels as indicated above.

Layering Glycolic Acid and Salicylic Acid Peels

Layering glycolic and salicylic acid peel preparations is an excellent choice for those clients who have tolerated these peels well individually and want to give their treatments a boost. Layered peels can also be alternated with individual peels of the same type. Using a layered approached with glycolic and salicylic acid peels is indicated for clients with age management issues and acne. As with all peels, home care compliance is necessary. This is an excellent choice for oily-rich, acneic, and topically dehydrated skin types that have been well prepared with home care containing AHA/BHA and retinoic acid ingredients in their products. The client should also have been using hydrating serums and environmental protection with an SPF of 30.

The Objective

Your objective in applying layered glycolic and salicylic acid peels is to perform a superficial exfoliation of the stratum corneum and to reduce oil and acneic conditions. While glycolic acid has the smallest molecular structure, it can reduce the amount of dead cellular debris. On the other hand, salicylic acid can work within the follicle to remove congestion and soften impactions, thus easing the evacuation process. It is necessary to perform a layered peel with just one layer of the glycolic acid preparation and one to two layers of the salicylic acid preparation, depending upon the skin thickness and level of acne that you are treating. For example, for thicker skin at an acne level 2, two layers of salicylic may be most beneficial. As with all peels, be conservative until you are acquainted with the skin you are peeling and have experience with your peeling solutions.

The peel has reached its optimum benefit when the skin has an even, slightly pink tone. If some areas are turning red faster than the skin overall, then they are peeling at a faster rate than the other areas and it is important to neutralize them with the manufacturer's recommended neutralizing product. The glycolic peel may show a slight frosting in some areas, particularly around acne lesions. Neutralize those areas, as you will be applying the salicylic acid peel layer next for follicular decongesting. If the client shows an extreme erythema reaction to the glycolic acid peel layer, it may be best to postpone the salicylic acid peel layer. There may be other factors in play, such as improper preparation in home care, client stress, or a stronger effect of the peel. As always, patch testing is necessary for all peels. Make certain to test both peel preparations in the patch test.

The more preparation you do before the peel in home care and patch testing, the better your results will be. This is true for all peels.

fyi

Some manufacturers recommend leaving on peel preparations. Always follow the manufacturer's protocols.

Follow all indications, contraindications, preparation, and protocols for the glycolic and salicylic acid peels described above.

Layering Glycolic Acid and TCA Peels

Clients concerned with age management but who do not have the downtime associated with ablative types of procedures may prefer the combination of glycolic acid and TCA. As with all peels, however, the results depend upon preparation and home care compliance. This client should have had peels preceding the layered peel and developed a tolerance to the peels. A good home care program for a client preparing for layered glycolic and TCA peels should include a combination of hydrators, antioxidants, AHAs, BHAs, retinoic acid, lighteners, and environmental protections with an SPF of 30.

The Objective

Your objective in applying layered glycolic and TCA peels is to perform a superficial exfoliation of the stratum corneum, to reduce hyperpigmentation, and to increase tightening and smoothing of the skin. While glycolic acid has the smallest molecular structure, it can reduce the amount of dead cellular debris. TCA can generate smoothing and tightening of the epidermis. It is necessary to perform a layered peel with just one layer of the glycolic acid preparation and one to two layers of the TCA peel depending upon the skin thickness and condition of the skin type you are treating. As with all peels, be conservative until you are acquainted with the skin you are peeling and have experience with your peeling solutions.

The peel has reached its optimum benefit when the skin has an even, slightly pink tone. If some areas are turning red faster than the skin overall, then they are peeling at a faster rate than the other areas and must be neutralized with the manufacturer's recommended neutralizing product. The glycolic peel may show a slight frosting in some areas, particularly around acne lesions. Neutralize those areas, as you will be applying the TCA peel layers next. If the client shows an extreme erythema reaction to the glycolic acid peel layer, it may be best to postpone the TCA peel layers. There may be other factors in play, such as improper preparation in home care, client stressed, or a stronger effect of the peel. As always, patch testing is necessary for all peels. Make certain to test both peel preparations in the patch test.

The more preparation you do before the peel in home care and patch testing, the better your results will be. This is true for all peels.

fyi

As mentioned previously in the text, it is imperative that you use esthetician-approved peeling preparations and work within your scope of practice. The TCA peels discussed here are of a lower level and not considered a medical grade. It you are using higher-level TCA preparations, do so only under the direction of qualified medical personnel. As always, check with your state licensing requirements.

CAUTION!

Some manufacturers recommend leaving on peel preparations. Always follow the manufacturer's protocols.

Follow all indications, contraindications, preparations, and protocols for glycolic and TCA acid peels, as listed above.

Layering Salicylic Acid and TCA Peels

The combination of salicylic acid and TCA is excellent for the client concerned with age management and acne but who does not have the downtime to recover from other ablative types of procedures. Another benefit is that it is not as expensive as treatments that use more costly technology. As with all peels, however, the results depend upon preparation and home care compliance. This client should have had peels preceding the layered peel and have developed a tolerance to the peels. A good home care program for a client preparing for layered salicylic acid and TCA peels should include a combination of hydrators, antioxidants, AHAs, BHAs, retinoic acid, lighteners, and environmental protections with an SPF of 30.

The Objective

Your objective in salicylic and TCA peels is to perform a superficial exfoliation of the stratum corneum, to reduce hyperpigmentation and acne; and to increase tightening and smoothing of the skin. Salicylic acid is excellent for reducing bacteria in the hair follicle, and provides decongestion, and TCA can generate smoothing and tightening of the epidermis. Use just one layer of the salicylic acid preparation and one to two layers of the TCA peel, depending upon the skin thickness and condition of the skin type you are treating. As with all peels, be conservative until you are acquainted with the skin you are peeling and have experience with your peeling solutions.

The salicylic peel has reached its optimum benefit when the skin has an even, slightly pink tone. If some areas are turning red faster than the overall skin, then they are peeling at a faster rate than the other areas and must be diluted with water or with the manufacturer's recommended neutralizing product. The salicylic acid peel may show a slight frosting (whitening) in some areas, particularly around acne lesions. Dilute or neutralize those areas, as you will be applying the TCA peel layers next. If the client shows an extreme erythema or frosting reaction to the salicylic acid peel layer, it may be best to postpone the TCA peel layers. Other factors may be in play, such as improper preparation in home care, client stress, or a stronger effect of the peel. As always, patch testing is necessary for all peels. Make certain to test both peel preparations in the patch test. The more preparation you do before the peel in home care and patch testing, the better your results will be. This is true for all peels.

Follow all indications, contraindications, preparation, and protocols for salicylic acid and TCA acid peels, as described above.

> **CAUTION!**
>
> Higher-level and nonbuffered peels are to be performed in a medical setting only, with qualified medical training and certification.

PEEL COCKTAILS

Many peel ingredients offer a completely new level of skin rejuvenation when combined with additional peeling products; antioxidants; and antibacterial, antiseptic, and cell and tissue support ingredients.

For years, we have seen the many benefits of layering peels (as we have just discussed). Now peel manufacturers and suppliers have infused ingredients to serve as a one-step peeling solution, with layered applications or passes. Many peel cocktails will include combinations of lactic, salicylic, glycolic, TCA, and phenol acids along with resorcinol.

Phenol acid peels have been modified and reconstituted for use in lighter peel applications—in contrast to how phenol peels were once used. Historically, the phenol acid peel was considered the deepest acting peel and required hospitalization. Today, with the synergistic benefits of combined acids along with cell protectants, tyrosinase inhibitors, and hydrating ingredients, the skin benefits from the new technologies in blended peeling solutions with minimal expense and down time. Often a peel cocktail will be a fraction of the price of four to five laser treatments and will provide great results. Depending upon the skin type, skin condition, and desired results, the peels can be applied routinely or as minimally as once or twice annually.

Pre- and Post-peel Care

The pre-peel preparation is often the same as it is for any peel that combines home care products—such as retinoic acid, hydroquinone, or skin lightening agents—AHAs, and BHAs for exfoliation and conditioning, hydration products with antioxidants, and environmental products with an SPF of at least 30. The post-peel phase requires that you do not use retinoic acid or retinol (unless it is a part of the manufacturers protocol), AHAs, BHAs, or other performance ingredients. Hydrators; antioxidants; calming and soothing ingredients, such as allantoin and azulene; and gamma linoleic acid for lipid replacement are excellent for post-peel phases. Again, you must follow the instructions as directed by the manufacturer or physician or as dictated by training and certification protocols.

PEEL SOLUTIONS AND PRE- AND POST-PEEL HOME CARE PRODUCTS

All clients or patients prone to herpetic outbreaks (cold sores) are required to take an antiviral medication prior to and during the healing phase of a chemical peel. Make sure that you include this on your informed consent document. Clients must initial the sentence that states that they visited their physician for a prescription and will use the medication prior to the peel (Table 4–4).

As with all peels, it is important to make sure that clients fully understanding the following:

- Have they planned for enough recovery time? They do not want to plan a weekend in the sun after a Friday afternoon peel.
- Do they understand that they are to use the prescribed home care products and applications? We do not want them to use products that may create a caustic reaction with their peel. It is best to have a clause on your informed consent document that they initial in which they accept this responsibility.
- If clients are anxious or undergoing a particularly stressful time in their lives, some peels can be more unpredictable. It may be better to wait to do a peel until things have stabilized for them.
- Do they fully understand that there is pre- and post-peel preparation that will directly influence the results of the peel? (Have them initial this sentence on the informed consent document.)

Table 4–4 Peel Pre- and Post-care

Skin Type or Condition	Peel Solutions	Ingredients to Include for Optimal Pre-peel Home Care Products	Ingredients to Include for Post-peel Home Care Products
Hyperpigmentation	lactic acid, glycolic acid, Jessner's solution, TCA	antiviral medication if client is prone to cold sores; Kojic acid, arbutin, hydroquinone, licorice extract, glycolic, lactic, malic, tartaric acids	allantoin, azulene, antioxidants such as ergothioneine, licochalcone (licorice extract), sunscreen ingredients such as zinc oxide and titanium dioxide
Normal/Aging/ Mature	glycolic acid, Jessner's, solution, TCA, resorcinol	antiviral medication if client is prone to cold sores, glycolic acid, hydroquinone, retinol, retinoic acid	emollient-based products with sodium hyaluronate, GLA (gamma linoleic acid) for lipid replacement, sunscreen ingredients such as zinc oxide and titanium dioxide
Dry/Dehydrated/ Pigmented/ Sensitive	lactic acid, glycolic acid, salicylic acid, papaya enzyme	antiviral medication if client is prone to cold sores, lactic acid, glycolic acid, papaya enzyme, retinol	emollient-based products, azulene, acetyl dipeptide, sunscreen ingredients such as zinc oxide and titanium dioxide
Oily/Acne prone	glycolic acid, salicylic acid, Jessner's solution, TCA	antiviral medication if client is prone to cold sores, glycolic acid, salicylic acid, Kojic acid, licorice extract, retinoic acid	gel-based products with hyaluronic acid, sunscreen ingredients such as zinc oxide and titanium dioxide

- Have they signed the informed consent document, and do they understand that there is a possibility of scarring, PIH, herpetic outbreak, erythema, and dehydration?
- If they are prone to herpetic outbreaks (cold sores), have they visited their physician for appropriate antiviral medication? (Have them initial the sentence on the informed consent document that states that they understand the importance of obtaining this medication and are using it.)

SUMMING IT UP

The rationale for performing a chemical peel varies from expense, skin type, and skin condition, or esthetician preference and experience. Three major considerations with chemical peels are as follows:

- Know and understand the skin you are peeling
- Know and have training and experience with the peel product you are using
- Know and comply with your state regulations

As we know, chemical peeling dates back to ancient Egyptian times, and has been successfully used with proper pre- and postcare. Be sure to purchase reputable products and train with a reputable company that has educators with field experience. It is important to work with professionals who have done thousands of peels and understand how the peel products affect various skin types and conditions. Do not perform peels that are out of your scope of practice. Perform advanced peels only under the direct supervision of a qualified physician or medical personnel.

ESTHETICIAN **PROFILE**

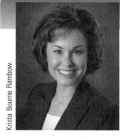

Krista Bourne Rambow.

Krista Bourne Rambow, LE
Episciences, Inc.

Dermatologist Carl Thornfeldt, MD

I am 48 years old and originally from California. I am currently the esthetics education director for Episciences, Inc., in Boise, Idaho, which manufactures and distributes Epionce skin care. I have worked for Episciences since 2006. I have been extremely fortunate to work closely with dermatologist Dr. Carl Thornfeldt, the founder and CEO of Episciences.

I coordinate training materials, including presentations, webinars, and advanced education training events held around the country. With Dr. Thornfeldt, I help create clinical and home care protocols for our skin care products and provide input for new product development. I manage our in-house clinical studies, performing clinical treatments and documenting our participants' progress with our computer imaging system. I organize our trade show schedule and help man the booth at various trade shows throughout the year. Additionally, I write articles for trade magazines and assist as part of the marketing team. Dr. Thornfeldt and I cowrote the book *The New Ideal in Skin Health: Separating Fact from Fiction,* which was published in 2010 by Allured Books.

I believe my interest in esthetics began in junior high or high school, although I didn't know it was called esthetics back then. Having personally struggled with acne issues and the horrid "hook" eyebrows as a teen, I have always been a little obsessed with skin and eyebrows.

I was a flight attendant for a major U.S. carrier for several years. At one point, one of my (nonflight attendant) friends was very excited about her new job. She was a licensed cosmetologist and had just been hired to work at a plastic surgeon's office. Her job was to help patients prepare their skin for a deep chemical peel treatment—to actually apply the chemical peel to their skin—and to help their skin recover after their peel. I was fascinated by this. After taking a voluntary furlough with the airline, I enrolled in an esthetic school. I received my esthetics license in 2003.

Training

I attended Idaho's First European Academy for Advanced Esthetics. I was very fortunate to find an esthetic school in my area, since there had not been one locally available for several years. We started with a class of eight students. In the end, seven graduated. (And I was very glad to have the Milady online study guide with all the practice tests to help me through the written exam.)

Practice Demographic

I work with people in their young teens (13) and older, and on all skin types, depending on what we are studying. My work has morphed into in-house clinical studies that are more specifically regimented and focuses on acne treatment, pigmentation, psoriasis, and skin redness/rosacea.

Services/Treatments Offered

- Signature and clinical facials
- Microdermabrasion
- Chemical peels and ultrasonic facials
- Waxing
- Computer imaging for before and after image photography

Personal Philosophy

I love connecting with people, developing that trusting relationship with someone and helping them conquer their biggest skin issues. I love to get out of my office and work with my hands on someone, then travel a bit, and personally talk to people about their skin and our skin care line. I love to answer the difficult questions about the challenging clients that our accounts sometimes encounter. Having that personal hands-on experience is a huge plus for me, to be able to help clients, and to relate to them what has worked successfully for me.

I do my best to stay on top of industry changes with my spa forums, trade magazines for estheticians, consumer beauty magazines, skin and beauty-related books, and magazines that target healthy aging and cosmetic surgery. I am currently studying to become NCEA certified, which is an excellent national organization for estheticians and a great source for industry trends, and education and governmental standards.

Additional Contributions to the Industry

Publishing our book gave me a wonderful platform for writing and publishing articles. I've written and published several in the past couple of years in a few trade magazines. The book has also given me a long list of subjects I would like to speak about to fellow estheticians—whether they are students or licensed estheticians. We are also working with our local junior college to help develop medical aesthetic training for nurses who wish to go into the aesthetic or plastic surgery field.

I created two classes for our community education offerings here in Boise that I teach on a volunteer basis. One is on aging gracefully without surgery; it helps consumers wade through all the misinformation out there about cosmetic products. The other class is on skin cancer awareness.

I speak about skin cancer awareness in high school health classes, and someday hope to convince school board authorities that it is a class that should be taught on a regular basis—at every junior high and high school health class in the state of Idaho. I have also presented on skin cancer awareness at a health fair sponsored by the Boise State nursing program.

Technology-Focused Facials and Treatments

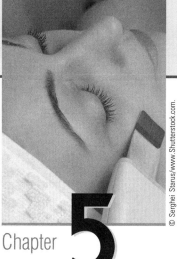

© Serghei Starus/www.Shutterstock.com.

> "If I were to say which skin type I treat most often, it would be in the anti-aging range ... I feel like a sculptress. After seeing a client's face, I know instantly how to "tailor make" the treatments in order to get the best results."
>
> —Alexandra Cole, Face Facts Face Studio, Buckinghamshire, UK

Chapter **5**

Chapter Capture

After completing this chapter, you will be able to:

- Have fun with technology.
- Understand technology facial protocols.
- Layer technology and understand the applications.
- Incorporate express or mini services in your menu.

EXPLORING NEW IDEAS IN ESTHETIC TECHNOLOGY

Esthetician-directed technologies have expanded dramatically over the last decade, and there is no indication that the desire for newer, more compact technology will slow down. In fact, the desire for smaller, more agile, and intelligent esthetic technology is as pervasive in the skin care industry as it is in the computer industry. Today, we are seeing these two industries merging in the development of smart devices, which frees up our time, space, and mobility. We know that nothing will replace the need for human touch. Thus, the more efficient use of technology will help ensure that the hands-on portion of services will always give the perceptive technician a leading role in the lives of his or her clients (Figure 5–1).

Estheticians want more value out of each dollar that they spend. Complicated navigation in a device is a good reason for *not* making a purchase today, as time, energy, and capital are all at a premium for both the skin therapist and the consumer. We have all discovered that complex, large, and cumbersome does not mean that a device is more efficacious.

Tried and true therapies continue to rule in many spas, salons, skin care clinics, and esthetic medical centers. Clients seek them because they work. The difference today is in the technological developments for these treatments. Microdermabrasion, ultrasonic, microcurrent, galvanic, LED (light-emitting diode), lasers, IPL (intense pulsed light) radio frequency, and oxygen treatments are all very much a part of the landscape for professional estheticians today and in the future. These devices are continually being upgraded and redesigned as they come to the market. We have also

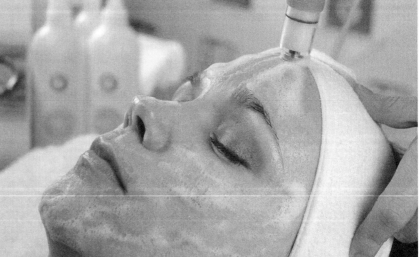

Courtesy of Bio-Therapeutic, Inc.

Figure 5–1 Wet–dry microdermabrasion, a newer concept in exfoliation.

seen that manufacturers are making mini end-consumer versions of professional esthetic devices. This development has kept clients involved in **home care compliance**. However, when they do not obtain the same results as they do from a professional, they return to their faithful esthetician, at the first opportunity. Another interesting and noteworthy point is that the devices made today do not look like those of the past. Some are quite fun and exciting to use. This is great for the skin care and beauty professional, as it fosters learning and the need for applying new techniques.

home care compliance
Clients or patients using products at home in a manner consistent with a plan created by an esthetician and physician.

Having Fun with Technology

Esthetic device manufacturers are taking tips from the computer industry in the design and styling of professional models. Many newer skin care devices look like toys. This is interesting to note if we follow the thoughts of marketing genius Harry Beckwith in his latest book, *Unthinking, the Surprising Forces Behind What We Buy* (*Business Plus*, 2011). Beckwith has worked with *Fortune* 500 companies such as Target® and Microsoft®, coaching them on business practices and looking at the philosophical concepts that explain why we buy certain products. Beckwith says that elements of play and fun are often associated with a technology purchase. Looking at the success of the iPod, iPhone, and iPad—and the fun and exciting colors available for their accessories—we see that this fever is also moving into the worldwide esthetic industry. Cosmetologists know this very well and are typically having fun in their work. On your next visit to your stylist or colorist, take a look at his or her assortment of gadgets, products, and implements. There is no end in sight for new equipment and products.

Many estheticians got started in the industry by viewing their work and tools as fun. This is not to demean the importance of our work or of our equipment, but often we will hear a colleague say, "Come by and look at my new toy." We like the sense of play, and are continually in awe of what we are able to do in skin care with new technology. As the technology improves, so do we, and so does the fun we are having. It keeps us going back to work day after day.

In this chapter, we will look at devices and protocols individually and then explore the layering of technology. The first facial that we review is a simple protocol that uses galvanic and high-frequency therapies Then we move to wet–dry microdermabrasion, oxygen therapy, microcurrent treatment, and LED treatment. We take a look at hand-held devices. We will also discuss how to layer these devices in a comprehensive technology treatment. As with all treatments, it is important to set up a good home care plan for the client.

Home Care Compliance

All clients should be on a skin-type- and condition-specific home care plan prior to receiving treatments in the salon, spa, or clinic. At a minimum, you will learn much about a client's habits and willingness to be compliant if you start them out with a simple, systematic, instructional skin care program. This will also help develop client loyalty and support what you are recommending in the treatment room. If you cannot control what a client is using at home, it may slow and alter the results of your treatment plan and applications.

BASIC FACIAL USING GALVANIC AND HIGH-FREQUENCY TECHNOLOGY

The best choice for some clients may be to offer a simple exquisite European facial that features cleansing, steam, galvanic current, minimal to no extractions, high-frequency technology, a wonderful massage, a masque, and a hydrating finish. This basic facial can be performed as pre- and post-operative care, or combined with other technologies in more comprehensive treatments (Figures 5–2 and 5–3).

To perform a basic facial using galvanic and high-frequency technology, you will need a magnification light or LED visor, steamer, galvanic and high-frequency devices, and towel warmer.

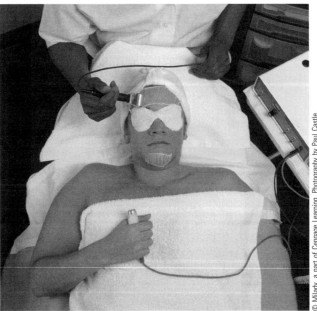

© Milady, a part of Cengage Learning. Photography by Paul Castle.

Figure 5–2 Galvanic machine in use.

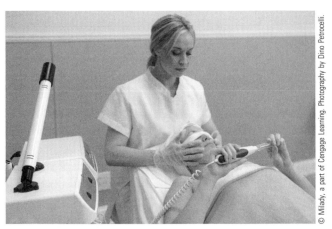

Figure 5–3 High-frequency in use.

The Objective

The objectives of a basic facial using galvanic and high-frequency devices include stimulation, relaxation, exfoliation, product penetration, deep pore cleansing, reducing acne level 1 or 2 lesions, and increasing hydration.

Indications

Clients who have the following conditions are the best candidates for a basic facial using galvanic and high-frequency devices:

- Acne level 1 or 2
- Dryness/dehydration
- Pre-operative condition
- Post-operative condition (for at least one month or as indicated by physician)
- Congestion

Contraindications

Clients who have the following conditions are not candidates for using galvanic and high-frequency in a facial.

- Pacemaker
- Neurostimulation devices
- Epilepsy
- Bleeding disorders
- Cancer
- Herpetic outbreak
- Viral warts

eczema

Inflammatory, painful itching disease of the skin, acute or chronic in nature, with dry or moist lesions. This condition should be referred to a physician. Seborrheic dermatitis, mainly affecting oily areas, is a common form of eczema.

dermatitis

Any inflammatory condition of the skin; various forms of lesions, such as eczema, vesicles, or papules; the three main categories are atopic, contact, and seborrheic dermatitis.

- Open lesions
- Sunburn
- **Eczema**
- **Dermatitis**
- Bacterial infections
- Conjunctivitis

PROCEDURE: BASIC FACIAL USING TECHNOLOGY

Supply List
- EPA-registered disinfectant
- Hand sanitizer/antibacterial soap
- Bowls
- Spatulas
- Fan and mask brush
- Implements (including lancet or extracting device)
- Sharps container
- Hand towels
- Clean linens
- Blanket
- Headband
- Client gown or wrap
- Tissue
- Gloves/finger cots
- Informed consent document
- Client charts

Products
- Cleanser
- Exfoliant
- Desincrustation fluid
- Masque
- Massage cream
- Toner
- Serum
- Moisturizer
- Environmental protection product with SPF 30 with antioxidants

Procedure

1. The client signs the informed consent document.
2. Cleanse the client's skin with a light foaming gel cleanser and remove all residues.
3. Apply an enzymatic exfoliant or exfoliating masque and steam for 7 to 10 minutes.
4. Remove all traces of the masque with warm towel or sponges.
5. Apply a desincrustation fluid and perform desincrustation/negative ionization with the galvanic device.
6. Perform extractions and then remove the desincrustation gel and debris.
7. Apply high–frequency for reducing bacteria.
8. Apply a skin-type- and condition-specific masque with brushes or your hands. Leave on for five to eight minutes.
9. Remove the masque with warm towels or sponges.
10. Apply toner.
11. Apply a skin-type- and condition-specific serum and moisturizer and ionize with a microcurrent or galvanic device.
12. Apply an environmental protection product with a minimum SPF of 30.
13. Cleanse your hands.
14. See the client to the retail area. Make product recommendations, sell through, and reschedule his or her next appointment.
15. Clean and disinfect the work area and equipment.
16. Make chart notes.

MICRODERMABRASION

Initially described as a trend, but continuing to evolve today, microdermabrasion has decidedly turned into an essential technology in the work lives of most estheticians. Even those who have opposed the treatment or technology in the past have slowly begun to warm to its multiple benefits in age management. We have gleaned a great deal about applications, contraindications, protocols, and client selections from its debut back in the early 1990s.

The options in microdermabrasion devices continue to inundate the market today. Many devices now have various mediums for exfoliation, such as particle types, stainless hand pieces studded with

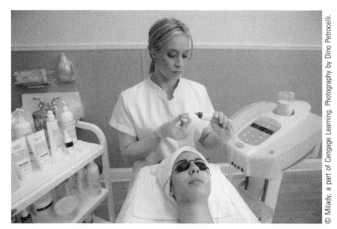

Figure 5–4 Microdermabrasion with particles.

industrial diamond particles, brushes, and even water. The newest devices include a solution infusion element or wet–dry microdermabrasion, which addresses one of the original issues we had with microdermabrasion: that it tended to dry out the skin. As we have learned, dryness, dehydration, and too much vacuum pressure can create elastosis and impaired barrier functions.

In all microdermabrasion devices, there is a direct relationship between the power of the vacuum, the number of passes, the speed of the passes, and the pressure applied by the esthetician. Client selection is also an important consideration for obtaining excellent results (Figure 5–4).

The Objective

The objective of microdermabrasion is to remove dead cellular debris at the level of the stratum corneum. Depending upon the devices used, hydration, skin lightening, and acne reduction may also be objectives, where specific solution-based products are used for target areas. Blood circulation and lymphatic fluid are stimulated with the vacuum pressure, and superficial hyperpigmented lesions can be reduced as the hand piece can provide the necessary exfoliation to lift some lesions. Client selection is important, as more pigment in upper Fitzpatrick skin types can be stimulated by too much pressure and aggressive microdermabrasion treatments (Figures 5–5 and 5–6).

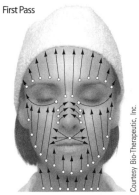

First Pass

Courtesy Bio-Therapeutic, Inc.

Figure 5–5 First pass
vertical movement chart.

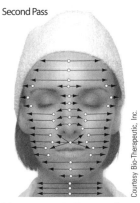

Second Pass

Courtesy Bio-Therapeutic, Inc.

Figure 5–6 Second pass
horizontal movement chart.

Indications

Clients who have the following conditions are the best candidates for microdermabrasion:

- **Rhytides**
- Photodamage
- Hyperpigmentation
- Sallow skin tone
- Rough, coarse skin texture
- Uneven skin tone
- Acne scarring
- **seborrheic keratosis**

Contraindications

Clients who have the following conditions are not candidates for microdermabrasion:

- **Isotretinoin** (formerly known as Accutane®) within the last year
- Rosacea
- Sensitive, reactive skin
- Bacterial infections, viral or fungal infections
- Open lesions, burns, or rashes
- Dermatitis
- Sunburn
- Active inflamed acne pustules, cysts, or nodules
- Immediate, post-operative cosmetic facial surgery (laser resurfacing, deep chemical peels, blepharoplasty, facelifts, neck lifts, liposuction)
- Pregnancy (may stimulate **melanocytes**)

rhytides
Wrinkles.

seborrheic keratosis
Crusty-looking, slightly raised lesions in mature, sun-damaged skin. They may be black, brown, gray, or flesh-toned. (They can be found all over the body.)

isotretinoin
Medication used for advanced cases of acne and extreme cases of rosacea formerly know as Accutane.

melanocytes
Cell that produces pigment granules/melanin in the basal layer of the epidermis.

PROCEDURE: MICRODERMABRASION

Supply List

- Device and accessories
- Facial bed/chair, client draping, and linen setup
- Eye protection for practitioner (safety goggles; crystal-free devices optional)
- Particulate mask (crystal-free devices optional)
- Eye protection for client (crystal-free devices optional)
- Gloves
- Disposable sponges or cotton pads
- Brush for removing crystals (not applicable with crystal-free devices)
- Water and bowl
- Cotton rounds

Products

- Cleanser
- Toner
- Particulate (if using particle version)
- Diamond tips (if appropriate to device)
- Solutions for device if using wet–dry diamond tip
- Solutions for device if using brush applicators
- Soothing serum, lotion, cream
- Environmental protection product with an SPF of at least 30 and antioxidants

Procedure

NOTE: In the first pass, use a microdermabrasion vertical movement chart.

1. The client signs the informed consent document.
2. Depending upon the type of microdermabrasion device, follow the manufacturer's recommendations for skin preparation and setup.
3. Apply protective eye pads to the client's face.
4. Put on protective eye goggles, protective apparel, and gloves.
5. Follow the manufacturer's recommendations for pressure settings, time exposure, and treatment protocol.
6. Perform a test patch along the client's mandible. Start with low settings, increasing them as you determine the client's tolerance level.

7. If you are using a wet–dry microdermabrasion device, apply products or solutions topically or simultaneously with the device for each pass, as indicated. If you are using a dry diamond tip or particle device, follow the manufacturer's recommendations accordingly.

8. Start the procedure on the client's forehead.

9. With all types of devices (wet–dry, diamond tip, particle), use vertical strokes on the entire width of the forehead, starting at the center just above the eyebrow and working toward the hairline above the temple.

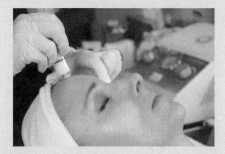

10. Repeat on the other side.

11. Apply vertical strokes to the client's temples and around the eye areas, cheeks, upper lip, chin, and nasal region.

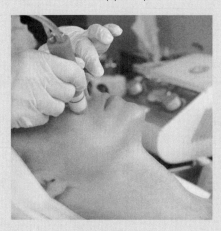

12. Repeat on the other side.

13. Apply vertical strokes on the neck and décolleté areas.

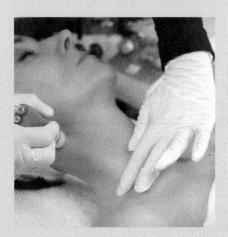

14. Repeat on the other side.

NOTE: In the second pass, use a microdermabrasion horizontal movement chart.

15. If you are using a wet–dry microdermabrasion device, apply topical solutions to target specific areas of concern, such as acne, aging, or hyperpigmentation. If the solutions are infused within the device, follow the manufacturer's recommendations.

16. Apply a horizontal movement, starting on the right half of the forehead. Hold the skin taut with your free hand.

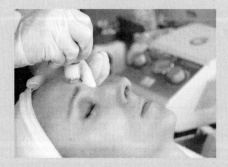

17. Make horizontal strokes on the entire width of the forehead, starting above the eyebrow, and applying the first "row" in the direction of the temple. Work row by row as you move toward the hairline.

18. Repeat on the other side.

19. Apply horizontal strokes to the temple and around the eye areas, cheeks, chin, upper lip, and nasal region.

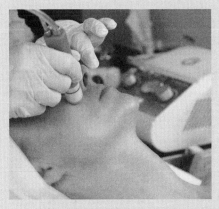

20. Gently apply a horizontal pass to the neck and décolleté.

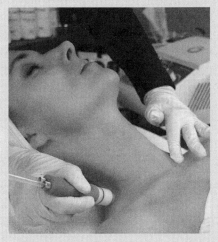

21. If using particles, remove all residue.

22. Conclude the treatment with soothing serum, lotion, or cream and an environmental protection product with an SPF of 30 or higher as well as antioxidants.

23. Cleanse your hands.

24. Send your client home with written instructions on avoiding AHAs, BHAs, retinoic acid, and other aggressive exfoliants for four to five days or as recommended by the manufacturer. Include a list of products that the client should use at home, such as gentle cleansers, serums, moisturizers, and environmental protection with an SPF of 30 or higher and antioxidants (for daily use). Have

the client sign a document stating that he or she will follow the home care protocols.

25. See the client to the retail area, sell through on product recommendations, and schedule his or her next appointment. Microdermabrasion can be performed every four weeks or as indicated for specific conditions, such as acne (which may be treated weekly).

26. Clean and disinfect the work area, device, accessories, and hand piece.

27. Make chart notes.

See Color Insert for full color photos.

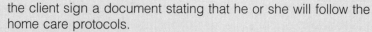 OXYGEN FACIALS

Oxygen facials have proven to be beneficial for infusing product into the skin; increasing ATP (adenosine triphosphate), which is referred to as the body's energy packet; and improving barrier functions. When applied topically, we can increase the oxygen and respiration uptake in the cells, and thus improve cell metabolism. According to Craig Wenborg, MD (*Esthetic Benefits of Oxygen Skin Care*, Skin Inc., April 2006), many oxygen skin therapies are based on the premise that using stable, natural oxygen acquired from the ambient air—consists of two atoms bound together by a stable chemical bond known as a **covalent bond** (which are atoms created by sharing electrons)—increases skin cell metabolism. This is not to be confused with unstable forms of oxygen molecules which are known as free radicals. Free radicals are most commonly a single oxygen atom (molecule/part) with unpaired electrons in their outer shell. This causes oxidation and ultimately begins to destroy the cells, one by one, if they are not neutralized by antioxidants.

It is, however, important to use antioxidants in the process of applying oxygen therapy, as the debate continues on whether oxygen and other devices create free radicals. We do know that while we are living and breathing, we are creating free radicals. It suffices to say that we should be using antioxidants both internally and externally on a daily basis to slow the proliferation of free radicals and to neutralize their effects as much as possible.

Esthetically oriented oxygen devices purify the ambient air by removing impurities and other elements to increase the available oxygen by up to 95 percent. Topical skin care products can then be infused through the purified air within the delivery systems on the device, to areas such as fine lines and wrinkles, dull, dehydrated, or in acneic skin.

 covalent bond
A form of chemical bonding characterized by the sharing of pairs of electrons between atoms.

Oxygen-device accessory packages offer various delivery systems, including air-brush wands that infuse the product with a fine spray or mist for general use; pulsating jets that deliver spot-specific product; and individual domes that can be applied over a skin-type- and condition-specific product-saturated mask. Each accessory functions independently and can be selected based on the specific needs of both the esthetician and client.

The Objective

The objective of an oxygen facial is to infuse product ingredients onto the skin, improve both lymph and blood circulation, and stimulate ATP—the body's energy source. Oxygen therapy revitalizes dull, dehydrated skin; when used with condition-specific ingredients within products, it can reduce acne lesion occurrence. It serves as a basic treatment for age management in routine monthly services, as a standalone service, or on combination with other technologies.

Indications

Clients who have the following conditions are the best candidates for oxygen facials:

- Dry, dehydrated skin
- Generalized aging
- Fine and deep lines
- Dull congested skin
- Acne
- Preapplication for other services
- Enlarged follicles

Contraindications

Clients who have the following conditions are not candidates for oxygen facials:

- Isotretinoin (formerly known as or Accutane®) use within a year (must obtain a physician's recommendation)
- Herpetic outbreak (cold sores)
- Open wounds (acne lesions or other bleeding lesions)
- Pregnancy
- Cancer
- Autoimmune disorders
- Sunburn
- Any contagious disease
- Dermatitis

PROCEDURE: OXYGEN FACIAL

Supply List

- Device and accessories
- Gloves
- Sponges
- Gauze
- Eye pads for spray-wand accessories
- Informed consent document

Products

- Cleanser
- Individual dome (if applicable)
- Product-infused paper mask
- Skin-type- and condition-specific serum, lotion, or cream
- Environmental protection product with an SPF of 30 and antioxidants

Procedure

1. The client signs the informed consent document.
2. Cleanse with a skin-type- and condition-specific product.
3. Exfoliate with a manual or mechanical product or device such as an exfoliating mask, enzyme peel, ultrasonic peeling, or microdermabrasion.
4. Cover the client's eyes with eye protection.
5. Apply a specific condition serum or ampoule to affected areas. This could be an acne product to lesions, a muscle-relaxing serum to expression aging areas (forehead, periorbital region), or a lightener to hyperpigmented areas.

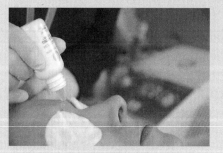

Courtesy of Bio-Therapeutic, Inc.

6. Blend the serum gently into the skin.

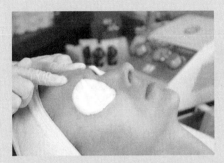

7. Apply pulsating jets to infuse the product directly onto the area. Adjust the device according to the manufacturer's specifications.

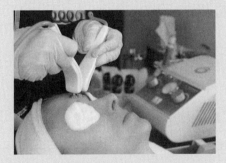

8. Apply the serum and pulsating jets to another area.

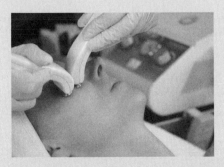

9. Fill the wand reservoir with a serum or solution that is specific to the client's condition—such as hyaluronic acid, peptides, and antioxidants for dry or dehydrated skin—and spray the serum or solution over the client's face. Adjust the device according to the

manufacturer's specifications. Apply the oxygenated product with the wand.

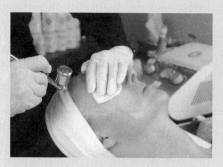

10. Spray over the neck and décolleté.

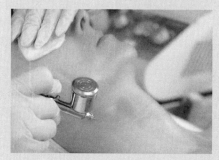

11. Apply a skin-type- and condition-specific masque and cover with an oxygen dome (for product infusion) for approximately 15 to 20 minutes.

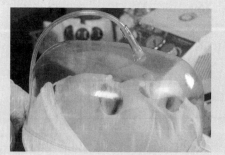

12. Remove the masque and dome.

13. Apply appropriate skin-type- and condition-specific hydration products and an environmental protection product with an SPF of 30 or higher and antioxidants.

14. Cleanse your hands.

15. Send your client home with written instructions on avoiding AHAs, BHAs, retinoic acid, and other aggressive exfoliants for four to five days or as recommended by the manufacturer. Include a list of products that the client should use at home, such as gentle cleansers, serums, moisturizers, and environmental protection product with an SPF of 30 or higher and antioxidants (for daily use). Have the client sign a document stating that he or she will follow the home care protocols.

16. See the client to retail area, sell through on product recommendations, and schedule his or her next appointment. Oxygen facials can be performed every four weeks or as indicated for specific conditions such as acne (which may be treated weekly).

17. Clean and disinfect the work area, device, accessories, and hand piece.

18. Make chart notes.

See Color Insert for full color photos.

 # MICROCURRENT THERAPY

Microcurrent services were once considered alternative but are now mainstream. They are found on the service menus in most salons, spas, and clinical settings. Microcurrent treatment is a low-level electrical current that mimics the body's own natural electrical rhythms. Nearly all the studies that demonstrated benefits of microcurrent treatment used current with less than 400Ua. This is opposed to other electrotherapies which use much higher levels of current, which may reduce benefits to the skin. Microcurrent acts as an external source of energy that the body can use to accelerate, healthier looking skin; ionizing product with microcurrent shows immediate hydration in the skin.

Muscle Memory and Re-education

Microcurrent is beneficial in strengthening and tightening musculature while firming and lifting. Just as we can lengthen and shorten muscles with massage, we can apply the same theory to using microcurrent in muscle reeducation. By simulating a massage technique while penetrating a low level of electrical current, we can see great results in muscle firmness and the reduction of atrophy. Microcurrent has been used in medicine and physical therapy for many years. We have recently begun to understand the many benefits and uses for age management through improving mitochondrial activity and cellular restoration.

Objective

The objective of a microcurrent facial is to perform a firming and toning treatment and to provide an excellent medium for iontophoresis and desincrustation. Microcurrent improves both lymph and blood circulation, stimulates ATP—the body's own natural energy source—and improves muscle memory. Through stimulating circulation and ATP, microcurrent increases fibroblast activity and thus upregulates collage and elastin production. It improves oxygenation and respiration in the cells and supports muscle movement and DNA replication. Microcurrent serves as a basic treatment for age management in routine monthly services, and in pre- and post-operative phases as a standalone service or in combination with other technologies (Figure 5–7).

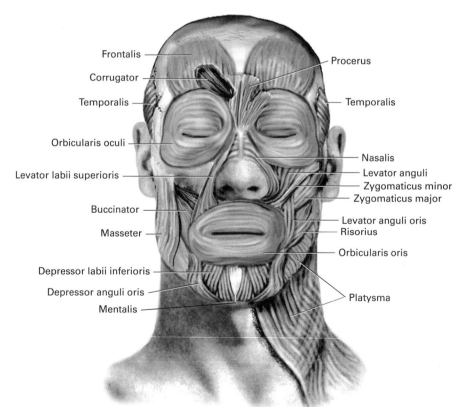

Figure 5–7 Facial Muscle chart.

Indications

Clients who have the following conditions are the best candidates for microcurrent:

- Dry, dehydrated skin
- Generalized aging
- Fine and deep lines
- Dull, congested skin
- Acne
- Preapplication for other services
- Enlarged follicles

Contraindications

Clients who have the following conditions are not candidates for microcurrent:

- Isotretinoin (formerly known as Accutane®) use within a year (must obtain a physician's recommendation)
- Herpetic outbreak (cold sores)
- Open wounds (acne lesions or other bleeding lesions)
- Pregnancy
- Pacemaker or neurostimulation implanted devices
- Epilepsy
- Bleeding disorders
- Cancer
- Autoimmune disorders
- Sunburn
- Any contagious disease
- Dermatitis
- Eczema

PROCEDURE: MICROCURRENT

Supply List
- Device and accessories
- Gloves
- Sponges
- Gauze
- Sponges or towels
- Informed consent document

Products
- Water-based cleanser
- Conductive solution

- Water-based serum
- Water-based moisturizer
- Environmental protection product with an SPF of 30

Procedure

1. The client signs the informed consent document.
2. Cleanse the skin using a gentle, water-based cleanser.
3. Exfoliate with a manual or mechanical product or device, such as an exfoliating mask, an enzyme peel, an ultrasonic peeler, or microdermabrasion.
4. Apply the conductive gel or manufacturer's recommended product along the area that you will be treating.

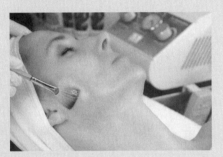

5. Moisten the metal conducting probes with the manufacturer's recommended conductive product. Some manufacturers recommend electric gloves for this purpose.
6. Set the device for the service that you will be performing, as recommended by the manufacturer.
7. Press "run" or "start."
8. Starting in the area of the lower **masseter**, place one stationary probe below the **zygomatic bone** and slowly pull the masseter upward with your other hand and the other probe, or "moving probe."

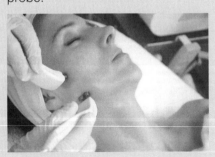

masseter
Muscle that coordinates with the temporalis, medial pterygoid, and lateral pterygoid muscles to open and close the mouth and bring the jaw forward; sometimes referred to as the chewing muscle.

zygomatic bone
Also known as malar bone or cheekbone.

9. Hold for the amount of time specified by the manufacturer.

10. Move toward the upper portion of the masseter above the zygomatic arch with the stationary probe, and slowly pull at the base of the masseter with your other hand and the other probe. Hold as recommended by the manufacturer.

11. Place the stationary probe at the **auricularis anterior**, and the moving probe with your other hand at the insertion of the **buccinator** and **risorius** region. Slowly pull back and hold.

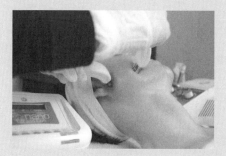

12. Place the stationary probe at the lower **orbicularis oculi**, and the moving hand and probe at the insertion of the **zygomaticus major**. Pull up toward the origin and hold.

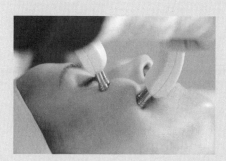

auricularis anterior
Muscle in front of the ear that draws the ear forward.

buccinator
Thin, flat muscle of the cheek between the upper and lower jaw that compresses the cheeks and expels air between the lips.

risorius
Muscle of the mouth that draws the corner of the mouth out and back, as in grinning.

orbicularis oculi
Ring muscle of the eye socket that closes the eyelid.

zygomatics major and minor
Muscles on both sides of the face that extend from the zygomatic bone to the angle of the mouth. These muscles elevate the lip and pull the mouth upward and backward in a laugh or smile.

nasalis
A two part muscle that covers the nose.

levator labii superioris
Muscles that elevate the lip and dilate the nostrils.

corrugators
Facial muscle that draws eyebrows down and wrinkles the forehead vertically.

13. Place the stationary probe at the position of the inner portion of the **nasalis** and the moving hand and probe at the insertion point of the **levator labii superioris**. Pull and hold.

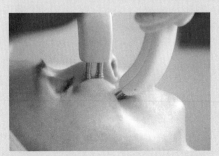

14. Place the stationary probe at the frontalis and the moving hand and probe at the insertion of the **corrugator**. Gently pull up and hold.

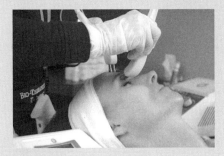

15. Place the stationary probe above the middle point of the eyebrow, and the moving hand and probe below it on the inner upper orbicularis oculi. Gently pull up and hold.

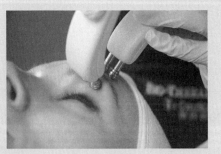

16. Place the stationary probe above the outer area of eyebrow, and the moving hand and probe below it on the inner upper orbicularis oculi. Gently pull up and hold.

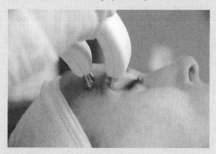

17. Repeat all these movements on the other side of face.
18. Ionize serum, as recommended by the manufacturer.

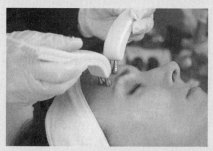

19. Ionize the cream. Penetrate a water-based cream into the skin to retain moisture and hydration.
20. Ionize the eye cream. Penetrate a water-based eye cream to hold in moisture and to protect the eye area.

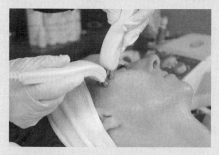

21. Apply an environmental protection product with an SPF of at least 30 and antioxidants.
22. Cleanse your hands.
23. Send your client home with written instructions on avoiding AHAs, BHAs, retinoic acid, and other aggressive exfoliants for two to three days or as recommended by manufacturer. Include a list of

products that the client should use at home, such as gentle cleansers, serums, moisturizers, and environmental protection with an SPF of 30 or higher and antioxidants (for daily use). Have the client sign a document stating that he or she will follow the home care protocols.

24. See the client to the retail area, sell through on product recommendations, and schedule his or her next appointment. Microcurrent facials can be performed every four weeks or as indicated for specific conditions, such as an introductory series. Acne may be treated weekly or as indicated by the manufacturer.

25. Clean and disinfect the work area, device, and accessories.

26. Make chart notes.

See Color Insert for full color photos.

photons
A particle of energy that has motion and travels in waves.

waveform
The form or shape of a wave of light.

wavelength
the measured distance between one wave of light and another.

nanometers
the actual measurement of the wavelength at a billionth of a meter.

light therapy
the use of a variety of types pf light to treat skin conditions (also called phototherapy).

phototherapy
the use of a variety of types light to treat skin conditions (also called light therapy).

blue light
Light-emitting diode for use on clients with acne.

 ## LED (LIGHT-EMITTING DIODE)

In brief, there are three types of light energy: visible light, invisible infrared light, and invisible ultraviolet light. They make up the electromagnetic spectrum of radiation. These forms of light are composed of small particles called **photons.** Photons travel at the speed of light in the form of a wave. Each type of light, depending upon whether it is visible or invisible, has its own form of wave, known as a **waveform.** A waveform is measured from the distance of one wave to another, which is called a **wavelength.** Wavelengths are also described as **nanometers.** Nanometers are a billionth of a meter (nm).

Nanometers also relate to the depth or distance in which the light can travel in light therapy, such as in the case of using lasers in surgical procedures and in using LED in skin care treatments. There is also a frequency component to light: longer wavelengths have low frequency, meaning the number of waves is less frequent (fewer waves) within a given length. Short wavelengths have higher frequency because the number of waves is more frequent (more waves) within a given length.

Light Therapy

Skin care professionals who use **light therapy** (also called **phototherapy**) have seen it evolve over time. From dermatologists using ultraviolet rays for treating psoriasis, to estheticians using **blue light** therapy for acne, to surgeons using the most high-tech lasers for advanced surgical procedures, the power of light is here to stay. We have barely scratched the surface of what can be done with LED in the field of esthetics.

LED works by releasing light onto the skin to stimulate specific responses at precise depths of the skin. LED devices are commonly used to treat photodamaged skin, mild to moderate acne, **erythema** from laser/light therapies, and for wound healing and the improvement of skin tone and texture. Studies show that LED therapy increases ATP, which increases fibroblast activity and thus upregulates collagen and elastin production. Here are some options for use of LED and the beneficial effects of each (Figure 5–8).

- **Red light** 600–660 nm: Increases cellular processes, stimulates ATP, boosts collagen and elastin production, and stimulates wound healing
- **Yellow light** 580–600 nm: Reduces inflammation, improves lymphatic flow, and detoxifies while increasing circulation
- **Green light** 500–530 nm: Lessens hyperpigmentation, reduces redness, and calms and soothes
- **Blue light** 410–470 nm: Reduces bacteria and is excellent for acne and rosacea

While the light color selection will change depending on whether the client is being treated for signs of aging, acne, or inflammation, the basic steps remain the same. Each manufacturer will have specific recommendations for individual devices.

Objective

Depending upon the skin type and condition you are treating, and the nanometer range that you are using, the objective of an LED service is specific to the needs of the client. Red light is used in age management, as it improves lymph and blood circulation and increases collagen and elastin production. Yellow light improves skin tone and texture and calms irritated and erythema (redness) skin. Green light lessens hyperpigmentation. Using blue light on clients with acne helps reduce lesions, kills bacteria, and slows sebaceous activity in oiler skin types. Blue and green light help reduce rosacea flare-ups.

Indications

Clients who have the following conditions are the best candidates for light therapy:

- Acne
- Age management
- Rosacea
- Dull, dehydrated skin

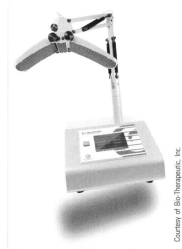

Figure 5–8 A four-color panel LED device.

Courtesy of Bio-Therapeutic, Inc.

erythema
Redness caused by inflammation.

red light
Light-emitting diode for use on clients to stimulate circulation and in collagen and elastin production.

yellow light
Light-emitting diode that aids in reducing inflammation and swelling.

green light
Light-emitting diode for use on clients with hyperpigmentation or to detoxify the skin.

- Hyperpigmentation
- Post-operative condition (as directed by a physician)

Contraindications

Clients who have the following conditions are not candidates for light therapy:

- Epilepsy
- Open or unidentified skin lesions
- Autoimmune disorders (i.e., HIV/AIDS, hepatitis B or C, lupus)
- Using photosensitive medications
- Pregnancy
- Bleeding disorders
- Cancer

PROCEDURE: LED

Supply List

- LED device
- Facial lounge, client draping, and linen setup
- Disposable sponges, cotton pads, or facial cloths
- Water and bowl or sink
- Cotton rounds or gauze pads
- Gloves
- Eye protection, as recommended by the manufacturer
- Informed consent document

Products

- Water-based cleanser
- Toner
- Serums or ampoules based on skin conditions and manufacturer's recommendations
- Environmental protection product with an SPF of at least 30 and antioxidants

Procedure

1. The client signs the informed consent document.
2. Cleanse with a water-based cleanser.
3. Perform a gentle exfoliation with an enzyme peel, ultrasonic peeler, or microdermabrasion.
4. Put on appropriate eyewear and provide the same for the client (following manufacturer's guidelines).

5. Program the device for the skin type and condition that you are treating according to the specific manufacturer's protocol for the treatment.

6. Position the unit.

7. If you are working with a panel device, program the unit for the treatment. Position the panels close to the client's face and press "start."

8. For age management (dull, dehydrated, and aging skin) use red light. Refer to color insert.

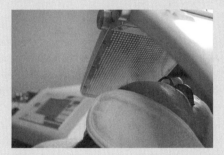

9. For clients with sensitive, irritated skin, use yellow light. Refer to color insert.

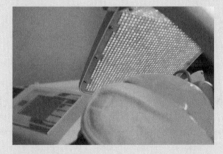

10. For hyperpigmentation and rosacea, use green light. Refer to color insert.

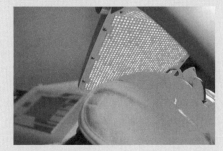

11. For acne, oily skin types and rosacea, use blue light. Refer to color insert.

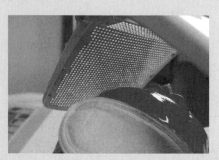

12. If you are using a handheld device, work around the face, holding the hand piece so that the light strikes the skin. Hold it in position for specified intervals. During the treatment, move from the forehead to the right side of the face, then to the left side of the face, and finally proceed to the upper lip and chin area.

13. Apply skin-type- and condition-specific serum, moisturizer, and an environmental protection product with an SPF of at least 30 and antioxidants.

14. Cleanse your hands.

15. Send your client home with written instructions on products to be used at home, such as gentle cleansers, serums, moisturizers, and environmental protection with an SPF of 30 or higher and antioxidants (for daily use). Have the client sign a document stating that he or she will follow the home care protocols.

16. See the client to the retail area, sell through on product recommendations, and schedule his or her next appointment. LED services can be performed every four weeks or as indicated. Specific conditions such as acne may be treated two to three times a week or as recommended by the manufacturer, estheticians, or a physician.

17. Clean and disinfect the work area, device, and accessories.

18. Make chart notes.

See Color Insert for full color photos.

Courtesy of Bio-Therapeutic, Inc.

 # LAYERING TECHNOLOGY PROTOCOL

All technologies can be combined and layered. Depending upon the skin type and condition of your client, multiple modalities may be used and strategically positioned for optimum benefit. Clients interested in age management often prefer a comprehensive approach to treatments and enjoy multiple technologies in each session.

PROCEDURE: LAYERED TECHNOLOGY FACIAL

Microdermabrasion Layer
First Pass

1. The client signs the informed consent document.
2. Depending upon the type of microdermabrasion device you are using, follow the manufacturer's recommendations for preparation and setup.
3. Provide the client with protective eye pads if you are using particulate (crystal or other product).
4. Put on protective eye goggles, protective apparel, and gloves.
5. Follow the manufacturer's recommendations for pressure settings, time exposure, and treatment protocol.
6. Perform a test patch along the mandible. Start with low settings, increasing them as you determine the client's tolerance level.
7. Start the procedure on the right half of the forehead. Hold the skin taut with your free hand.
8. Make vertical strokes on the entire width of the forehead, starting at the center just above the eyebrow and working toward the hairline above the temple.
9. Repeat on the other side.
10. Repeat vertical applications on the temples; cheeks; chin; and nasal, neck, and décolleté regions.
11. Gently apply microdermabrasion to the orbital region below the eye from the inside out toward the zygomatic bone.

Second pass

12. If a second pass is warranted, use a horizontal movement, starting on the right half of the forehead. Hold the skin taut with your free hand.
13. Make horizontal strokes on the entire width of the forehead, starting above the eyebrow. Apply the first "row" toward the temple. Work row by row toward the hairline.
14. Repeat on the other side.
15. Repeat horizontal applications on the temple, cheeks, chin, upper lip, and nasal regions.
16. Angle the hand piece slightly toward a horizontal orientation and apply gently to the neck and décolleté.
17. Gently apply microdermabrasion to the orbital region below the eye from the inside out toward the zygomatic bone.
18. If using particles, remove all residues.

Oxygen Layer

19. Cover the client's eyes with eye protection.

    For steps 21, 22, or 23 choose one of the three delivery systems of the oxygen device, depending upon the skin type and condition that you are treating. For "spot-specific" areas, use the pulsating jets; for general application of oxygenated product misting, use the airbrush wand; or for a hands-free oxygenated masque, use a condition-specific paper masque and the oxygen dome.

20. Apply a skin-specific condition serum or ampoule to affected areas. This could be an acne product to lesions, a muscle-relaxing serum to expression aging areas (forehead, periorbital region), or a lightener to hyperpigmented areas. Apply pulsating jets to infuse the product directly onto the area. Adjust the device according to the manufacturer's specifications.

21. Fill the wand reservoir with serum or solution that is specific to the client's condition—such as hyaluronic acid, peptides, and anti-oxidants for dry or dehydrated skin—and spray the serum or solution over the face, neck, and décolleté. Adjust the device according to the manufacturer's specifications.

22. Apply a product-saturated paper mask according to skin type and condition, and cover with an oxygen dome for product infusion for approximately 15 to 20 minutes.

23. Remove the dome.

Microcurrent Layer

24. Moisten the metal-conducting probes or the cotton swabs that are inserted into the conducting probes with the manufacturer's recommended product.

25. Set the device for the service that you will be performing as recommended by the manufacturer.

26. Press "run" or "start."

27. Starting at the upper masseter, place one stationary probe at the zygomatic arch. with the other probe slowly pull up from the lower portion of the masseter (below the mandible). Hold for the amount of time as specified by the manufacturer.

28. Move toward the upper portion of the masseter above the zygomatic arch with the stationary probe. Slowly pull at the base of the masseter with the other probe. Hold as recommended by the manufacturer.

29. Place the stationary probe at the auricularis anterior, and the moving probe and hand at the insertion of the buccinator and risorius region. Slowly pull back and hold.

30. Place the stationary probe at the lower orbicularis oculi, and the moving hand and probe at the insertion of the zygomatic major. Pull up and hold.

31. Place the stationary probe at the nasalis and the moving hand and probe at the insertion point of the levator labii superioris. Pull and hold.

32. Place the stationary probe at the frontalis and the moving hand and probe at the insertion point of the corrugator. Gently pull up and hold.

33. Place the stationary probe above the middle point of the eyebrow on the frontalis, and the moving hand and probe below it on the inner upper orbicularis oculi. Gently pull up and hold.

34. Place the stationary probe above the outer area of eyebrow on the frontalis, and the moving hand and probe below it on the inner upper orbicularis oculi. Gently pull up and hold.

35. Repeat all movements on the other side of the face.

LED Layer

36. Put on appropriate eyewear and provide the same for the client (following manufacturer's guidelines).

37. Program the device for the skin type and condition that you are treating according to the specific manufacturer's protocol for performing the treatment.

38. Position the unit.

39. If you are working with a panel device, program the unit for the treatment. Position the panels close to the client's face, and start.

40. For handheld devices, work around the face, holding the hand piece so that the light strikes the skin. Hold it in position for specified intervals. During the treatment, move from the forehead to the right side of the face, then to the left side of the face, and finally proceed to upper lip and chin area.

41. Conclude the session with a skin-type- and condition-specific serum, moisturizer, and environmental protection product with an SPF of at least 30 and antioxidants.

42. Cleanse your hands.

43. Send your client home with written instructions on products that he or she should use, such as gentle cleansers, serums, moisturizers, and environmental protection product with an SPF of 30 or higher and

antioxidants (for daily use). Have the client sign a document stating that he or she will follow the home care protocols.

44. See the client to the retail area, sell through on product recommendations, and schedule his or her next appointment. Combination services can be performed every four weeks or as indicated for specific conditions. This could include providing an introductory series or repeating a combination series, which can be done weekly for 8 to 10 services and then resumed on a monthly basis.

45. Clean and disinfect the work area, device, and accessories.

46. Make chart notes.

 # MINI SERVICES WITH HANDHELD DEVICES

Talk about fun! Handheld devices are certainly fun, and with good-quality products, there is no limit to what we can do with them. The market has driven the demand for smart devices, which can be used in or out of the treatment room. There are devices which use ultrasonic alone for iontophoresis; microcurrent and ultrasonic for peeling and iontophoresis and desincrustation; and galvanic for iontophoresis. These devices have been developed to perform mini services and services at home in between esthetic appointments.

Some estheticians feel that smaller, retail devices may compete with their own practices, but this is not a threat to us in any way. The end consumer and our clients will be exposed to these devices available OTC (over the counter), and many will receive them as gifts. Thus, it is imperative that we become familiar with these devices to determine which ones are of superior quality, manufactured for the professional, and perhaps consider selling them to our clients. That way, our customers can acquire the best possible devices on the market rather than purchasing a nonperforming or poor-quality model.

Ultrasonic and Microcurrent Handheld Devices

Handheld devices for use in mini services or "micro services" can be provided in a "lounge type" setting or area near your retail area to stimulate excitement, product sales, and service introductions in the salon or spa. They can also serve as a bridge and selling tool for more comprehensive services provided in treatment rooms. Newer devices use a combination of ultrasonic and microcurrent, which allow peeling or exfoliation and

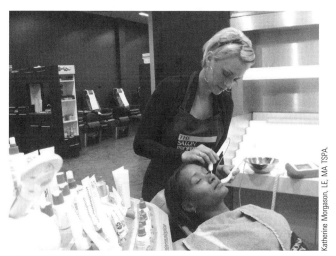

Katherine Morgason, LE, MA TSPA.

Figure 5–9 Working in a MicroZone lounge.

product penetration or iontophoresis. These devices appeal to both veteran estheticians and students and are well suited for use in a variety of service settings in or out of the treatment room (Figure 5–9).

The Objective

The objective of using an ultrasonic peeling and penetrating device is to reduce and remove sebum and surface debris; improve congestion; and penetrate ampoules, serums, and creams into the skin for hydration and barrier improvements.

Indications

Clients who have the following conditions are the best candidates for microcurrent:

- Dry, dehydrated skin
- Dull, congested skin
- Acne
- Preapplication for other services
- Enlarged follicles
- Preparation for another service

Contraindications

Clients who have the following conditions are not candidates for microcurrent:

- Isotretinoin or Accutane® use within a year (must obtain a physician's recommendation)

- Herpetic outbreak (cold sores)
- Open wounds (acne lesions or other bleeding lesions)
- Pregnancy
- Pacemaker or neurostimulation implanted devices
- Epilepsy
- Bleeding disorders
- Cancer
- Autoimmune disorders
- Sunburn

PROCEDURE

Ultrasonic Peel and Iontophoresis Treatment

Ultrasonic peeling and iontophoresis treatment supplies:

- Chair or facial lounge
- Ultrasonic peeling with iontophoresis device
- Gauze
- Cotton rounds
- Sponges
- Bowl

Product Supplies:

- Water-based cleanser
- Water-based toner
- Water-based masque or product for peeling
- Water-based serum or ampoule
- Water-based cream and eye cream
- Environmental protection with SPF of at least 30 and antioxidants

1. Have the client read and sign a consent form.
2. Cleanse with water-based cleanser.
3. Apply a light, low-viscosity masque or product for peeling.

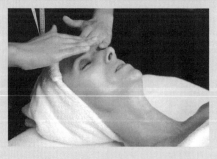

Courtesy of Bio-Therapeutic, Inc.

4. Turn on the device and choose the "peel mode."

5. Begin ultrasonic peeling; using a 45-degree angle, start at the neck and work upward.

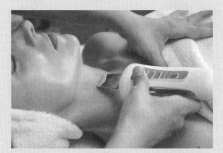

6. Continue to work upward on the chin.

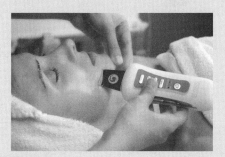

7. Continue working upward on the sides of the face; wipe the blade free of dead cellular debris and product with each pass.

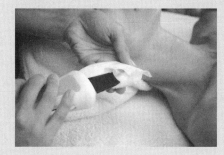

8. Carefully peel the nasal region.

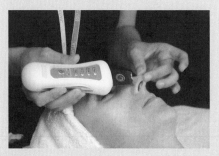

9. Continue to peel both sides of the face and the **periorbital region**. Finish at the forehead.

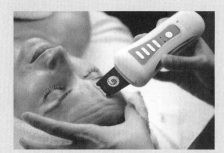

10. Remove all remaining traces of the masque or product with warm water.
11. Apply a desincrustation solution or product in oily areas.
12. Choose the –ion (negative ionization) mode for microcurrent and ultrasonic technology combined. Flip the device over. Holding your free hand within two inches of the blade (this serves as the ground), perform desincrustation, using upward movements.

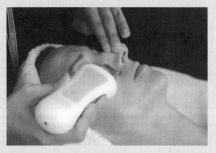

13. Remove the desincrustation solution or product and debris.
14. Apply an ampoule or serum to the entire face and throat.

periorbital region
Area around the eye; periorbital bone.

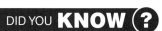

DID YOU **KNOW** ?

To perform mechanical extractions with your ultrasonic device, apply more desincrustation solution or product to the areas where you have performed negative ionization, and go back to the ultrasonic peel mode for mechanical extractions. With gentle upward strokes, carefully push the sebum up out of the hair follicles.

Courtesy of Bio-Therapeutic, Inc.

15. Choose +ion 1 mode for microcurrent and ultrasonic technology to penetrate the ampoule or serum into the skin. Flip the handheld device over. Holding your free hand within two inches of the blade, gently ionize in the product. Start at the neck, using upward movements.

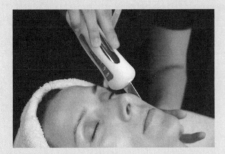

16. Continue to ionize the ampoule or serum into the skin in all areas.

17. Continue to ionize the product in upward movements on both sides of the face.

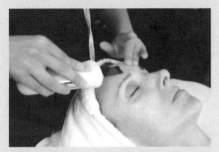

18. Choose +ion 2 mode for applying facial and eye creams. Holding the free hand within two inches of the blade, gently ionize in the product. Start at the neck, using upward movements

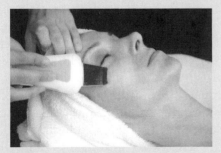

19. Apply environmental protection with an SPF of at least 30 and antioxidants.

20. Cleanse your hands.

Mini services such as ultrasonic facials may be a precursor to another service, can be a standalone service in a mini facial lounge near the retail area.

21. Send your client home with written instructions on home care, including a list of products that he or she should use, such as cleansers, serums, moisturizers, and environmental protection with an SPF of 30 or higher and antioxidants (for daily use).

22. See the client to the retail area. Sell through on product recommendations and schedule his or her next appointment. Mini ultrasonic facials can be performed two to three times a week or as indicated for specific conditions (such as acne, which may also be treated daily at home).

23. Clean and disinfect the work area and device.

24. Make chart notes.

See Color Insert for full color photos.

 # SUMMING IT UP

While technology does not take the place of the human touch, by any means, we continue to find that clients demand excellent results through the use of devices in the marketplace. The most important choices that we make as estheticians are to determine what type of technology we plan to employ and to buy devices wisely. It is necessary to look at your service menu, your objectives for services, and the type of clients that you want to attract and retain. Here are a few points to remember while looking at traditional esthetic services and newer technology:

- Microdermabrasion continues to be a strong tradition for exfoliation. As we see, it continues to evolve: from the earliest devices using corundum or particles, to particle-free diamond-tip hand pieces, to the newest in solution-infused devices that may combine diamond tip or plastic exfoliation tips.
- Oxygen therapy is loved by celebrities. It is becoming better understood by practitioners as an excellent modality for infusing products and increasing oxygen and respiration to the cells.
- Microcurrent has been around for decades. Once considered an alternative therapy, it is now used for multiple purposes, including iontophoresis, muscle reeducation, relaxation, and healing.
- The health benefits for LED services are far reaching, and we have just begun to discover applications for its multiple uses in skin health. We know of its reparative benefits and regeneration in wound healing, but its uses in combating aging issues are on the

rise. We need more published studies and documentation for the positive results we are witnessing for LED use in esthetics.

- New handheld devices will continue to be good choices for estheticians and will work synergistically with other modalities while freeing valuable space and time. The enterprising professional esthetician or skin therapist may practice from any location imaginable today. This may better serve the client and can generate more income, which may have been incomprehensible just a few years ago.

- All we need is the drive to succeed, routine education and upgrades, and dependable equipment along with a backup plan. As always, it is good planning to think of the old adage, "If I have two of something, I now have one … and if I have one, I have none." Remember to have back stock in products, extra accessories, and possibly an additional device.

ESTHETICIAN **PROFILE**

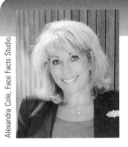

Alexandra Cole, Face Facts Studio.

Alexandra Cole
Beauty Therapist, Face Facts Face Studio

Buckinghamshire, UK

My name is Alexandra Cole. I was born in London and lived there for the first 30 years of my life before moving to Buckinghamshire, where I now live. My business, Face Facts Face Studio, first opened its doors in 1997. Since then, I have built up expertise and a national reputation as a facialist. I have done this by following my passion for the face, and showing women how to lift their self-esteem, and their faces, the nonsurgical way.

My inspiration was my mother, the late Countess of Balfour, who was Elizabeth Arden's right-hand woman in the 1930s and 1940s. I grew up fascinated by how important it is for women to feel facially good about themselves through skincare and make-up.

Face Facts Studio's reputation rests on providing the latest and most beneficial antiageing facial treatments, which are holistic and destressing, and offering only the best of treatments and products. All of these must be "results driven."

Training

I continually train, and am certified and trained in the following:

- Microdermabrasion
- Ultrasonic technology
- Microcurrent
- Facials
- Makeup
- Products: Murad, ESPA, Jane Iredale, Glo Minerals, Arbonne

Services Offered

I chose these treatments and products because I wanted to treat the face in a nonsurgical way and help my clients' skin to be at optimum health. All the chosen treatments and skin care ranges are result driven, the best quality, at the cutting-edge of technology, and updated regularly.

As a facialist, the range of treatments I offer includes:

- Microcurrent facial toning: including face and eye masks
- Hand treatments: a perfect addition to a treatment.
- Ultrasonic facials with handheld devices
- Wet–dry microdermabrasion with solutions and diamond tip
- Crystal microdermabrasion
- Facials using products by Dr Howard Murad, Espa, and the Swiss skincare range Arbonne

Personal Philosophy

As a facialist, and against the backdrop of my mother's inspiration, I am passionate about helping women feel good about themselves and raising their self-esteem by feeling good about themselves facially.

I keep what I offer in my studio updated by having a good relationship with suppliers and other companies. They keep me informed as to the latest and best that they offer.

As a makeup artist, I offer my clients makeup tutorials. I teach them how to update their existing look or how to create a completely new look. This is the "icing on the cake" after skin treatments. The makeup ranges I offer are Glo Minerals, Jane Iredale, and Arbonne.

To sustain my studio, in what are not the easiest of times, I am very active in my marketing, which I do myself. I make sure that I always offer the best and give the highest standard of treatment and service to my clients. Plus, I give my clients "good value" by offering only excellence in everything I do.

Additional Contribution to the Industry

I am very proactive in both national and local media, which has included appearances on morning television shows and radio programs (where I have been a regular guest, speaking about facial beauty). I also write regular lifestyle articles for local business journals and have contributed to magazines and newspapers. I am also involved in local women's charities, again helping them raise their confidence by feeling good about themselves.

- I have been voted a Murad "Salon of Excellence"
- I have been named as a Salon of Excellence in Bio-Therapeutic Technology
- Carlton TV's Lifeline program promoting an awareness of the benefit of camouflage cover for scarring was filmed at Face Facts Studio

I am presently very involved with the Swiss skin care company Arbonne and offer workshops in its makeup at my studio.

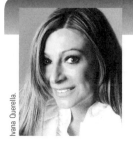

ESTHETICIAN **PROFILE**

Ivana Querella
Beauty Therapist, Manicurist, Owner, Kosmetikstudio, Salon

Munich, Germany

I was born in Turin, Italy. I finished my degree in business economics with a diploma in microeconomics. I worked in London for two years as a secretary for a Swedish paper company. I then began my career in Germany at Escada Fashion. I worked as an export manager for Escada Fashion for the last four years of my time there. I was very good in my job but had no free time. I worked until late in the night, on Saturdays and Sundays, and traveled through Europe and Canada.

I decided to start my own business. I spent one very challenging year attending school at night in Munich, Germany, to become an esthetician. I thought it would be a nice job and I wanted to be my own boss. I speak five languages, and as Munich is an international city, I knew that I could attract many foreign customers. I enjoy meeting people. My clients' parents, family members, and friends visit me when they are in Munich. They all love to come to see me for treatments. They come from Paris, Vienna, Italy, and England. It is as if you went to Paris to see the Eiffel Tower; when they come to Munich, they come to see me for a skin care treatment. It is amazing! I love the contact I have with people. I have such great clients; it is a pleasure to work with them.

Training

Initially I trained at the Medi Care Institute, in Munich, Germany. It is a large beauty center, with a large perfumery. I worked with a variety of products and perfumes on the market. This helped me greatly later, when I needed to choose products for my own business. I have been trained in the following:

- Laser therapies
- Microdermabrasion
- Microcurrent
- LED
- Permanent makeup
- Various nail technologies

Practice Demographic

My base client is a middle-aged woman. There is a great deal of focus on age management here in Germany. Everyone wants to look beautiful and to prevent lines and wrinkles and aging in general. They start taking care of their skin early in Germany. I have younger clients, from 17 to 29, and older clients, from 60 to 80. My treatments cover a broad range of issues, and I can serve most necessities.

I sell a special series of 10 treatments plus one for free. If a client brings me one new client, I give her a free treatment. I am always acquiring new clients that way. I also have a special where I offer a treatment at a special price that includes a product.

I also treat clients who are referred from a plastic surgeon. I perform lymphatic drainage of the face and neck post-operatively. When the operation is scheduled, the surgeon's secretary schedules the first two treatments with me. If the patient lives in Munich, he or she begins to see me for regular microcurrent treatments, which help maintain the tone and elasticity of the muscle and skin.

Services/Treatments Offered

I perform treatments from head to toe. This is great because I can do a variety of treatments, and there is always something new to prepare for and to learn. I like the mix of change and diversity. It is wonderful for the client, because he or she does not have to go to several difference locations for services. I can do it all. This was part of my business plan 17 years ago.

I perform the following technology facials:

- Microdermabrasion
- Ultrasonic technology, and perform
- Infrared cold laser with hyaluronic acid (instead of injections)
- Microcurrent device
- LED
- Nail services with an LED device
- Permanent makeup

Personal Philosophy

I believe in education. I am always learning new services and continue to learn with my current service options to improve and remain up-to-date. I recommend that all professional estheticians continue to study, read trade journals, and attend classes, seminars, and trade shows. It is important to remain current and to know your business. One important way for me to acquire new clients is to get out and meet new people. I speak 5 languages so that I have French, English, Spanish, German and Italian clients, so this gives me an opportunity to use my language skills, while connecting with potential clients. I recently learned how to play golf and have a few new clients as a result. It's all fun!

Additional Contributions to the Industry

I am a judge for the Munich Esthetics Fair nail competition and have participated for 10 years. I am a certified and authorized trainer for nail design in south Germany, with Light Concept Nails Company (LCN).

Medical Practices

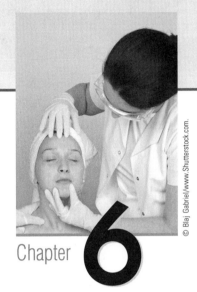

> " I love to hear testimonials about how I have changed someone's life by using lasers for removing unwanted facial hair, reducing folliculitis, and removing leg veins and tattoos. "
>
> —Debbie Caddell, RE, LE, CLS, CPE

Chapter **6**

Chapter Capture

After completing this chapter, you will be able to:

- Perform protocols for hair reduction using lasers and intense pulsed light (IPL).
- Perform protocols for photorejuvenation using IPL.
- Understand injectables.
- Understand physician-performed procedures.
- Understand pre- and post-operative stages.

Esthetician-Performed Treatments

Section Outline

- ESTHETICIAN-PERFORMED AND PHYSICIAN-DIRECTED PROCEDURES

- LASER OR IPL HAIR REMOVAL TREATMENT PROTOCOLS

- IPL PHOTOREJUVENATION TREATMENT PROTOCOLS

ESTHETICIAN-PERFORMED AND PHYSICIAN-DIRECTED PROCEDURES

Physician-directed treatments have been successfully performed by well-trained estheticians for nearly two decades. Estheticians serving in a medical setting have experienced a tremendous opportunity to use devices and technologies that are not available to those estheticians practicing in a salon, spa, or skin care center without a qualified medical professional on staff. Most states require a physician to be within a certain proximity of the esthetician using class II devices or above. It is vital to have as many qualified, licensed, and certified professionals present while training with and using lasers. People have health issues that may be unknown at the time of the service, practitioners make mistakes, and devices can fail. Plan for everything; practice with a focus on all going well; and remember: when in doubt, don't.

Estheticians are well suited for working with lasers, intense pulsed light (IPL), and other types of light therapies, as we tend to be meticulous and are focused on the health of the surrounding tissue. Experienced estheticians tend to take conservative approaches to working with technology and are aware of many potential issues that may arise concerning scarring, infection, and pain control; therefore, they take the least amount of risk for a positive outcome. We tend to refer our client to another, more qualified practitioner earlier in the process rather than later if we become aware that the condition is beyond our scope of practice. All of these points make for an ideal esthetician and technician working with technology.

 # LASER OR IPL HAIR REMOVAL TREATMENT PROTOCOLS

Laser or IPL hair treatment has easily become the gold standard for hair removal in the last decade. As devices have improved, more studies have been performed, and the marketplace has driven home the hair-free culture for those dealing with excessive hair or interested in the convenience of not having to shave. This option of hair removal has represented freedom for many who suffered years of embarrassment and humiliation from hirsutism and hair growing in places where they feel it should not. This protocol serves as a general guide to laser or IPL hair removal and should not supercede the directions and recommendations of a qualified physician or the manufacturer's recommendations (Figure 6–1).

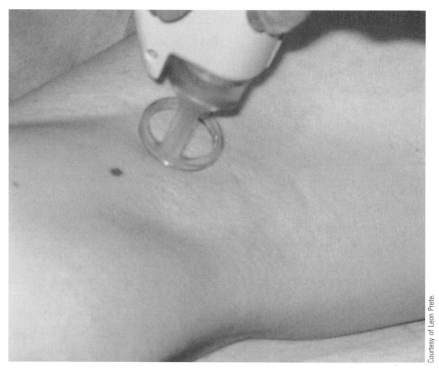

Courtesy of Leon Prete.

Figure 6–1 Laser hair removal.

The Objective

To remove unwanted hair with light therapy.

Indications

Clients who have the following condition are the best candidates for laser or IPL hair removal:

- Excessive or unwanted hair

Contraindications

Clients who have the following conditions are not candidates for laser or IPL hair removal:

- Herpetic outbreak
- Autoimmune diseases (lupus or arthritis, in which the body identifies its own cells as foreign bodies)
- Photosensitizing medications
- Cancer
- Skin cancer

- Diabetes
- HIV/hepatitis
- Pregnancy
- Tanning or tanned skin
- Bleeding disorders
- Keloid or connective tissue conditions
- Isotretinoin (formerly known as Accutane®) use within one year (or otherwise indicated by a physician)
- Pacemaker or neurostimulation device
- Epilepsy

PROCEDURE: LASER HAIR REMOVAL

Supply List
- Laser or IPL unit
- Key to laser or IPL unit
- Treatment lounge
- Paper towels
- Laser or IPL "In Use" sign, following Occupational Safety and Health Administration (OSHA) guidelines
- Protective eyewear for client
- Protective eyewear for technician
- Protective eyewear to hang outside room
- Gloves (as recommended)

Products
- Pre-treatment cleansing product
- Topical anesthetic (if recommended by the manufacturer or a physician)
- Soothing lotion
- Disinfecting lotion

Preparation
1. Set up the treatment room, per the manufacturer's guidelines.
2. If you are using a laser device, cover the windows and all reflective surfaces.
3. Test your equipment to ensure proper operation.
4. Gather and set up supplies.
5. Remove your jewelry and have the client remove his or her jewelry.
6. Counsel the client and ensure his or her suitability for the procedure.
7. Have client read the home care instructions and sign an informed consent.

fyi

The client or patient will typically undress just next to the area that is being treated. We do not use linens while operating lasers to minimize fire hazards, and regulations require that a fire extinguisher be within reach.

8. Shave the hair in the areas to be treated.

9. Apply a topical anesthetic (if recommended by the equipment manufacturer).

10. Have the client put on the appropriate treatment gown, if necessary.

Procedure

11. Unlock the laser device.

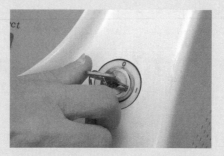

12. Put on gloves and safety goggles. Have the client put on safety goggles also.

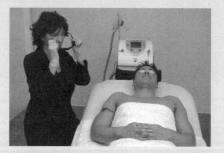

13. Apply gel, as recommended by the manufacturer.

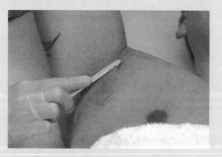

14. Set the treatment parameters. Follow the manufacturer's guidelines or charted settings from a previous treatment for the area, hair, and skin and according to the response at the test site.

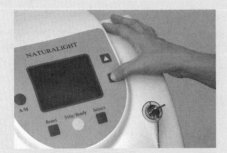

15. Perform the treatment at the highest fluence that the skin can tolerate and in accordance with the manufacturer's recommendations for the most effective hair reduction. The time needed to cover the area depends on the spot size of the beam and the scanning pattern of the hand piece.

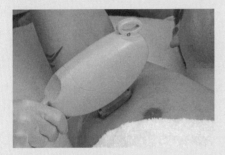

16. Compress the skin firmly with the hand piece to disperse the oxyhemoglobin (a chromophore that competes with melanin) away from the treatment area. (Doing so allows for greater absorption of the laser light, reduces the risk of epidermal damage, and maneuvers the dermal papilla closer to the surface, which makes for a more effective treatment.)

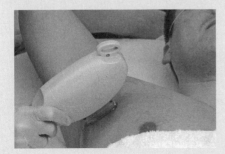

17. Select a starting spot and do a test pulse to ensure that the client can tolerate fluence.

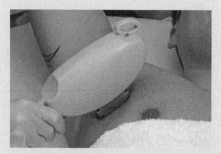

18. Following a well-defined pattern, work across the area where hair is to be removed, administering a single pulse per area.

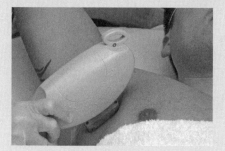

19. During the treatment, between some of the pulses, clean the hand piece with a mild cleaning solution to free it of the carbonized hair that collects on the window. The buildup makes the window feel hot and impedes the flow of the laser beam. Some laser device manufacturers recommend the use of ultrasonic gel on the skin to prevent accumulation of burnt hair on the lens.

20. If topical anesthesia and cooling remedies have not reduced the client's discomfort, make adjustments.

21. Remove any gel that may have been used with the device.

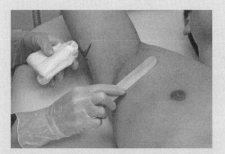

22. After treating the entire area, wipe the skin with a soothing antiseptic lotion.

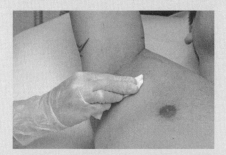

Post-procedure

23. At the end of the treatment, turn off the laser device and remove the key.

24. Provide the client with home care guidelines. Counsel him or her on using a soothing moisturizer and environmental protection with an SPF of 30 in all areas that are exposed to light and other natural elements.

25. Schedule the client for his or her next visit.

IPL PHOTOREJUVENATION TREATMENT PROTOCOLS

As with all devices, whether they are class I or above, it is vital to train extensively on theory, protocols, and practical applications. If you are working with IPL or laser devices, you must work within your scope of practice and under the direction of a physician. IPL has been used for

© Milady, a part of Cengage Learning. Photography by Rob Werfel.

> ⚠ **CAUTION!**
>
> **Cleanup and Disinfection**
>
> Because the hand piece comes into contact with the skin, wipe it clean with a disinfectant between treatments or soak the distance gauge in disinfectant according to OSHA and the manufacturer's directions.

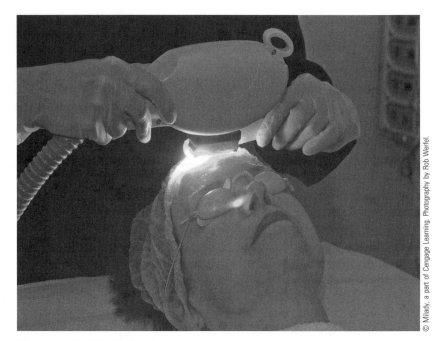

Figure 6–2 IPL photorejuvenation.

many years for hair removal and facial rejuvenation. It is efficacious for vascular lesions, and remains among the best light therapies for diffuse redness in the case of rosacea (Figure 6–2).

IPL is a nonablative skin rejuvenation technique that uses high-intensity, pulsed light to reform pigmented lesions, vascular lesions, and fine lines and wrinkles. It improves conditions such as rosacea, hyperpigmentation, and uneven texture by emitting light over many wavelengths (lasers produce a single wavelength); this allows light to penetrate all levels of the skin and to reach target areas such as **melanocytes** and dilated vessels.

The Objective

The objective of using IPL for skin rejuvenation is to reduce pigmented lesions in cases of hyperpigmentation, vascular lesions such as in **telangiectasias**, and in general improve diffuse redness. It has also been recommended to boost collagen and elastin production, thus smoothing fine lines and wrinkles.

melanocytes
Cells that produce pigment granules/melanin in the basal layer of the epidermis.

telangiectasias
Small, dilated blood vessels; also called spider veins.

Indications

Clients who have the following conditions are the best candidates for IPL photorejuvenation treatment:

- Rosacea
- Photoaging
- Hyperpigmentation
- Poikiloderma
- Telangiectasias
- Cherry angiomas
- Elastosis

Contraindications

Clients who have the following conditions are not candidates for IPL photorejuvenation treatment:

- Herpetic outbreak
- Autoimmune diseases (lupus or arthritis, in which the body identifies its own cells as foreign bodies)
- Photosensitizing medications
- Cancer
- Skin cancer
- Diabetes
- HIV/hepatitis
- Pregnancy
- Tanned skin, or self-tanning within two weeks (may cause scarring)
- Bleeding disorders
- Keloid or connective tissue conditions
- Isotretinoin (formerly known as Accutane®) use within one year (or otherwise indicated by a physician)
- Pacemaker or neurostimulation device
- Epilepsy

IPL Pre-treatment Protocols

The pre-treatment for an IPL phase is important for the conditioning of the skin. Common ingredients and products for use in a home care plan include alpha or beta hydroxy acids (AHAs and/or BHAs) for exfoliation and increased cellular production. **Tretinoin** (retinoic acid) is often used to increase fibroblast activity, increasing collagen and elastin production and further exfoliation. (This is left to the

Tretinoin
Derived from vitamin A, also known as retinoic acid. Used to increase collagen and elastin production.

tyrosinase
Enzyme that synthesizes tyrosine and L-dopa to create melanosomes.

discretion of the physician, as it is a prescription and can become irritating to some patients.)

Skin lighteners can be added to the plan. These may include hydroquinone, Kojic acid, arbutin, and licorice extracts (to inhibit **tyrosinase**, an enzyme located in melanocytes, which are specialized cells that produce the pigment). These types of skin lighteners slow down melanin production. The following products can be added to the mix for optimum pre-treatment measures:

- Hydrators and moisturizers with amino acids, hyaluronic acid, and/or sodium hyaluronate; antioxidants such as ergothioneine and superoxide dismutase to enhance hydration levels and combat free radical proliferation respectively.
- Serums with ingredients used in tissue support, such as those that work as an anti-inflammatory and encourage cell renewal, such as Syn-Tacks®, acetyl-dipeptide, and Matrixl® 3000: these are all peptides used in quality age-management products.
- Environmental protection products with an SPF of at least 30 and broad spectrum chemical sunscreen ingredients, such as octyl methoxycinnamate and benzophenone-3, and the physical sunscreen ingredients zinc oxide and titanium dioxide; it is also advisable to include products that contain antioxidants such as cassia ala leaf extract, superoxide dismutase, and polyphenols (copper and resveratrol).

A simple home care regimen is used as follows:

A.M.
1. Cleanse with an appropriate skin type and condition cleanser.
2. Apply a lightener or other tyrosinase inhibitor: hydroquinone or Kojic acid, vitamin C, arbutin, or licorice extract (licochalcone or glabridin).
3. Apply a moisturizer/hydrator with AHA or BHA.
4. Apply sunscreen with an SPF of least 30.

P.M.
1. Cleanse with an appropriate skin type and condition cleanser.
2. Apply a lightener or other tyrosinase inhibitor: hydroquinone or Kojic, vitamin C, arbutin, or licorice extract (licochalcone or glabridin).
3. Apply Tretinoin/retinoic acid (at the discretion of a physician).
4. Apply a moisturizer/hydrator.

PROCEDURE: IPL PHOTOREJUVENATION

Supply List

- Treatment bed or chair
- Disposable sponges and tongue blades
- Cleansing cloths and towels
- Gloves
- Disposable hair bonnet or headband
- Water and bowl or sink
- Gauze pads or cotton rounds
- Protective eyewear for client
- Protective eyewear for esthetician/technician

Products

- Gentle cleanser
- Post-treatment serum
- Sunscreen
- Water-soluble gel

Preparation

Set up the general treatment room (this will vary depending on the unit):

1. Prepare the treatment lounge and client gown.
2. Assemble towels and disposables.
3. Set up products and protective devices.
4. Have the appropriate sign for the outside door ready.
5. Cleanse the client's face; if you are using a topical anesthesia, apply it with time for absorption prior to the treatment. (Some devices require no anesthetics.)
6. Review the postcare instructions with the client. These can be discussed while any anesthetic absorbs.
7. Close the doors, cover the windows, and hang the "IPL in Use" sign on the treatment room door.

Procedure

8. Hang the appropriate eyewear on the door for staff who may enter.
9. Turn on the IPL device. The device will undergo a self-test.
10. Perform device calibration as the manufacturer recommends.
11. Replace any IPL hand pieces or filters that need replacing.
12. Pull back and secure the client's hair away from his or her face.

fyi

Goggles or green eyewear with an **OD (optical density)** of 3 is appropriate for staff and operators. It is imperative that the client wears the approved eyewear for IPL treatments. Always follow manufacturer's recommendations for specific IPL eyewear for clients.

 OD (optical density)
Measurement of how much light an object absorbs and how much of the light passes through the object.

CAUTION!

Topical anesthesia should always be applied by qualified medical personnel, who must follow the manufacturer's recommendations. It should be applied in select treatment zones, not over extensive areas. If in doubt, always ask the supervising physician or qualified medical personnel. Increased absorption of topical anesthesia can lead to toxicity and possible death.

13. Precleanse and remove all makeup and anesthetics.

14. Assess the client as a Fitzpatrick skin type I–V. (Some devices are only approved for clients skin types I–IV, so check the manufacturer's specifications.)

15. Ask the client if he or she has tanned recently or used a self-tanner within the last month. This can drastically affect the outcome, and there is a potential for scarring with skin that is compromised from tanning. Treatments should be rescheduled if the client has recently tanned or is using a self-tanner.

16. Turn on the device.

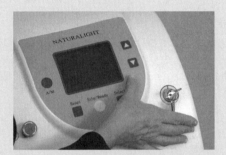

17. Reconfirm the areas of treatment and the client's goals.

18. Take photographs for the client's file.

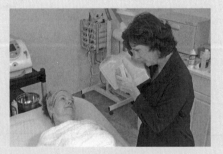

19. Enter the client's demographic data into the IPL system, if so required by the device.

20. Select the appropriate treatment mode, filter, and parameters on the screen and make sure that the corresponding filter is inserted into the treatment head.

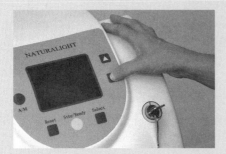

21. Double-check all parameters before beginning the treatment.
22. Place protective eyewear on the client and yourself.

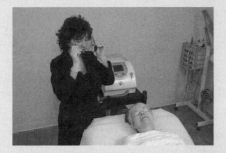

23. Put on gloves.

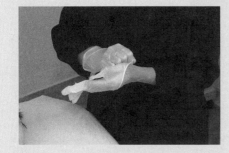

24. Apply gel coolant, if appropriate for the device.

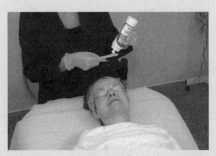

25. Test a spot on the side of the client's face in front of the ear (periauricular area), as directed by the manufacturer's guidelines.

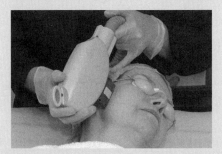

26. Float the filter in the gel, if this is appropriate for your specific device. The degree of floating in the gel will vary based on the type of device and if the filter has a chilled sapphire window.

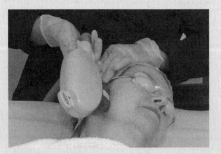

27. After testing the spot on the side of the face, assess the clinical end points:
    a. Observe for slight erythema.
    b. Observe for darkening of a vessel or vasospasm.
    c. Observe for darkening or redness of a lentigo.

28. If the test response is acceptable, continue the treatment with the same settings. If not, raise or lower the joules accordingly or switch to a different parameter or filter.

29. Start treatment with the forehead. Be careful of the hair line and eyebrows: protect them with a tongue depressor.

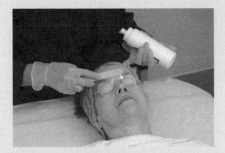

30. Follow the manufacturer's device recommendations for the amount of passes on all the treatment areas.

31. Place the hand piece perpendicular to the skin so that it is floating in the gel (if required by the manufacturer).

32. Fire the trigger.

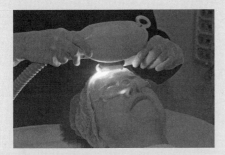

33. Shift the hand piece to an adjacent area of the skin, with no overlap.

34. Fire the trigger.

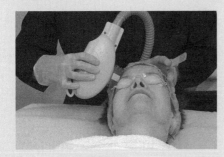

35. Repeat the process across the forehead, working in a systematic manner.

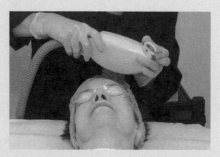

36. Continually assess the reaction and tolerance of the client's skin.

37. Move to the nose, upper lip, and chin in a systematic manner. Then move below and above the lips, being careful not to work over the lip vermillion.

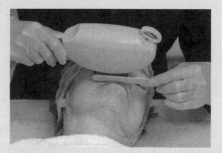

38. Progress to the cheeks and treat across the cheeks in a systematic manner.

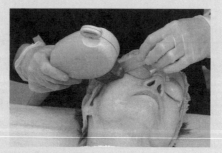

39. Remove any residual gel.

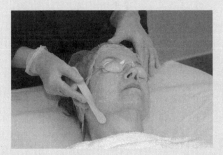

40. Cleanse the client's skin.

41. Apply a soothing gel, as recommended by the manufacturer, and protective sunscreen.

Post-procedure

42. Supply the client with an ice pack, if recommended or needed.

43. Escort the client to the front office for processing and scheduling of additional treatments and/or follow-ups. Instruct him or her to use the post–IPL treatment home care protocol.

44. Instruct the client to call the office to provide information on his or her condition the following day or if he or she has questions and/or concerns.

45. Complete the documentation on the procedure and place photos in client's file.

Cleanup and Disinfection

46. Turn off the device with the key, following the manufacturer's guidelines.

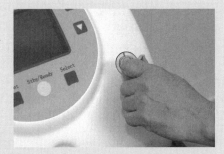

47. Wipe down the device with germicidal wipes.

48. Remove and store the key.

49. Clean the hand piece and filters per the manufacturer's guidelines.
50. Follow clean up and disinfection procedures in accordance with OSHA and/or state guidelines.

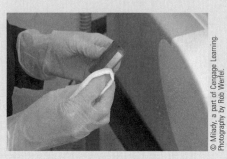

© Milady, a part of Cengage Learning. Photography by Rob Werfel.

51. Reset and prepare the room for the next client.

IPL Post-treatment Protocol

As with all treatments, it is important to follow your physician's protocol and that of the manufacturer for optimum post–IPL treatment results. In general, healing, soothing, and calming ingredients and products are appropriate after IPL treatments for up to two to three weeks following the procedure. Here are some general guidelines for home care:

A.M.
1. Cleanse with a gentle cleanser without AHA/BHA or any active ingredients.
2. Apply a moisturizer/hydrator with aloe, azulene, or allantoin.
3. Apply sunscreen with an SPF of at least 30.
4. Use good quality mineral makeup (if worn).

P.M.
1. Cleanse with a gentle cleanser.
2. Apply a soothing moisturizer/hydrator with aloe, azulene, or allantoin.

As with all devices, it is important to follow the manufacturer's recommendations and protocols, to follow the protocols of your physician, and to have been trained under a qualified health care professional. This protocol serves as a guideline and should not be used in place of the standard, which has been recommended by the manufacturer.

Physician-Performed Procedures

Section Outline

- INJECTABLES: NEUROTOXINS AND SOFT-TISSUE FILLERS

- THE ESTHETICIAN AND NEUROTOXIN INJECTIONS

- SOFT-TISSUE FILLERS

- THE ESTHETICIAN AND SOFT-TISSUE FILLERS

- THE ESTHETICIAN'S ROLE IN PRE- AND POST-OPERATIVE CARE

- SKIN RESURFACING

- RHYTIDECTOMY (FACELIFT)

- BLEPHAROPLASTY (EYELIFT)

INJECTABLES: NEUROTOXINS AND SOFT-TISSUE FILLERS

According to the American Society of Plastic Surgeons (ASPS), neurotoxins and soft-tissue fillers are the most sought-after procedures today. The use of neurotoxins and soft-tissue fillers and laser hair removal continue to show annual increases. In 2011, Botox® was up 5% and soft-tissue fillers showed a 7% increase from the year before. A total of $10.4 billion was spent on cosmetic procedures. There were a total of 1,579,079 cosmetic procedures (facelifts, liposuction, breast augmentation), and 12,249,647 minimally invasive procedures (laser hair removal, neurotoxins, soft-tissue fillers, microdermabrasion) performed in 2011. Laser hair removal, soft-tissue fillers, neurotoxins (Botox®), and microdermabrasion all continue to make the list of noninvasive procedures annually. This data demonstrates the continued interest in noninvasive procedures and the public's perennial willingness to spend their salaries on their appearance.

Esthetician Responsibility

As with all procedures—whether invasive or noninvasive—it is of great importance to learn about them in order to best support your client (or patient). Regardless of whether we are working with a physician, we are in fact supporting one the moment that we work with a client who is having procedures. We need to be armed with knowledge and understanding in order to avoid complications and adverse reactions. Below, we discuss some of the most commonly used neurotoxins and soft-tissue fillers, indications for their use, and what we need to know as estheticians to support clients who are using these injections to improve their appearance.

Warning: Do Not Perform Injections

With our current licensure, training, and laws in the United States, estheticians are not allowed to perform injections and must instead refer their clients to reputable, qualified physicians, ARNPs, PAs, and nurse injectors. If you do choose to perform injections, you will be held liable. There are two known cases before the courts today in which estheticians were alleged to have performed injections that resulted in disfiguring, life-changing events for the patient. In one case, the esthetician was allegedly selling the injection serums to a client for home use. The ethical implications in these cases, and abhorrent disregard for human beings, do not speak well to the intentions of estheticians in a broad sense, lowers the standards of professionalism for all esthetic practitioners, and forces irreparable damage upon our industry.

Neurotoxins

Neurotoxins referred to as **Botox®** and **Dysport™** are botulinum toxin type A. Neurotoxins have been available and used for a variety of applications in patients for over 50 years. Two earliest uses were to treat patients with spasmodic vocal cords (**spasmodic dysphonia**) and crossed, or excessively twitching eyes. In the case of the vocal cord rehabilitation, the patients would receive small amounts of botulinum toxin injected into the muscle surrounding their vocal cords to relax spasms and normalize high-pitched, squeaky voices. Historically, the relaxing effects of botulinum toxin muscle have been used in ophthalmological practices for **strabismus** (misaligned eyes) and **blepharospasm** (uncontrollable blinking). This has been of great help to these patients, who have felt embarrassed and self-conscious, and given them freedom from jokes and ridicule.

Through the use of botulinum toxin for strabismus, Jean Carruthers, MD (a Canadian ophthalmologist), with her dermatologist husband Alastair Carruthers, discovered that a type of botulinum toxin type A called Oculinum removed the lines around the eyes of a patient. That patient asked in a later visit if she could have the same treatment applied to her forehead, because the wrinkles around her eyes had disappeared. This surprised Dr. Carruthers, and was the impetus to study the serums effects on wrinkles.

Through subsequent studies by her dermatologist husband, Alastair Carruthers, real, and definite lasting effects were demonstrated with the use of the serum. Botox® was born, and later approved by the Food and Drug Administration (FDA) for the treatment of wrinkles.

Botox®

Allergan, the makers of Botox®, received FDA approval for its use for wrinkles in 2002. Other **off-label** uses include the treatment of migraine headaches (it relaxes the muscles that create the headaches) and excessive sweating (hyperhidrosis) in the hands, feet, scalp, and axilla (under arms). It is also used to relax tense neck muscles (neck bands) as well as the muscles of the chin, such as the tightening or puckering caused by the **depressor labii inferioris** or the **mentalis** or **depressor anguli oris**. One must see an experienced injector for this type of application, as restricting the muscle activity using neurotoxins can go terribly wrong. It can paralyze the muscles of the chin, creating a crooked smile, or reduce one's ability to smile, which may last for three to four months. Clients must do their homework in finding an expert (see Color Insert, Figures 6–3 and 6–4).

Botox®
Botulinum toxin type A that, when injected into a muscle, restricts its movement.

Dysport™
Botulinum toxin type A that, when injected into a muscle, restricts its movement.

spasmodic dysphonia
Voice disorder, often leading to a squeaky or high-pitched sound.

strabismus
Eyes that are misaligned or crossed.

blepharospasm
Uncontrollable blinking.

off-label
Product or device being used for purposes other than its intended use.

depressor labii inferioris
Muscle found in the chin, depresses lower lip and allows movement form side to side.

mentalis
Muscle found on the chin, which raises and protrudes the lower lip, as in drinking from a glass.

depressor anguli oris
Muscle found on the chin, which the corners of the mouth depresses, also called the triangularis.

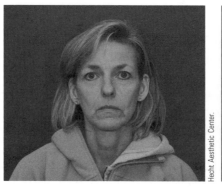

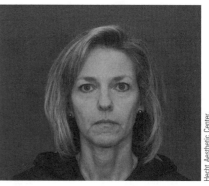

Figure 6–3 Patient, before Botox.   **Figure 6–4** Patient, after Botox.

Indications

While the FDA has approved the use of Botox® for the lines and furrows between the brows, the indications and multiple uses for the treatment of Botox® are as follows:

- Wrinkles
- Relaxing overly tight muscles of the face and neck
- Migraines
- Excessive sweating (hyperhidrosis)
- Voice rehabilitation (spasmodic dysphonia)
- Ocular applications (strabismus, blepharospasm)

Contraindications

Contraindications for Botox® are varied as follows:

- Herpetic outbreak
- Autoimmune diseases
- Cancer
- Communicable diseases
- Diabetes
- Bleeding disorders
- Keloid or connective tissue disorders
- Isotretinoin (within two to three years or as directed by a physician)
- Neurological disorders and diseases

Dysport™

Dysport™, also known as Reloxin®, is a newer neurotoxin, botulinum toxin type A. It has been approved by the FDA for its use on wrinkles in the **glabellar lines** (between eyebrows) and for **cervical dystonia**

glabellar lines
Vertical and horizontal forehead lines found between the eyebrows and across the forehead.

cervical dystonia
Neck muscles that contract abnormally, causing pain.

(neck pain and abnormal head positioning). Many physicians have found it to be less expensive, to perform muscle relaxation more quickly, and to last longer than Botox® in some cases. One study showed a great improvement in reducing the lines in the lateral periorbital region (crow's feet) in a shorter amount of time.

As with all injectables, it is of vital importance that you have an experienced medical provider injecting the product into the patients and clients, as the dosing and mixture combinations are different from Botox®. Furthermore, if you are medical personnel and purchasing these products, be sure you get from a reputable source.

THE ESTHETICIAN AND NEUROTOXIN INJECTIONS

As with all medical procedures, the esthetician's role must be within the scope of his or her licensure and practice at all times. Many estheticians serve as assistants to physicians or other qualified medical provider by cleansing the areas to be treated, obtaining ice when appropriate, and setting up the room. Camouflage makeup can be applied once the physician or medical provider gives the go-ahead. Fine-grade mineral powders are best for this application. The esthetician may also provide patient education, such as reminding the client not to drink alcohol, take unapproved drugs, go running, or have an extensive facial treatment immediately after a neurotoxin injection. Scheduling recurrent appointments may also be a part of the duties and details of the esthetician.

> **CAUTION!**
>
> Estheticians do not compound or mix Botox or doses of other injectables. Licensed, qualified medical personnel must mix the products. Medical practices found to be employing estheticians for these applications are at risk for litigation.

> **DID YOU KNOW ?**
>
> As with all innovations, there are those working diligently on all matters of facial aging, and those directly associated with wrinkles specifically on the face, neck, and décolleté. As estheticians, we know these areas are target zones for prevention of premature aging and in the rehabilitation of the skin, and we are focused on bringing forth the most natural effects and products for our clients. There has been much research into topical applications of materials that will be safe and effective for reducing wrinkles and smoothing skin. While interesting, an understanding of the implications of applying a topical neurotoxin is in the formative stages. Until these materials can remain isolated and not travel into the bloodstream and other tissues (which could be of great harm to the health of the individual), we await studies and findings that will tell us more.

SOFT-TISSUE FILLERS

The success of soft-tissue fillers has been evident for nearly two decades now; beneficiaries include those seeking age management techniques and reconstructive work related to scars, birth defects, and illness. Fillers have proven to be inexpensive and do not require the healing of a surgical procedure. New and improved soft-tissue fillers are released onto the market annually, and many are less irritating and have fewer adverse reactions than those of the past. As with all procedures, it is important to work with qualified, licensed, and certified medical professionals, who are experienced in injecting these materials. If materials are injected into a vein or into tissue for which it is not designed, there can be grave circumstances that may result in **necrosis** or death of the tissue, and eventually organ death.

Technically, there are two categories of soft-tissue fillers: semipermanent, which may last 3 to 12 months, depending upon the client's metabolism, the injector, and the materials; and permanent soft-tissue fillers, which may last indefinitely. Before the injections have been performed, it is important to weigh the benefits of the choices carefully and make sure that the indications match the conclusion of choice material to be injected. Often a physician or qualified medical injector will use a semipermanent material to determine whether the effects are what the patient is looking for; this is better than applying a permanent solution prematurely. The most common fillers used in cosmetic applications are listed below.

Semipermanent Soft-Tissue Fillers

Hyaluronic acid is a popular base for soft-tissue fillers, as it poses little to no sensitivity issues in most people and mimics our own hyaluronic acid, as found in the extracellular matrix. Common brands are: Restylane® and Perlane® (nonanimal derived) from Medicis; Prevelle® Silk (nonanimal derived) from Mentor; Juvederm® from Allergan; Captique™ (nonanimal derived), and Hylaform® (animal derived, rooster combs) from INAMED Aesthetics.

Indications
- Defining jaw line
- Nasolabial folds
- Marionette lines
- Thin or small lips
- Scars
- Glabellar lines
- Lower-lid eye troughs

necrosis
Death of cells in living tissue.

Hyaluronic acid
Hydrating fluids found in the skin and around joints for lubrication; also a hydrophilic agent with water binding properties found in skin care products.

Contraindications

- Herpetic outbreak
- Autoimmune diseases
- Cancer
- Communicable diseases
- Diabetes
- Bleeding disorders
- Keloid or connective tissue disorders
- Isotretinoin (within two to three years or as directed by a physician)
- Neurological disorders and diseases

Radiesse

Radiesse is a calcium-based gel with microspheres used as a soft-tissue filler. Manufactured by Merz Pharmaceuticals, Radiesse has been used for over 20 years in medical applications for incontinence, breast reconstruction, and vocal cord rehabilitation. It has been used to successfully treat facial muscle and fat atrophy from HIV and other chronic illnesses. It lasts longer than hyaluronic acid fillers, in some cases one to two years. Its cosmetic uses are varied; it is not recommended for lips, however, as it may create **granulomas** (spherical nodes).

It works like other fillers by laying down scaffolding for collagen to build upon, thus making the treated area fuller and plumper. Some physicians may opt for a hyaluronic acid filler, with shorter-term effects, to ensure that the patient is happy with the results prior to committing to a longer-lasting material. Remember that fillers are not recommended for those with allergies to any of the material parts. But how can we know whether a client is allergic to a given material? Recommending or conducting a pre-injection test to determine compatibility in an inconspicuous area is a good idea. Do not be in a rush to have a new material implanted: take your time in the discovery phase and recommend that your clients do the same.

Indications

- Glabellar lines
- Nasolabial folds
- Nasal contour
- Upper lip (oral commissures)
- Marionette lines
- Chin depressions
- Acne scars
- Volumizing an atrophied face

Radiesse
Soft-tissue filler used for wrinkles, and an increase in facial volume. Also used in medical applications for incontinence, breast reconstruction, and vocal cord rehabilitation.

granulomas
Nodular lesion on the skin.

> **CAUTION!**
>
> Many of us have experienced less-than-favorable outcomes when there is a rush to try a new injectable. Ask to conduct a test patch in an inconspicuous area, using the dose match for a given area, before injecting it into the face. Even the most commonly tolerated products can be an allergen for some. Be cautious!

Contraindications
- Herpetic outbreak
- Autoimmune diseases
- Cancer
- Communicable diseases
- Diabetes
- Bleeding disorders
- Keloid or connective tissue disorders
- Isotretinoin (within two to three years or as directed by a physician)
- Neurological disorders and disease

Collagen

The use of collagen soft-tissue fillers dates back many years. The material was among the first used for wrinkles and lip atrophy. Compared to many of the fillers today, however, collagen-based fillers are reported to have a shorter lifetime. They are also more likely to create allergies, as collagen is animal derived (either porcine, from a pig; or bovine, from a cow).

Other collagen formulas are created either from the patient's own tissue or from another human. Many physicians have used these materials and found consistent, excellent results. As in all products use, the physician determines what best works in his or her practice through education, experience, exposure, and personal preference. With collagen soft-tissue fillers, it is recommended that patients have an allergy test. The physician will determine what pre-treatment options are necessary for collagen injections.

Indications
- Nasolabial folds
- Marionette lines
- Thin or small lips
- Scars
- Glabellar lines

Contraindications
- Allergies to animal or collagen-based by-products
- Herpetic outbreak
- Autoimmune diseases
- Cancer
- Communicable diseases
- Diabetes
- Bleeding disorders

- Keloid or connective tissue disorders
- Isotretinoin (within two to three years or as directed by a physician)
- Neurological disorders and diseases

Fat Transfers

Another option is to harvest and inject stomach, thigh, or buttocks fat into the facial tissue to improve volume. As with all procedures, this must be performed by an experienced, qualified physician with a proven record of favorable results with this procedure.

Once the fat is taken from one area, the physician or medical personnel uses a centrifuge process to remove blood and excess fluids. The fat is then placed into another syringe and relocated via injection into the desired area, such as the nasolabial folds, lips, or tear troughs.

There is a risk of infection and a slight risk to rejection of the fat cells in the new location.

Indications
- Defining jaw line
- Nasolabial folds
- Marionette lines
- Thin or small lips
- Scars
- Glabellar lines
- Lower-lid eye troughs

Contraindications
- Allergies to fat material (test patch)
- Herpetic outbreak
- Autoimmune diseases
- Cancer
- Communicable diseases
- Diabetes
- Bleeding disorders
- Keloid or connective tissue disorders
- Isotretinoin (within two to three years or as directed by a physician)
- Neurological disorders and diseases

Permanent Soft-Tissue Fillers

Sculptra

Sculptra is injected deep into the dermis to stimulate collagen growth by the host at the injection site. It does not fill the wrinkle, as in the

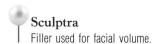
Sculptra
Filler used for facial volume.

poly-L-lactic acid
A synthetic material used as a facial volumizer to build collagen that has been lost due to aging or weight loss.

case of other soft-tissue fillers, but rather stimulates a response from the individual's own growth factors.

Sculptra is made from a synthetic material called **poly-L-Lactic** acid to build collagen that has been lost due to aging, illness, and weight loss. It is applied in three to four injections over a certain period of time, such as once every two to three months, or as determined by the attending physician or qualified injector. It has been used in other applications for many decades to anchor implants and the surgical mesh used as a foundational material to which tissue adheres and grows. Sculptra has been reported to last for two to three years; however, as with all reports, there are variances. Make sure that Sculptra is the best material for the application before having it (or any filler) injected by a qualified medical professional.

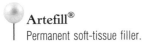

Artefill®
Permanent soft-tissue filler.

Artefill®

Manufactured by Suneva Medical Inc., **Artefill®** is a permanent soft-tissue filler that consists of collagen and polymethylmethacrylate (PMMA) microspheres in a gel base. It is necessary to test all patients prior to injecting Artefill®, as the collagen is bovine in origin, and may reveal allergies (see Color Insert, Figures 6–5 and 6–6).

More than one injection may be necessary to meet the objectives; however, it is important to note that once the material is injected into the tissue, it is permanent. The only way to remove Artefill® is through surgical methods. It is not recommended for lips, as it can become lumpy and thus result in painful granulomas.

Suneva Medical is conducting ongoing studies to determine the use of this product for facial volume in the malar region, scar revision, and nonsurgical rhinoplasty. Many products on the market are being used

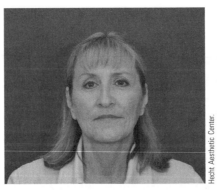

Figure 6–5 Patient, before soft-tissue filler.

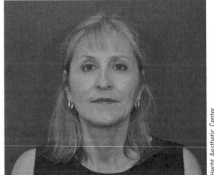

Figure 6–6 Patient, after soft-tissue filler.

for these applications, and most often the materials are absorbed by the body. Artefill® is not absorbed and the microspheres are in place permanently. As with all medical procedures, it is vitally important to seek the service, council, and support of a qualified medical professional before embarking on soft-tissue fillers.

THE ESTHETICIAN AND SOFT-TISSUE FILLERS

Estheticians can offer much support to patients and clients undergoing treatment for wrinkles via soft-tissue fillers. Whether they are receiving neurotoxins or soft-tissue fillers, it is necessary to know when the client is having their injections. A general rule of thumb (which is often documented in protocols), for injections and facial services, is to allow for two weeks on either side of an injection. This is conservative. You may see some physicians and other qualified injectors make other decisions: they know their product and the patient they are treating. However, it is always best to check with the attending provider, as there may be extenuating circumstances that may preclude a client or patient from having an esthetic service.

Estheticians can be of great support to clients with both in-office and home care protocols prior to and after a procedure. Here are key action items that estheticians can do to support clients and medical personnel during injectable procedures:

- **Follow up with clients on over-the-counter (OTC) use prior to injections.** If you are working closely with the patient and a physician, make certain that the client is following the home care protocols: this includes not using blood thinners and OTC medications such as aspirin and ibuprofen before and after injection appointments. Remind clients to follow the physician's instructions on what they can and cannot take before and after any medical procedure including injections.
- **Keep abreast of new materials coming onto the market.** With new fillers and neurotoxins on the rise, learn as much as you can about new products; liaise with a nurse injector, PA-C (physician assistant, certified), or physician for new product information.
- **Determine the placement of your treatment options.** For example, if a client has just had a neurotoxin placed into a muscle, we do not want to apply a rigorous microdermabrasion application in that area on the same day. Some physicians may state that a

microdermabrasion service could be performed prior to the injections, but always check with the client's physician if you are unsure.

- **Transparency is best**. Tell your clients to ask their injector when they should resume facial treatments in their given circumstances. Most physicians recommend waiting two weeks after injections before having a facial treatment.

- **Recommend and sell home care products**. This is an untapped opportunity for most estheticians to educate and offer products for use, specifically for procedures such as fillers and neurotoxins. Offer simple cleansers with little to no performance ingredients that may stimulate activity. Offer products with tried and true ingredients that are calming and soothing to the tissue, such as those with allantoin, azulene as an anti-inflammatory, or acetyl dipeptide for reducing stress on the skin. Make sure that clients leave your premises with a good environmental protection product with antioxidants and an SPF of at least 30. You could make up a pre- and post-procedure kit for your clients, whether you work in a medical setting, salon, spa, or skin care center.

THE ESTHETICIAN'S ROLE IN PRE- AND POST-OPERATIVE CARE

As estheticians assisting in pre- and post-operative phases with patients, we work much more closely with the physician than we do while attending to our routine treatments. Whether you work in or outside a medical facility, it is vital to the well-being and health of the patient to follow the physician's direction and to be in direct and constant contact with the medical team.

For those of us who have experience working with a patient throughout a surgical procedure, we have found that it provides a connection to another human, which encompasses a full range of emotion for both the patient and the esthetician. It is necessary to remain professional at all times and to stay closely connected to the medical team from the pre-surgical skin care consultation to following the treatment plan; applying treatments; making certain that the patient is using proper home care protocol and products; and then, finally, to the post-operative and healing phase. It is legally necessary to maintain full and complete chart writing, whether you are using electronic or paper files.

Each procedure has specific protocols, which are fundamental to obtaining the desired results, and each physician will have his or her own protocols determined by extensive research, education, and practice experience. Well-designed pre- and post-operative treatment plans will facilitate conditioning the skin to heal at its optimum capacity. Pre-operative plans will focus on stimulating and increasing the skin metabolism and reducing photodamage and dead cellular buildup. Post-operative stages will focus on decreasing inflammation and swelling, soothing and calming the skin, and increasing hydration and moisture levels.

Noncompliance

If at any time, you as an esthetician hear from the patient that he or she is not following part of the plan, or is having problems with any phase of the preparation, it is important to share that information with the physician or medical personnel. It is common for patients to be anxious and nervous about undergoing a procedure; however, if you see that clients are noncompliant, it may affect the surgical outcome measurably. On occasion, surgeries are rescheduled if, for example, a patient has not discontinued a certain type of a prescribed medication, is using drugs and alcohol, or has not modified his or her diet as directed by the doctor. This can be quite costly to the physician or the client both financially and in the outcome of the procedure, so it is necessary to report any variances.

SKIN RESURFACING

Whether using Fraxel®, CO_2, CO_2 fractionated, an Erbium-YAG, or one of the many other ablative laser resurfacing options in the market today, there are as many pre- and post-operative skin care programs as there are devices. Taking it a step further, each physician will have his or her own specifications for in-office and home care protocols as well. Treatment plans run the gamut from physicians recommending little or no preparation to the skin before or after a procedure to a very intensive program in which the physician has the patients see the esthetician weekly and follow systematic instructions at home for weeks in advance.

Here is a compilation of tried-and-true protocols that have yielded excellent results for many years. It is necessary to follow the instructions as determined by the patient's physician, however, and details may vary. As we know, the more skin conditioning preparation there is before a procedure, the better the outcome. This protocol begins at eight weeks prior to surgery; however, in some cases this period may be modified. All medications are prescribed and dispensed by the attending physician (Figures 6–7 and 6–8, see Color Insert).

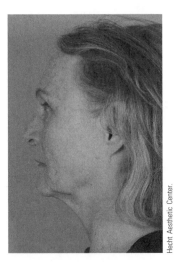

Figure 6–7 Patient, before skin resurfacing.

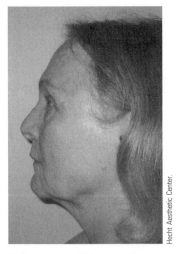

Figure 6–8 Patient, after skin resurfacing.

Indications

- Rhytides (wrinkles)
- Hyperpigmented lesions
- Photodamaged skin
- Light scarring due to acne
- Elastosis
- Seborrheic keratosis

Contraindications

- Pacemaker, neurostimulation device
- Pregnancy/lactation
- Patient with unrealistic expectations
- Patient who develops keloids easily
- Infectious disease
- Isotretinoin within one year (a determination made by a physician)
- Immune disorders
- Tanning/sunburn

Pre-operative Skin Resurfacing Home Care Plan

The pre-laser phase is important for the conditioning of the skin. Here are common ingredients and products used for the pre-laser home care plan:

- AHAs and/or BHAs for exfoliation and increased cellular production.
- Tretinoin (retinoic acid) to increase fibroblast activity, increasing collagen and elastin production, and further exfoliation. (This is left to the discretion of the physician, as it is a prescription and can become irritating to some patients.)
- Skin lighteners, such as hydroquinone, Kojic acid, arbutin, and licorice extracts, for use as tyrosinase inhibitors and melanocyte suppressants.
- Hydrators and moisturizers with amino acids, hyaluronic acid and/or sodium hyaluronate, and antioxidants such as ergothioneine and superoxide dismutase—to enhance hydration levels and combat free radical proliferation, respectively.
- Serums with ingredients used in tissue support, such as those that work as an anti-inflammatory and encourage cell renewal, such as Syn-Tacks®, acetyl-dipeptide, and Matrixl® 3000.
- Environmental protection product with an SPF of at least 30 and broad spectrum chemical sunscreen ingredients such as octyl

methoxycinnamate and benzophenone-3 and the physical sunscreen ingredients zinc oxide and titanium dioxide. It is also advisable to include products containing antioxidants such as cassia ala leaf extract, superoxide dismutase, and polyphenols (copper and resveratrol).

A simple home care regimen is used as follows:

A.M.
1. Cleanse with an appropriate skin type and condition cleanser.
2. Apply a lightener or other tyrosinase inhibitor, such as hydroquinone or Kojic acid, vitamin C, arbutin, or licorice extract (licochalcone or glabridin).
3. Apply a moisturizer/hydrator with AHA or BHA.
4. Apply a sunscreen with an SPF of at least 30.

P.M.
1. Cleanse with an appropriate skin type and condition cleanser.
2. Apply a lightener or other tyrosinase inhibitor: hydroquinone or Kojic acid, vitamin C, arbutin, or licorice extract (licochalcone or glabridin).
3. Apply Tretinoin/retinoic acid.
4. Apply a moisturizer/hydrator.

Pre-operative Skin Resurfacing Treatments

Eight weeks before surgery, you may begin a treatment plan, under a physician's direction, that will change and adapt according to the patient's needs. If you are not working within a physician's office, make sure to coordinate your plan with the patient's physician. The plan will follow through to the post-operative phase, although products and in-office treatments will be more suited to healing and involve patient participation in the recovery phase.

Depending upon the patient's skin type, classification (level or degree of photodamage), and condition prior to surgery, there are various options for pre-skin resurfacing treatments. These options are listed below. These may be alternated or combined depending upon the protocol of the physician and medical team. A combination of chemical or enzyme peels, microdermabrasion, and LED therapy makes an excellent conditioning program in addition to a skin type and condition-specific home care program.

See Chapters 4 and 5 for step-by-step protocols for peels and technology facial treatments.

Superficial Chemical Peels

- Lactic acid
- AHA/BHA (these can be combined)
- Jessner's solution (traditional or modified)
- Peel cocktails, such as combinations of all peels at a low concentration (lactic, glycolic, salicylic acid; light TCA)

To stimulate the home care program, peels exfoliate the upper layers and add an additional medium for skin lightening. Make sure that the patient stops using Tretinoin/retinoic acid three days prior and three days after the peel to avoid irritation. Always check with a physician if an irritation does occur: you do not want your patient to have inflamed, uncomfortable skin throughout the pre-surgical phase. A slight erythema (redness) and light itching while acclimating to the change in home care products may be apparent; this may be treated with a low-level hydrocortisone cream or other soothing product, such as calendula, azulene, or chamomile cream, until it is resolved. The skin must be intact for laser resurfacing of any type for the surgery to proceed.

Microdermabrasion

Whether particle, nonparticle, or water, microdermabrasion supports the exfoliation and skin conditioning process of the pre-skin resurfacing plan. The patient must stop using Tretinoin three days before and three days after microdermabrasion. Microdermabrasion provides an excellent exfoliation treatment choice for oilier, thicker skin that is also photodamaged. Peels and microdermabrasion can be alternated; or in some cases, may be combined depending upon the skin type and condition, the physician's selection of peel products, and the esthetician's expertise.

Enzyme Peels

An enzyme peel may be substituted for a chemical peel for sensitive, reactive skin types. Enzymes such as papain (papaya), bromelain (pineapple), or pumpkin are proteolytic and thus will dissolve dead cellular debris to soften and aid in the hydration of the skin. Papaya is the most gentle of the three options.

LED Therapy

Light-emitting diode (LED) is an excellent device to include in in-office treatments for a patient preparing for a surgical procedure. Red light (approx 660 nm), yellow light (approx 590 nm), green light (approx 525 nm), and blue light (approx 470 nm) applied after a peel (whether it is chemical, mechanical, or enzymatic) enhance healing through stimulating adenosine triphosphate (ATP), the biocatalyst for all chemical processes in the body. Depending upon the specific skin type, you can choose your light accordingly. Here are some choices:

- Red light: Increases cellular processes, stimulates ATP, boosts collagen and elastin production, and stimulates wound healing. Red light is excellent for boosting sluggish, dry, and dehydrated skin.
- Yellow light: Reduces inflammation, improves lymphatic flow, and detoxifies while increasing circulation. Yellow light is of great support for a patient who is irritated and inflamed.
- Green light: Lessens hyperpigmentation, reduces redness, and calms and soothes. This is good to use on a patient with stubborn pigmented lesions.
- Blue light: Reduces bacteria, excellent for acne and rosacea. Use blue light on a patient struggling with acne during the preoperative phase.

If using LED therapy, it is important to observe contraindications such as epilepsy, pregnancy, cancer, bleeding disorders, under a physician's care for a chronic condition, and light sensitivity.

At Six Weeks Before Surgery
- Continue the home care plan.
- Continue the in-office treatment plan.

At Four Weeks Before Surgery
- Continue the home care plan.
- Continue the in-office treatment plan.

At One Week Before Surgery
- Home care change: Drop the lightener and Tretinoin from the plan. Continue using a skin type and current condition cleanser; a hydrator with light AHA ingredients, such as lactic or glycolic acid; and an environmental protection product with an SPF of 30 and antioxidants.
- Continue the in-office treatment plan.

At Three Days Before Surgery
- Home care: Add an antiviral and antibiotic, as recommended by a physician, to suppress the potential of herpetic outbreaks and infection. In addition, some physicians will use *Arnica montana* to reduce swelling. It is vital, however, that you follow the direction of the medical staff, as some medications including OTC may interfere and interact with existing medical condition that the patient may have of which you are unaware.

- In-office treatment may consist of a standard facial aimed at soothing and calming the skin along with a combination of red (healing) and yellow (reducing inflammation) light. Manual lymphatic drainage is also an option at this point, pre-operatively.

Post-operative Skin Resurfacing Care

Days 1–5

Depending upon their protocol, many physicians choose to use a dressing on the improved skin immediately after surgery. These may be silicone and polyurethane membranes, or semi-occlusive dressings that do not stick to the wound. It is advisable to remove the dressings after 48 hours, as the risk of infection increases. Medical personnel must remove the dressing. Then, an emollient ointment or salve such as Aquaphor® or petroleum jelly is used to keep the skin moist as it reepithelializes. This improves the patient's comfort and reduces vulnerability to postoperative infection. It is important that the skin does not dry out.

The patient continues to take all of the medications (including the antiviral) as prescribed and to return to the office for dressing removal on day 3. After the dressing is removed, the home care changes to a post-operative program, which includes the following:

- Apply solution soaks with $4'' \times 4''$ gauze pads every two to three hours. The solution can be made of vinegar and water (1 teaspoon of vinegar to 1 cup of water) or saline solution, depending upon the protocol.
- Follow soaks with a generous application of salve, emollient-based product, or Aquaphor®. Keep the skin well lubricated. The skin should be kept from drying out for two reasons: for patient comfort and to reduce the risk of the patient developing a secondary infection due to bacteria building up on the tissue.

Days 5–10

The home care program may change slightly depending upon the skin type, oil production, and healing. Product changes are made if it is determined that the patient needs a lighter product; this is especially true if the patient has very oily skin or is becoming congested. Some physicians may use a combination of copper peptides and amino acids for hydration. In general, however, this period is critical to the healing of the skin, and a positive outcome is dependent upon the following protocols. Very little deviation is necessary.

Days 10–15

Once the patient's skin has epithelialized (regained intact epidermis), the physician will dictate the next phase in healing: to begin the following home care plan:

- Use a gentle cleanser (no AHAs/BHAs or other acids or exfoliants).
- Apply triamcinolone or hydrocortisone for irritation or redness.
- Use a gentle moisturizer with sodium hyaluronate, silicones for moisture loss, and allantoin for soothing and healing.
- Use an environmental protection product with an SPF of 30 and zinc oxide and/or titanium dioxide.
- Mineral powders may be used at this time if the patient's healing is on track.

Days 15–30

- Continue the home care use of the cleanser; hydrators, such as hyaluronic acid; and lipid replacement products, such as gamma linolenic acid and squalane. Peptides, such as Palmitoyl Tripeptide-7 and copper peptide, can be introduced as an anti-inflammatory, and for cell renewal; environmental protection with antioxidants such as ergothioneine, superoxide dismutase, or green tea extract with an SPF of at least 30 must be used every day.
- Makeup can be introduced again; this may include mineral powders without irritating fillers or drying compounds. The use of natural pigments and professional products such as Color Science and Jane Iredale are preferred; the latter have been used successfully at postoperative stage for many years. Lycogel® is an option for makeup following laser treatment. It has great coverage and was created for post-procedure conditions, antiaging, and sensitive skin.

One Month After Laser Treatments

Most patients will tolerate a low-level AHA with a high pH one month after a laser treatment. Check with the physician before you add performance ingredients back into the program, however. Some patients will continue to peel into the second and third month post-operatively, and this will help reduce peeling. In-office treatments given by the esthetician, however, focus on soothing, calming, hydrating, and healing. LED therapy is excellent in all of the recovery phases, using red and yellow light combinations; and green and blue light for those patients who may be struggling with hyperpigmentation and acne.

Here are pre- and post-operative examples of treatment options for skin resurfacing based on skin types. Protocols for the treatments can be found in Chapter 4 on chemical peels and in Chapter 5 on technology-focused facials.

CAUTION!

Do not perform microdermabrasion or chemical peels again until indicated by the patient's physician. Some patients will not require further chemical peeling, as their skin's textural issues have improved. It is important to change the treatment plan accordingly. Look at other modalities for age management for these patients as they circle back to client status; these include such maintenance facial treatments as European facials, and technology facials using oxygen, microcurrent therapy, galvanic current, LED, and wet microdermabrasion (once full healing has taken place and the physician supports the treatment), with a focus on hydration.

Table 6–1 Pre- and Post-operative Treatment Options for Skin Resurfacing: Dry/Dehydrated/ Photodamaged Skin

Procedure: Skin Resurfacing	Pre-operative	Post-operative
Skin Type:	**Technology Facials**	**Recovery Healing Phase**
Dry **Dehydrated** **Photodamaged**	1. Microdermabrasion: One pass 2. Oxygen: Use airbrush wand to infuse skin with hydrators and lighteners 3. Microcurrent: Muscle reeducation and hydrating skin work 4. LED: Use red and yellow light *Technology can be layered	1. The medical team sees the patient. 2. The esthetician can give the client a shoulder/hand massage on the first visit. 3. The microcurrent is set to enhance/healing modes. 4. LED is administered in red and yellow light.
	Chemical Peel Options • Enzyme peels • AHA: Lactic, glycolic acids • Jessner's • Light TCA • Combination and layered peels	

*Do not apply chemical peels with microcurrent; alternate between visits.

Table 6–2 Pre- and Post-operative Treatment Options for Skin Resurfacing: Normal Skin

Procedure: Skin Resurfacing	Pre-operative	Post-operative
Skin Type:	**Technology Facials**	**Recovery Healing Phase**
Normal	1. Microdermabrasion: One pass 2. Oxygen: Use airbrush wand with hydrating serum 3. Microcurrent: Muscle reeducation and hydrating skin work 4. LED: Use red and yellow light *Technology can be layered	1. The medical team sees the patient. 2. The esthetician can give the client a shoulder/hand massage on the first visit. 3. The microcurrent is set to enhance/healing modes. 4. LED is administered in red light.
	Chemical Peel Options • AHA: Lactic, glycolic acids • Jessner's • Light TCA • Combination and layered peels	

*Do not apply chemical peels with microcurrent; alternate between visits.

Table 6–3 Pre- and Post-operative Treatment Options for Skin Resurfacing: Oily Skin

Procedure: Skin Resurfacing	Pre-operative	Post-operative
Skin Type: **Oily**	**Technology Facials** 1. Microdermabrasion: Two passes 2. Oxygen: Use airbrush wand with desincrustation product applied to reduce oil 3. Microcurrent: Apply desincrustation modes 4. LED: Use blue light *Technology can be layered	**Recovery Healing Phase** 1. The medical team sees the patient. 2. The esthetician can give the client a shoulder/hand massage on the first visit. 3. The microcurrent is set to enhance/healing modes. 4. LED is administered in red and blue light.
	Chemical Peel Options • AHA: Lactic, glycolic acids • Salicylic acid • Jessner's • Light TCA • Combination and layered peels • Peel cocktails: Combine multiple ingredients	

© Milady, a part of Cengage Learning.

*Do not apply chemical peels with microcurrent; alternate between visits.

Table 6–4 Pre- and Post-operative Treatment Options for Skin Resurfacing: Sensitive/Reactive Skin

Procedure: Skin Resurfacing	Pre-operative	Post-operative
Skin Type: **Sensitive/Reactive**	**Technology Facials** 1. Ultrasonic peeler 2. Microcurrent: Muscle reeducation and hydrating skin work 3. LED: Use red and yellow light *Technology can be layered	**Recovery Healing Phase** 1. The medical team sees the patient. 2. The esthetician can give the client a shoulder/hand massage on the first visit. 3. The microcurrent is set to enhance/healing modes. 4. LED is administered in red and yellow lights.
	Chemical Peel Options • Enzyme peel • Lactic acid • Ultrasonic peel	

© Milady, a part of Cengage Learning.

*Do not apply chemical peels with microcurrent; alternate between visits.

RHYTIDECTOMY (FACELIFT)

As with skin resurfacing, the patient tolerates the post-operative phase of a facelift more easily if the skin is well prepared and in optimum condition, with well-orchestrated, comprehensive in-office and home care protocols. Additionally, the pre- and post-operative care will be determined by the physician—his or her training, exposure to technology, and preferences. This protocol offers some guidelines; however, it is not meant to supersede the directions of the physician whom you are supporting, whether in the office or at another location (see Color Insert, Figures 6–9 and 6–10).

It is beneficial to start protocols 8 to 10 weeks ahead; however, if time does not allow, they can be modified and abbreviated. Not that if the patient were to have a combination of procedures such as laser work in addition to a facelift, you would combine both protocols.

Pre-facelift Home Care at Eight Weeks, as Provided by the Esthetician

Depending upon the patient's skin type, classification, and condition, have him or her use a combination of the following for optimum skin conditioning:

- AHAs and/or BHAs, for exfoliation and increased cellular production; *Chlorella vulgaris* extract, for cell stimulation; and antiglycation

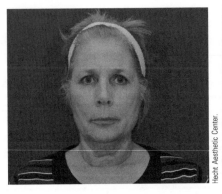
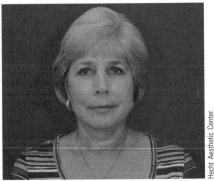

Figure 6–9 Patient, before facelift.   **Figure 6–10** Patient, after facelift.

(which reduces glycation, where a sugar molecule attaches itself to proteins such as collagen and elastin, creating brittle fibers and a loss in elasticity).

- Tretinoin (retinoic acid) to increase fibroblast activity, increasing collagen and elastin production and further exfoliation. (This is left to the discretion of the physician, as it is a prescription and can become irritating to some patients.)
- Skin lighteners, such as hydroquinone, Kojic acid, arbutin, and licorice extracts, for use as tyrosinase inhibitors and melanocyte suppressants.
- Hydrators and moisturizers with amino acids, hyaluronic acid, and/or sodium hyaluronate; antioxidants such as ergothioneine and superoxide dismutase to enhance hydration levels and combat free radical proliferation, respectively.
- Serums with ingredients used in tissue support, such as those that work as an anti-inflammatory and encourage cell renewal, such as Syn-Tacks®, acetyl-dipeptide, and Matrixyl® 3000.
- Environmental protection product with an SPF of at least 30 and broad spectrum chemical sunscreen ingredients, such as octyl methoxycinnamate and benzophenone-3, and the physical sunscreen ingredients zinc oxide and titanium dioxide. It is also advisable to include products that contain antioxidants such as cassia ala leaf extract, superoxide dismutase, and polyphenols (copper and resveratrol).

A simple home care regimen is used as follows:

A.M.
1. Cleanse with an appropriate skin type and condition cleanser.
2. Apply a lightener or other tyrosinase inhibitor: hydroquinone or Kojic acid, vitamin C, arbutin, or licorice extract (licochalcone or glabridin).
3. Apply a tissue-support serum with peptides.
4. Apply a moisturizer/hydrator and eye cream with AHA or BHA.
5. Use sunscreen with an SPF of a minimum of 30 and antioxidants.

P.M.
1. Cleanse with an appropriate skin type and condition cleanser.
2. Apply a lightener or other tyrosinase inhibitor: hydroquinone or Kojic acid, vitamin C, arbutin, or licorice extract (licochalcone or glabridin).
3. Apply Tretinoin/retinoic acid (if recommended by a physician).

4. Apply a moisturizer/hydrator and eye cream with Chlorella vulgaris extract, for antiglycation, and Matrixyl® 3000.

Pre-facelift Treatments

Eight Weeks Before Surgery

Using Technology

The treatments best suited for facelifts provide rejuvenation, stimulation, and nourishing elements to both the skin and muscles. Contouring and smoothing ahead of the surgery are vital goals, and patients take better care of their skin when they have been educated on the merits of pre- and post-surgery home care and treatments. Having a facelift is a major event for most patients. They need to know that in addition to selecting a good surgeon, their adherence and compliance to protocols will determine the outcome of the surgery. A combination of microdermabrasion for exfoliation, oxygen therapy for barrier improvements, microcurrent muscle reeducation, and LED services are excellent choices for prepping a patient for such an extensive surgical procedure.

Using Chemical Peels

Chemical peels provide excellent skin rejuvenation. They may be used pre-operatively or alternated with technology facials. This means that during one visit, the esthetician gives the client a technology facial; on the next visit, he or she applies a chemical peel, depending upon the client's skin type and condition, and the goals of the attending physician.

Make certain that your client or patient does not have health issues that are contraindicated for microdermabrasion, oxygen therapy, microcurrent, LED services, or chemical peels.

Here are pre- and post-operative treatment options for a rhytidectomy (facelift), according to skin type. See Chapters 4 and 5 for step-by-step protocols.

Between Six and Three Weeks Before Surgery

- Continue the home care regimen.
- Continue in-office treatments weekly or biweekly (whether for layered facials or peel/facials).

Two Weeks Before Surgery

- Continue the home care regimen.
- Continue in-office treatments (whether for layered facials or peel/facials).

Table 6–5 Pre- and Post-operative Treatment Options for Rhytidectomy: Dry/Dehydrated/Photodamaged Skin

Procedure: Rhytidectomy (Facelift)	Pre-operative	Post-operative
Skin Type: **Dry** **Dehydrated** **Photodamaged**	**Technology Facials** 1. Microdermabrasion: One pass 2. Oxygen: Use hydrating masque and dome 3. Microcurrent: Muscle reeducation and hydrating skin work 4. LED: Use red and yellow light *Technology can be layered **Chemical Peel Options** • Enzyme peels • AHA: Lactic, glycolic acids • Jessner's • Light TCA • Combination and layered peels	**Recovery Healing Phase** 1. The medical team sees the patient. 2. The esthetician can give the client a shoulder/hand massage on the first visit. 3. Manual lymphatic drainage is performed. 4. The microcurrent is set to enhance/healing modes. 5. Hydrating, relaxing facials are given. 6. LED is administered in red and yellow light.

© Milady, a part of Cengage Learning.

*Do not apply chemical peels with microcurrent; alternate between visits.

Table 6–6 Pre- and Post-operative Treatment Options for Rhytidectomy: Normal Skin

Procedure: Rhytidectomy (Facelift)	Pre-operative	Post-operative
Skin Type: **Normal**	**Technology Facials** 1. Microdermabrasion: One pass 2. Oxygen: Use masque and dome 3. Microcurrent: Muscle reeducation and hydrating skin work 4. LED: Use red and yellow light *Technology can be layered **Chemical Peel Options** • AHA: Lactic, glycolic acids • Jessner's • Light TCA • Combination and layered peels	**Recovery Healing Phase** 1. The medical team sees the patient. 2. The esthetician can give the client a shoulder/hand massage on the first visit. 3. Manual lymphatic drainage is performed. 4. The microcurrent is set to enhance/healing modes. 5. Hydrating, relaxing facials are given. 6. LED is administered in red light.

© Milady, a part of Cengage Learning.

*Do not apply chemical peels with microcurrent; alternate between visits.

Table 6–7 Pre- and Post-operative Treatment Options for Rhytidectomy: Oily Skin

Procedure: Rhytidectomy (Facelift)	Pre-operative	Post-operative
Skin Type: **Oily**	**Technology Facials** 1. Microdermabrasion: Two passes 2. Oxygen: Use airbrush wand with desincrustation product 3. Microcurrent: Apply desincrustation modes and muscle reeducation 4. LED: Blue light *Technology can be layered **Chemical Peel Options** • AHA: Lactic, glycolic acids • Salicylic acids • Jessner's • Light TCA • Combination and layered peels • Peel cocktails: Combine multiple ingredients	**Recovery Healing Phase** 1. The medical team sees the patient. 2. The esthetician can give the client a shoulder/hand massage on the first visit. 3. Manual lymphatic drainage is performed. 4. The microcurrent is set to enhance/healing modes. 5. LED is administered in red and blue light.

© Milady, a part of Cengage Learning.

*Do not apply chemical peels with microcurrent; alternate between visits.

Table 6–8 Pre- and Post-operative Treatment Options for Rhytidectomy: Sensitive/Reactive Skin

Procedure: Rhytidectomy (Facelift)	Pre-operative	Post-operative
Skin Type: **Sensitive/Reactive**	**Technology Facials** 1. Ultrasonic peeler 2. Microcurrent: Muscle reeducation and hydrating skin work 3. LED: Use red and yellow light *Technology can be layered **Chemical Peel Options** • Enzyme peel • Lactic acid	**Recovery Healing Phase** 1. The medical team sees the patient. 2. The esthetician gives the client a shoulder/hand massage on the first visit. 3. Manual lymphatic drainage is performed. 4. The microcurrent is set to enhance/healing modes. 5. LED is administered in yellow light.

© Milady, a part of Cengage Learning.

*Do not apply chemical peels with microcurrent; alternate between visits.

One Week Before Surgery

- Continue the home care regimen; remove Tretinoin and hydroquinone if they are part of the home care plan.
- Provide a final in-office treatment before the surgery date: focus on calming, soothing, and hydrating applications. Stop all peels, Tretinoin, and aggressive applications. Manual lymphatic drainage may be applied at this point.

Note: Patients with rosacea are to remain on their topical medications throughout the preparatory phase as indicated by their physician.

Post-operative Care

One Week After Surgery

Home Care Immediately After Surgery

Medical personnel provides all immediate care to the patient after surgery. Depending upon how extensive the surgery was, some physicians opt to use bandages; others may not. This is strictly up to the attending physician. The patient can clean exposed areas with a warm, soft cloth. It is important for the patient to follow the protocols and post-operative plan, as the recovery and results depend upon strict adherence to the directions. Medication is often recommended for pain, and the patient is instructed to rest, sleeping with his or her head up on stacked pillows. The client must avoid using products and water near the suture sites and make sure not to do any heavy lifting, not to bend over, and not to increase body stress levels or overstimulation.

In-Office Visits

- Physicians typically see patients within 48 hours of surgery for follow-up. Bandages may be replaced and sutures inspected and cleaned.
- The esthetician could give a light shoulder or hand massage at this visit, if approved by the physician.

4 to 15 Days After Surgery

Home Care Once the Bandages Are Removed

- Instruct the patient to maintain a gentle cleansing regimen (avoiding the use of products on all sutures and staple sites).
- Remind the patient to follow his or her physician's recommendation for cleaning the suture sites. It is imperative that these areas be kept clean and are well protected.

- Moisturize and hydrate the skin in all other areas (avoid the sutures).
- Use sunscreen with an SPF of 30 if the client is going outside (avoid the sutures).

In-Office Visit

- The patient sees his or her physician and nurse for suture removal, as directed by the physician.
- The patient sees the esthetician for manual lymphatic drainage, gentle massage, and camouflage therapy (makeup). LED can be used if allowed and/or recommended by the physician. Consult with the client to begin to add regular home care products back into his or her regimen, avoiding AHAs and aggressive active agents.

Two Weeks After Surgery

Home Care

- Continue with home care.
- Apply camouflage makeup.
- Medical personnel instructs the patient to maintain good scar management, including recommendations on as the use of scar tapes and silicone products.

In-Office Treatments

- Continue light facials and light or gentle massage or manual lymphatic drainage twice a week, three days apart; LED can be used for healing. Avoid all chemical peels, microdermabrasion, heat or steam, or other aggressive treatments at this time.
- The physician will see the patient at this time to check on his or her progress.

Three Weeks After Surgery

Home Care

- Most patients care return to their presurgery home care regimen at this point. They can use AHAs, BHAs, hydrators, moisturizers, and sunscreens. They must avoid scar sites with acids, however, as those areas will be sensitive and may be reactive.
- The patient's physician may recommend that he or she increases activity.

Esthetic Treatments

- Resume treatments at four weeks. *Do not use* heavy microdermabrasion techniques, aggressive chemical peels, or microcurrent muscle reeducation within the first three weeks after surgery. Use ultrasonic peeling (see Chapter 5 for options), enzymes, or manual exfoliation; use microcurrent therapy for product penetration and healing modes. Use LED for continued healing. Some patients will have numbness at the scar sites: this is normal.
- Review all products to determine if a change is needed in the protocol. This often happens after a procedure, as the surgery may have resolved older concerns. This is especially true in the case of makeup, so give the patient a new makeup plan. Patients will usually be more objective about their new look by now, and will need some support from you. Old makeup applications can pull down the appearance of a fresh new face.

BLEPHAROPLASTY (EYELIFT)

Eyelifts are among the highest-sought-after surgical procedures for both men and women, and with good reason. The eyes, neck, and the back of the hands are often the first to show age as a result of little to no oil in those areas, thinner skin, and constant environmental exposure. The pre- and post-operative phases for an eyelift are similar to those of the facelift. Treatments can be modified if they are performed in conjunction with another procedure such as a face/forehead lift, laser work, or chemical peeling. If multiple procedures are be combined, infuse the protocols for those procedures as well (see Color Insert, Figures 6–11 and 6–12).

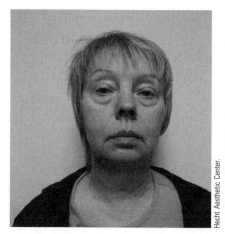
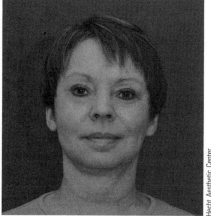

Figure 6–11 Before blepharoplasty.   **Figure 6–12** After blepharoplasty.

Pre-operative Blepharoplasty Home Care

Home Care at Six Weeks Before Surgery

Use routine skin care on the face as you would for a face and forehead lift. Use an eye cream with peptides, arnica, hyaluronic acid, and hesperidin methyl chalcone to help stimulate blood and lymphatic circulation, reduce swelling, and hydrate and protect delicate tissue around the eye area. If the patient is having a chemical peel or a skin resurfacing application in addition to the eyelift, add a skin lightener and Tretinoin as recommended by the physician to the evening home care program.

Pre-operative Treatments for Blepharoplasty

Add to the layered facial a second round of muscle reeducation movements to the microcurrent-specific protocol to further stimulate the eye area. This extra focus in the orbicularis oculi area can help stimulate cell renewal and ultimately support the post-operative healing phase.

If using chemical peels, use a light peel for exfoliation, lightening, and hydrating. If this is not tolerated, apply a hydrating stimulating facial. Depending upon skin type and classification, follow up with appropriate hydrators and sunscreen.

Three Weeks Before Surgery

Home Care

- Continue with home care.

Esthetic Treatment

- Continue with in-office treatments.

Two Weeks Before Surgery

Home Care

- Continue with home care.

Esthetic Treatment

- Continue in-office treatments.

CAUTION!

Do not mix chemical peels and microcurrent in the same treatment. Make certain that the patient does not have any contraindications for electrical devices. If they do, use chemical peels or follow the basic facial protocols in Chapter 5 for use in pre- and post-operative phases.

One Week Before Surgery

Home Care

- Continue home care. Stop using Tretinoin or hydroquinone if this is used in laser or chemical peel prep.

Esthetic Treatment

- Continue in-office treatment but switch to lymphatic drainage or a traditional hydrating facial. Stop all peels and technology facials.

Post-operative Care for Blepharoplasty

Days 1–7 After Surgery

Home Care

- Apply topicals, eye drops, and protocols as directed by a physician.
- Take medication for pain as directed by a physician.

In-Office Visit

- A nurse or physician removes the sutures at five to seven days after the procedure.
- If a laser or chemical peel was applied, medical personnel will clean the abraded area and apply a lubricating product.

Days 7–12 After Surgery

Home Care

- Continue to follow the protocol as directed by the physician.
- Apply a lubricating product, as recommended.
- Camouflage therapy can be applied typically, but check with the physician. Fine mineral products work best for this.

In-Office Treatment

- The client has a follow-up visit with the physician to check his or her progress.
- Perform manual lymphatic drainage for healing or microcurrent therapy in healing modes.
- Administer LED (red light 620 nm) for healing. Check with the manufacturer's and physician's recommendations.
- Apply camouflage therapy (makeup) for bruised areas.

Two to Three Weeks After Surgery

Home Care

- If a laser or chemical peel was applied, continue with the protocol as directed by the physician.
- Transition to routine skin care.

In-Office Treatment

- Client pays a follow-up visit to the physician.
- With the physician's consent, treatments may resume. Start with an LED session in red or yellow light for healing and anti-inflammatory work, and then move toward full treatments on a monthly basis. Perform manual lymphatic drainage or microcurrent therapy in healing modes.
- Apply camouflage therapy (makeup).

Here are pre- and post-operative treatment options according to skin type.

> **CAUTION!**
>
> If the patient has had a chemical peel, laser work, or other aggressive surgical procedure, *do not* use microdermabrasion or apply other chemical peels until the client has fully recovered and his or her physician has been consulted. As always, check with a physician on any and all applications prior to performing esthetic services on patients.

Table 6–9 Pre- and Post-operative Treatment Options for Blepharoplasty: Dry/Dehydrated/Photodamaged Skin

Procedure: Blepharoplasty (Eyelift)	Pre-operative	Post-operative
Skin Type:	**Technology Facials**	**Recovery Healing Phase**
Dry Dehydrated Photodamaged	1. Microdermabrasion: One pass 2. Oxygen: Use pulsating jets with hydrating product around the eye area 3. Microcurrent: Muscle reeducation and hydrating skin work focus on eye area 4. LED: Use red and yellow light *Technology can be layered	1. The medical team sees the patient. 2. The esthetician can give the client a shoulder/hand massage on the first visit. 3. Manual lymphatic drainage is performed, with a focus on the eye area. 4. The microcurrent is set to enhance/healing modes. 5. LED is administered in red and yellow light.
	Chemical Peel Options • Enzyme peels • AHA: Lactic, glycolic acids • Jessner's • Light TCA • Combination and layered peels	

*Do not apply chemical peels with microcurrent; alternate between visits.

Table 6–10 Pre- and Post-operative Treatment Options for Blepharoplasty: Normal Skin

Procedure: Blepharoplasty (Eyelift)	Pre-operative	Post-operative
Skin Type: Normal	**Technology Facials**	**Recovery Healing Phase**
	1. Microdermabrasion: One pass	1. The medical team sees the patient.
	2. Oxygen: Use pulsating jets with hydrating product around the eye area	2. The esthetician can give the client a shoulder/hand massage on the first visit.
	3. Microcurrent: Muscle reeducation and hydrating skin work around the eye area	3. Manual lymphatic drainage is performed, with a focus on the eye area.
	4. LED: Use red and yellow light	4. The microcurrent is set to enhance/healing modes.
	*Technology can be layered	5. LED is administered in red light.
	Chemical Peel Options	
	• AHA: Lactic, glycolic acids	
	• Jessner's	
	• Light TCA	
	• Combination and layered peels	

*Do not apply chemical peels with microcurrent; alternate between visits.

Table 6–11 Pre- and Post-operative Treatment Options for Blepharoplasty: Oily Skin

Procedure: Blepharoplasty (Eyelift)	Pre-operative	Post-operative
Skin Type: Oily	**Technology Facials**	**Recovery Healing Phase**
	1. Microdermabrasion: Two passes	1. The medical team sees the patient.
	2. Oxygen: Use pulsating jets with hydrating product around the eye area	2. The esthetician can give the client a shoulder/hand massage on the first visit.
	3. Microcurrent: Apply muscle reeducation and skin work, with a focus around the eye area	3. Manual lymphatic drainage is performed, with a focus on the eye area.
	4. LED: Blue light	4. Microcurrent is set to enhance/healing modes, with a focus around the eye area.
	*Technology can be layered	5. LED is administered in red and blue light.
	Chemical Peel Options	
	• AHA: Lactic, glycolic acids	
	• Salicylic acid	
	• Jessner's	
	• Light TCA	
	• Combination and layered peels	
	• Peel cocktails: Combine multiple ingredients	

*Do not apply chemical peels with microcurrent; alternate between visits.

Table 6–12 Pre- and Post-operative Treatment Options for Blepharoplasty: Sensitive/Reactive Skin

Procedure: Blepharoplasty (Eyelift)	Pre-operative	Post-operative
Skin Type: **Sensitive/Reactive**	**Technology Facials**	**Recovery Healing Phase**
	1. Ultrasonic peeler	1. The medical team sees the patient.
	2. Microcurrent: Muscle reeducation and hydrating skin work around the eye area	2. The esthetician gives the client a shoulder/hand massage on the first visit.
	3. LED: Use red and yellow light	3. Manual lymphatic drainage is performed, with a focus around the eye area.
	*Technology can be layered	4. Microcurrent is set to enhance/healing modes, with a focus around the eye area.
		5. LED is administered in yellow light.
	Chemical Peel Options	
	• Enzyme peel	
	• Lactic acid	

*Do not apply chemical peels with microcurrent; alternate between visits.

© Milady, a part of Cengage Learning.

 # SUMMING IT UP

Estheticians who have been well trained and are diligent about following protocols have successfully used lasers and IPL devices for nearly two decades. As with all medical devices in classification II and above, it is necessary to work under the direction/supervision of a physician or otherwise qualified medical personnel as dictated by your state regulations. Clients continue to seek laser hair removal and IPL treatments for skin rejuvenation. According to the ASPS, laser hair removal is routinely one of the top five minimally invasive procedures performed each year.

As we can visualize, there are multiple opportunities to serve the client who becomes a patient and then a client again. Interestingly, patients do not see themselves as patients, nor do they call themselves clients. They perceive themselves as people with a desire to feel and look their very best. By applying a few techniques and managing a healthy business, we can help them navigate through neurotoxins and soft-tissue fillers, surgical procedures, and facials and home care products. We can take them from consult to referral to facials, and then on to home care plans and use. Connecting and staying connected is the solution.

ESTHETICIAN **PROFILE**

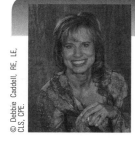

© Debbie Caddell, RE, LE, CLS, CPE.

Debbie Caddell, RE, LE, CLS, CPE

Caddell's Laser & Electrolysis Clinic, Inc., Bellevue, WA

I was born and raised in Seattle, Washington. From the beginning I have been attracted to hair removal because I was really hairy and always hated it! I began having electrolysis while in college. Six months after I graduated, I changed my career plan and became an electrologist. Since there were no schools in Washington, I went to California to receive my training and license. (Washington is still an unregulated state.) I became an electrologist in 1982. Eighteen years later, I decided to learn about laser hair removal. I attended Rocky Mountain Laser College (RMLC) in 2000. In just 10 years, my business grew from two employees and one treatment room to seven employees, four treatment rooms, and six lasers. In 2007, new laws were implemented by the Department of Health in Washington State. I could no longer work with lasers unless I became an esthetician. At that point, I knew that I loved what I was doing, and found an esthetics course at Clover Park Technical College in Tacoma, Washington. I fell in love with esthetics. I became a licensed esthetician and then continued on to become a certified medical esthetician.

Training

I am certified in the following modalities and devices: microcurrent, chemical peels, electrology, tattoo removal, microdermabrasion laser tattoo removal, and laser hair and vein removal. I am a laser safety officer and a certified laser specialist. I am a graduate of the California Institute of Electrology.

While attending laser training, my instructor demonstrated tattoo and vein removal. Fascinated by the technology, I realized during the session that I too could perform those treatments. The key to being a successful laser specialist is training. I have often asked if I should be working with lasers. When I question myself and my mentors, trainers, and colleagues about this, the answer

is always the same. Yes, estheticians can work with lasers if you have the proper training, are within the scope of the state licensing regulations, and are working under medical supervision.

Practice Demographic

My hair removal clients range in age from 14 to 80. People from all walks of life have unwanted hair. With laser and electrolysis, we are able to treat all skin types and all hair colors. I perform tattoo removal for former gang members, corporate people, tattoo artists, and lovers of tattoos who want to cover up an old tattoo. Women over 40 in the middle- to upper-income brackets are our target market. Fitzpatrick skin types I–III are the best candidates for my services, as they have less melanin and potential for scarring.

Services/Treatments Offered

I offer electrolysis, laser hair removal, laser vein elimination, laser tattoo removal, and facial rejuvenation using Erbium-YAG, or Fractional CO_2 lasers. Seventy percent of my business is from hair removal, which is great; as I have mentioned, it has been my passion for years.

Personal Philosophy

I am very enthusiastic about my work. I love to help people "enhance their beauty," and my mind is always racing ahead to the next laser I hope to purchase. I love to hear testimonials about how I have changed someone's life by using lasers for removing unwanted facial hair, reducing folliculitis, and removing leg veins and tattoos. Some women will not wear shorts or skirts because of the veins on their legs. Today, we can eliminate most of them. One of my first hair removal clients was 25 years old. She came in with long hair that hung over her cheeks. Her head was down. She was very shy and had never been on a date. She had very thick hair on her chin and full bushy hair as side burns. I watched her personality blossom as the hair began to go. A couple of years later, she married. Working with her was such a gratifying experience. She changed my life, as I had changed hers.

There are many challenges to running a business. I have to come up with ideas on how to grow the business. I deal with staff problems and clients who are unhappy with their results. Interestingly, fluctuations in the economy do not affect the electrolysis business. People will always find a way to obtain hair removal methods. The best way to increase your business is through referrals from happy clients.

Additional Contributions to the Industry

In addition to presenting and my work at the Northwest Aestheticians' Guild, I write articles on hair removal. I provide treatment for people interested in changing their lives by removing tattoos that no longer serve their best interests (such as former gang members) and for others whose early decision to apply a tattoo has limited their life choices. In some cases, I work with individuals who didn't truly choose to have a tattoo; rather, they were branded, in a sense. I have a great deal of compassion for these people and my skill has given them new opportunities in their lives. Having tattoos removed represents freedom to those individuals. I do much of this type of tattoo removal pro bono for these very special clients.

I am a member of the following associations:

- American Society for Lasers in Medical Surgery
- International Guild of Hair Removal Specialists
- Society of Clinical and Medical Hair Removal
- American Electrolysis Association
- eWomen Network
- State Liaison of the Society for Clinical and Medical Hair Removal

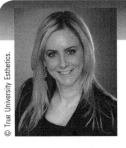

ESTHETICIAN **PROFILE**

Terri A. Wojak, LE
Licensed Esthetician, Author and Educator

Plastic Surgery Affiliation, Steven Dayan, MD; Cofounder of True University, Chicago, IL

© True University Esthetics.

I was born and raised in Chicago, Illinois. My very first job at 14 was as a shampoo girl at a salon down the street from my house. I loved the atmosphere, and ended up working there for several years. After finishing high school, I decided to go to college for business. I liked anything that had to do with business: balancing check books, paying bills, and managing schedules. When I started college, I was working at another salon, Mario Tricoci, as a nail assistant. I eventually started working there as a nail technician. One day, an esthetician asked me if I would like a facial. I knew nothing about what it entailed but said yes. To my surprise, it was at that moment that I decided to switch career goals and become an esthetician. The esthetician explained everything so thoroughly and technically, that it piqued my interest enough to want to change career paths! Within one hour, I went from going to school for business to becoming a skin care specialist.

Training

I decided to go to school at Pivot Point International Academy in 1995. I had researched several schools and heard it was the best, so I made the hour-and-a-half drive everyday to receive the best education available for my new career. After my initial training at

Pivot Point, I trained at Mario Tricoci for an additional three months. I have taken several other classes along the way, anything to do with medical esthetics, treatments for acne, and chemical peels. One of my favorite courses is the skin biology and chemical peel seminar from PCA Skin®. In fact, I liked the seminar so much that I have recently become a PCA®-certified trainer and now offer this class as part of the medical esthetics training that I provide. I go to as many trade shows as I can. I feel that estheticians must stay up on the changing trends in the industry. Besides going to shows, I read trade magazines to keep up with the latest news.

Practice Demographic

My client base consists of a little of everything, but I have always specialized in acne. I tend to get a younger demographic that has tried many different things in the past for acne treatments, with no success. I also perform a lot of chemical peeling treatments, especially for darker skin types. I feel that mild peeling is effective for many different skin conditions. A large part of what I do in treating clients' skin is product recommendation; if the client is not using the proper products at home, treatments will not be as effective.

Services/Treatments Offered

The services I offer include facials, microdermabrasion, chemical peels, dermaplaning, ultrasound treatments, oxygen treatments, and laser hair removal. Everyone has different skin; therefore, I offer a multitude of treatments to treat all skin types and conditions. Sometimes clients need a deep peeling treatment to give them a fresh new start to their skin, other times a simple cleansing facial may be all that is needed. I also offer oxygen treatments to help stimulate and revitalize dull skin. Ultrasound is great for post-op patients to reduce edema and stimulate collagen production. I often use microdermabrasion or dermaplaning as a nice surface exfoliation before a mild peel or facial to allow the other products to penetrate more effectively.

Personal Philosophy

I love my job, especially the education aspect of it. When I started working with Dr. Steven Dayan, I was able to take my career to a new level. Here, I have the ability to be creative and have started many new ventures with the support of my mentor.

When it comes to clients, I like making people feel better about themselves. To boost a client's self-esteem makes me feel that I can really improve people's lives. It's important to make clients happy. It doesn't matter what others think; what matters is how one perceives him- or herself. When I am teaching, I ensure that my students understand this concept. Too often providers will look at what they think can be improved for a client; but what matters is what the client would like to see improved.

To sustain our practice, we make sure to not only offer our clients the latest and greatest treatments but to also offer students the best in education. Every student is treated as a unique individual at True University. Because everyone has different learning styles, we keep our class sizes small. It is very rewarding when students tell me how much they learned in a short period of time. I am happy to share my experiences and my knowledge with anyone I can to make our business as a whole greater.

Additional Contributions to the Industry

I started working with Dr. Steven Dayan, FACS in 2006. I have exceeded any expectations I ever had for my career. Together, Dr. Dayan and I started an educational program called True University; it is a medically guided advanced education center for estheticians. We did this when we saw the need for this type of training through our own experiences with estheticians in the industry. We also wrote a book for the program called *Mastering Medical Esthetics*. The programs and the book include chemical peeling treatments, mechanical peeling treatments, pre- and post-operative treatments, how to assist with medical treatments such as injectables and lasers, and advanced training on skin conditions.

I have spoken at several skin care conferences around the country about what it is like to work in a medical practice as well as about the additional education that is needed to work in a medical facility. I also write articles for several magazines including *Skin Inc.* and *In with Skin.* I will continue to share my knowledge with students and clients for as long as I can.

The Business of Esthetics

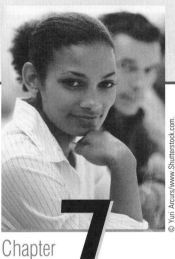

> "Although learning business skills is not nearly as much fun for most students or professionals as the latest new treatment protocol, it is a major part of what is needed to be a successful esthetician."
> *—Jesse Cormier, Executive Director ASCP*

Chapter Capture

After completing this chapter, you will be able to:

- Develop and implement a business plan.
- Take five simple steps to get started.
- Write your business plan.
- Minimize risks as an esthetician or beauty professional.
- Understand the risks involved for product and device manufacturers.
- Understand the types of insurance.
- Obtain the proper help and support for your business.
- Build and trust your intuition.

DEVELOP AND USE A BUSINESS PLAN

A business plan will pay off from the moment you implement it. The actual process of business planning generates finite, detailed action items and provides a big-picture perspective on your business. Daniel H. Pink, the author of *A Whole New Mind, Why Right-Brainers Will Rule the Future* (Riverhead Books, NY, 2006), states: "In general, the left hemisphere participates in the analysis of information ... while the right hemisphere specializes in putting isolated elements together to perceive things as a whole." As any entrepreneur will tell you, this is especially critical in business applications. As Daniel Pink brilliantly sums it up, it takes the whole brain to run a successful business. We must be able to measure and chart progress, provide structure and margins to our days, and use our energy efficiently to sustain a business. Ideas and concepts that emerge from excellent brainstorming sessions (whether alone or with team members and colleagues) are inspirational and necessary to create excitement and motivation. However, we have all run ourselves ragged on whims and fleeting ideas when a simple plan of action visually orchestrated would have provided the support and foundation for achieving our goals, and in turn making more money. Many of our colleague estheticians will say that making more money is not the only reason for being in the esthetic business; however, in order to stay in business making money is necessary for building a business, and we must have the capital to do so.

GUEST SPOT

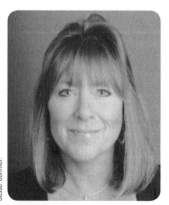

Jesse Cormier.

JESSE CORMIER, EXECUTIVE DIRECTOR, ASCP.

"I visit both students and instructors at skin care schools across the country as part of my work with Associated Skin Care Professionals. I often hear the frustration of instructors, who find that teaching the technical aspects of an esthetics career doesn't leave enough time to prepare their students for the business side of the equation. Although learning business skills is not nearly as much fun for most students or professionals as the latest new treatment protocol, it is a major part of what is needed to be a successful esthetician.

This five-step process to creating a business plan is a commonsense approach that is virtually foolproof, whether one is an independent practitioner or a salon owner. This approach breaks it down into manageable steps that eliminate the fear factor. The end result will be a viable, effective plan for any esthetician to attain professional goals.

Another subject that many estheticians find rather intimidating is risk management and liability insurance. Nobody likes to think that a client might be injured during a treatment, but as an insurance provider, ASCP regularly hears of cases where estheticians found out the hard way that accidents can happen and that they were not covered by the spa where they work. Estheticians need good, solid advice on how to manage their risk—using proper documentation and appropriate client treatment forms, seeking trustworthy counsel, and having individual liability insurance that covers both professional and general liability. These are all critical for protecting your business and future earnings."

There is a natural ebb and flow with any business, and having a written plan will guide you when you are at your peaks and get you back on track when challenges can feel threatening. A business plan should be a fluid body of work, subject to change with updates and room for market fluctuations. Evaluate it regularly to implement changes and goals (Figure 7–1).

Many plans are overly complicated. Often the net gain only benefits the person who wrote the plan, and for the time that he or she is creating it. If you hire a third party to write a plan for you, you will be completely cut out of the process and the valuable lessons learned from building it yourself. And the plan will be placed on a shelf or thrown into a drawer.

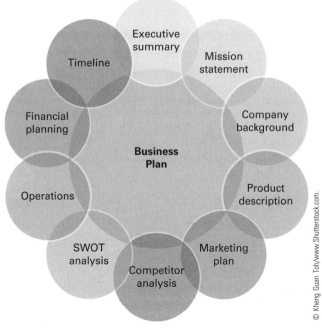

Figure 7–1 Business plan elements.

We need to use our plan every day; it is as ritualistic and natural as breathing in and out. Eventually, what was once awkward and time-consuming in the development of your business plan will become the infrastructure that provides the lifestyle, realization of dreams, and plans for your future.

Do Not Stress About Building a Business Plan

Making your business plan is simple, really. Our business plan serves as our global positioning system (GPS) for determining where we are at a given time; but more importantly, it continually reminds us of where we are going. It is essential that the plan be written in our own voice, with our own terms and growing knowledge of our business. Whether you are a solo practitioner or have 1,000 vital employees, you must have developed key elements so that at a glance, you and everyone on your team understands what role they play, what their goals are, and where they are going, today.

 ## USE A FIVE-STEP PLAN

As a solo practitioner, a new esthetician working in a spa, a long-term professional working with physicians in clinical setting; or the owner of a large salon with many moving parts, here is a five-step, straightforward preparatory approach to creating a live, working plan:

1. **Audit Your Business.** Where are you? Go through every receipt, look through your financials, review your marketing materials, consider every product and device company you are dealing with and categorize them instantly. At a blink, put them in two stacks and rate them according to their performance. Ask yourself two questions:
   a. Is this working for my business?
   b. Is this not working for my business?

   Next, go back through each stack and look carefully at the documents. Verify your instincts by looking at real numbers. How much have you sold of a product line? How do your clients like the devices that you use? Are they getting the results that they desire? (We rarely obtain this information, yet it is important.) Are your vendors or sales representatives providing the support that you need? Are they willing to help you with events and extra samples, or are they too busy for you when you call them? Is your Web site working for you? Does your business card need updating? Does it convey your message to

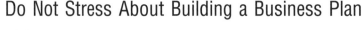

your target market? Does the paper look good? Is the color appropriate for your practice now? Who is your target market? Have many of your clients have retired or are reducing their amount of visits because they travel more now? How do you find new clients?

Looking at all of these questions can lead to finding new ways of doing business, building up your business for the future, and maintaining your business for stability. If a vendor, a service, or your bottom line is not what you want it to be, make a note of it. Sometimes we stay with practices because they are easy or comfortable even when they no longer serve a purpose.

If you are an employee, audit yourself as well. Become self-correcting and self-evaluating. Show your employer that you are taking initiative in all aspects of your work. In a respectful and timely manner, offer suggestions that will support the efforts of the team. Keep track of your goals and look for ways to improve your own performance and then share these with your employer. There is nothing more rewarding than to work with individuals for whom routine healthy, self-evaluation is standard practice. It makes business planning and work fun and achievable.

2. **Establish Goals**. Look at your business as if it were 36 months from now. Then 24 months from now, 18 months from now, 12 months from now, and in one month. Work toward the present day. It is easier once you have established the previous year's numbers; eventually you will be looking at last year's figures, which will drive your goals for the current year. This way you will develop a *master map* and the big picture view of your plan.

   In this section, you will develop your budget, which serves to provide the pathway to your purchasing power. This is true whether you are acquiring new or upgrading technology; adding or streamlining products; implementing a marketing plan; identifying and employing other business management techniques (such as evaluating your competition); and incorporating avenues for funding, if necessary.

   It will be easier to make more immediate decisions when they come up if you plan long range and chart your course. We do not feel as vulnerable if we are moving toward an objective. When we are tempted to go with an impulsive whim, we can assess the situation by asking, "Does this fit with my business plan?" If not, it is easier to let it go, even if it seems interesting. So much energy, time, and money are lost on trial and error. Remain true to your strengths and build on what is working for you. We cannot underestimate the value of doing our homework when it comes to evaluating potential risks to our business.

3. **Identify Roles and Responsibilities**. If you are the only one on your team, you may feel that this does not apply to you, as you are responsible for everything within your business. However, we are all dependent upon product and device manufacturers, bookkeepers/accountants, property owners or real estate brokers, insurance brokers and agents, and other professionals who make up the balance of our team. These partnerships must fuse seamlessly into our business profiles, and the professionals that you work with must have your interests as their priority.

   If you have employees, attention to this is immediate, as you are together daily. It is important to respect the talents of employees, but also to demand that individuals honor the culture and organizational pursuits of the business. Furthermore, employees must be fulfilling their roles and responsibilities in order to retain the integrity of the team.

4. **Create a One-Page Achievement Plan.** Build a *one-page* achievement plan. Make sure that everyone understands what your mission/vision statement is; name the team members; describe the tasks involved; and outline what the results should be (Figure 7–2). All assignments must be:
   a. Attainable: can be achieved
   b. Focused: directed toward the goal
   c. United: congruent with the business plan

5. **Work the Plan.** This final step can often be the most difficult part of business development, but is essential to your being able to measure how well your plan is serving you and to keep the practice on track. As a side note, it can serve as a distraction buster as well. As estheticians, we tend have an immeasurable amount of compassion for everyone within our reach. Most of us have spent an inordinate amount of time (which is expensive financially and emotionally) on solving other people's problems or putting out fires that may have very little to do with our own work lives. Many of us have repeatedly supported individuals by opening doors for them professionally and personally, only to find that, figuratively, they continue to jump out a back window. They, for whatever reason, are not ready to learn and grow.

   This is not to suggest that we ignore the needs of friends, employees, and colleagues; rather, if we focus on our own plan, we can be more effective all the way around. As estheticians, we are leaders, mentors, and coaches. We need to be the types of leaders that generate a healthy positive environment, rather than distraction and inappropriate attachments (codependence).

Karlee Jenson Skin Care

One-Page Achievement Plan

Audit	Working	Not Working
• Marketing Materials		X
• Products	X (60%)	X (40%)
• Treatments		
• Microdermabrasion	X	
• Chemical Peels	X	
• Waxing	X	
• LED	X	
• Skin tightening		X

GOALS:

$250,000.00 annually $20,833.00 monthly $5208.00 weekly
$1041.67 daily $148.81 hourly (based on a seven-hour day)

Identify Roles:

- Karlee Jenson: Owner/manager esthetician, age management specialist (full-time)
- Kristy Martin: Esthetician, waxing specialist (part-time)
- Jenna Wilson: Esthetician, chemical peel specialist, and general age management specialist (full-time)

Quick Analysis:

It appears the money spent on marketing has not been effective. Look at other methods, such as having events, networking (both social and direct as in leads groups), and increasing our online presence. It appears that 40% of the products are not selling. Determine why, and if they need to go, put them on sale or give them to a shelter to free up space for products that do sell. The team has determined that the skin-tightening device is not worth its presence in the skin care center. Look to see if more training is needed or find another service to offer in its place that will be lucrative. In order for each team member to meet her goals, and for us to meet our overall goals, it is important to determine how much each person is responsible for. Even if goals are not met every time, it provides a target that we can shoot for. If we do not have goals, we will not reach them.

Figure 7–2 An achievement plan.

Demonstrate good decision-making skills, a positive attitude, business acumen, and appropriate behaviors, and you will be a stronger, more constructive force in the lives of those you are leading than if you ride along their bumpy path each time they have an episode.

Some of us have not fully realized that a business plan is for our own practical use in designing and creating our future. It needs to be clear, concise, and make sense to us. Think of it as a conversation that you are having with your ideal team that has signed up to help you every step of the way. When we focus our thoughts and actions this way, great manifestations develop in all areas of our lives.

Make the Plan Yourself

Historically, business plans were simply multiple forms or templates with cumbersome, drawn-out explanations of mission/vision statements, executive summaries that bored us to tears, and financials that none of us could understand. Often, business plans are outsourced or developed by a third party (perhaps not even in the skin care industry) who has no idea what your business is about, and sadly, does not have your passion. The global "reset" that we are experiencing provides a rich environment and untold opportunities for estheticians to learn about business while planning for continued success. Success is within our reach, if we manage the items that we can control, we can then grow beyond our current circumstances.

THE BUSINESS PLAN

Creating a business plan takes discipline; however, it is far less discipline than it takes to become a successful esthetician in today's market. As professionals, many of us take for granted what we put into every day. Let us take a snapshot of any given day in the work life of the busy esthetician. Here are just a few action items and duties that we must do to remain in business:

- Client selection
- Client education
- Prepping for clients
- Performing treatments
- Cleaning and infection control management
- Chart writing
- Working with vendors and suppliers

- Scheduling
- Our own edification
- Laundry
- Selling/retailing products
- Merchandising
- Marketing
- Staff training/meetings
- Filling orders

For most estheticians, these details are taken care of before noon. This list does not include any of the things we do before getting to work. Even if you have a team of employees helping with all of the details of your business, you need to oversee their actions to make certain that they have been completed correctly. Our business plan helps us make every step count, applying purposeful intentions and providing the necessary structure and balance to achieve our objectives.

WRITING THE PLAN: EXECUTIVE SUMMARY

The **executive summary** is a condensed version of your business plan and includes your mission/vision statement. The most important part of the document, it answers the "who, what, where, why, and how" questions. While the executive summary appears in the front of the plan, it is useful to write it last, as you will have learned much about your business through the process of building the plan.

executive summary
The overview of a business in a business plan.

The executive summary can be brief, but it must have impact. If you are vying for financial support from a lender, it must be well organized and easy to read and follow. Beware of industry jargon and insider terms: you want your readers to understand it quickly without having to rely on lengthy explanations. (These people are busy too.) This is helpful to you and/or your staff as well; as you make additions and update your plan, it will seem less dated if you use more general terms.

Here are the key elements to the executive summary:

Business (Practice) Name, Company Description, and Management

It is important to describe the essentials of your business in simple terms. If you are starting a business, make sure that your name conveys the type of business you are establishing. People are too busy today to

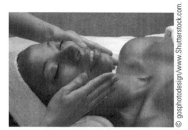

Figure 7–3 A client receives a facial massage.

try to figure out who are; we need to tell them. As tempting as it is to have an unusual or thought-provoking name such as "Exotica" or "Transformation," include the purpose of your business in the name, such as "Exotica: The Skin Care Center," or "Transformation Skin Health Clinic."

A word of caution: watch the use of the term *day spa*. This phrase has been highly overused. Every other skin care establishment includes the words "day spa" in their name today. Unless you truly are a day spa—meaning clients can come in for comprehensive treatments, such as body services, facials, manicures, pedicures, and products—you will attract more of your target market if you are clear about the services you offer in the name of your business. In reaching your target market, both you and your clients will have greater satisfaction, and you will not have to spend time telling people what you offer. People will not come in expecting one type of service and receive another. Be clear here. If you do only European facials, or specialize in a type of facial, put that in your name: "Anna Bromick European Facials" or "The Ayurvedic Facial Center." Your clients will not have to play a guessing game. The public will know who you are and what they can expect before even making contact with you (Figure 7–3).

Selecting a Name for Your Business

Before signing off on the perfect name, it is important to make sure that your name is uniquely yours and that you have the legal right to its use. A simple Google search can help you identify names that are already trademarked or used by others. Nor do you want to choose a name that is similar to many other names. You can go to Network Solutions (www.networksolutions.com) and do a more formal specific search to determine those domain names that are already in use. It is important to do your homework here, as there can be legal consequences for infringing on names that are already in use or for using a name that is too similar to a competitor's name. You will want to register your name with your state licensing agency. Next, you must choose a legal entity. Most businesses start as a sole proprietor (single owner) or as a partnership (more than one person).

Mission and Vision Statements

Incorporate your mission and vision statements into a paragraph in the part of your business plan where you describe your company. Mission statements are the foundational premises on which a business operates. Vision statements relate more to the application of plans. When creating or refining a mission statement, it is vitally important to communicate your philosophy within the declaration. Every word in your mission or vision statement counts. This is not a paragraph for fluff or flowery terms. Stick to the facts.

Whether you work in a team or are flying solo, one tried-and-true method for writing a successful mission statement is **mind mapping**. Make a circle in the center of a whiteboard, a large piece of paper, or on your computer. Write the name of your business in the middle of the circle. If you do not have a name yet, or are thinking about updating your business, just write the word *Name* in the circle. (This exercise can help you focus on discovering a name for your business as well.) Next, without thinking too much, draw a line from the center of the circle and make another circle. Inside that circle, write a word or phrase that describes the core mission/plan of for your business, or describe what you want to do.

Now, list everything that you are interested in doing with your business. Then weed out those ideas that are less interesting or that can be combined with others. Take your top solid four or five ideas and put them together on the map (Figure 7–4).

mind mapping
A diagram or graphic developed to link ideas, tasks, and information to help organize thinking on a specific theme.

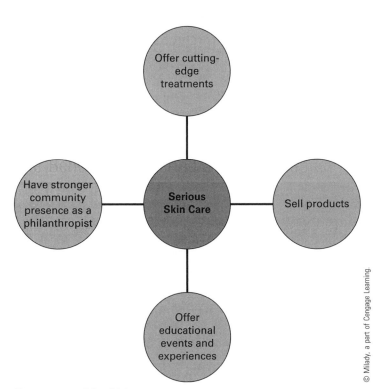

Figure 7–4 Mind Mapping.

Here are some examples of ideas for a mission/vision statement that might come up through mind mapping:

- Help people less fortunate
- Work with cancer survivors
- Introduce new products to the community
- Give skin care advice
- Apply peels, facials, and/or camouflage makeup
- Be a mentor
- Meet new people
- Be the expert in my field
- Obtain good clients who can pay for services and products
- Work with schools and student estheticians

mission/vision statement
Mission statement is the foundational premise on which a business operates; vision statement relates more to the application of plans.

A **mission/vision statement** compiled from these terms would read as follows:

At Serious Skin Care, we strive to offer compassionate skin care services for those who are serious and motivated to care for their skin health and its beauty (mission statement). We are committed to using products that feature the latest in technology in peels, facials, makeup, and in home care regimens (vision statement). Our estheticians also provide educational consultations to cancer survivors; this includes a full skin analysis for individuals whose skin has undergone changes due to medical treatments.

Products and Services

The product and services section of your business plan is your opportunity to name and refine the products and services you offer or plan to use. It can be a brief, straightforward overview. For example, if you are going to offer high-tech facials, then you want to state that you plan to offer European facials, dermaplaning, microdermabrasion, and microcurrent and LED services, along with products that support the services or that have been formulated for use with these technologies. You might state that the products you use have ingredients that are proprietary and/or are necessary to use for the function of the device—perhaps the products are conductive solutions for electrical current devices or enhance the use of LED services. Another example would be that you offer skin health products that contain antioxidants and cell protectants, and a variety of sunscreens for environmental protection.

Industry Analysis Information

Include a general recap of industry trends, growth, and profits. This section should include an overview of industry trends, mentioning those forces that may affect the industry as a whole. We often say that the beauty industry is impervious to a recession; however, in the most recent economic climate, both spa goers and estheticians made different choices about how they were going to spend money. This behavior forced adjustments in the types of services that the public received. We as an industry have outperformed most industries during this recession, but it would be good to note in this section that the economy can indeed have an effect on our business. You might state: "Recent changes in the economy have made it necessary for us to reformulate our service menu to include more value-conscious services and products." We have all seen changes in product purchases and requests for shorter services and a focus on value. It is vital that you acknowledge these trends in your business plan. It shows a lending institution good faith and it shows that you are doing your research. More directly, it shows that you are implementing changes that are necessary to remain in business. It is also important to show the size and growth of the skin care industry. For example, as estheticians and personal appearance professionals, we have historically seen steady growth increases in our industry and have outperformed other industries. Skin care, salon, and spa businesses have been good enterprises to fund, provided their practitioners were skilled at owning and managing the business. Include such statistics within industry analysis information if you can.

Industry Growth

The U.S. Department of Labor and the U.S. Bureau of Labor Statistics have data about industry studies. Share figures that show the growth rate during the sluggish years of late, and the potential for skin care professionals. Note the projections of 31 percent in our industry between the years of 2011 and 2018 (see Table 7–1).

Table 7–1 Industry Growth Information	
Occupation	**Job Growth 2011–2018**
Skin Care Specialists	51%
Hair Dressers, Hair Stylists, and Cosmetologists	31%
Manicurists and Pedicurists	24%
Makeup Artists, Theatrical and Performance	21%
Shampooers	20%
Barbers	12%
Total Personal Appearance Jobs	**31%**

© Milady, a part of Cengage Learning.

Professional Beauty Association (PBA)
Association that serves to advance the professional beauty industry by providing its members with business tools, government advocacy, education, and networking to ensure their success.

U.S. Deparment of Labor and Bureau of Labor Statistics
A government agency that produces economic data the reflects the state of the U.S. economy.

The Future of the Esthetic and Beauty Business

As provided by the **Professional Beauty Association (PBA)** and the **U.S. Department of Labor and Bureau of Labor Statistics** (2011 data) not only do salons and spas provide employment opportunities for individuals of all backgrounds, they also give individuals the experience to own businesses. This is an equal opportunity industry. An individual can really make an impact in the beauty business; with constant training and study, it is possible to earn a great income and help others do the same.

- Sixty-one percent of salon businesses are owned by women, compared to just 30 percent of businesses in the overall private sector.
- Twenty-one percent of businesses in the salon industry are black or African American owned, versus just 7 percent of total private sector businesses.
- Seventeen percent of salon businesses are Asian, nearly three times the 6 percent Asian-ownership rate for businesses in the private sector overall. Opportunities abound with business acumen.
- Nine percent of salon businesses are owned by individuals of Hispanic origin, matching the proportion of Hispanic business ownership in the private sector overall. This is also promising and can be increased.

When we consider the business potential that awaits industrious estheticians or beauty professionals, the future is as bright as these statistics reveal. We might also consider the possibility of connecting and collaborating with like-minded individuals with an interest in the industry, thus sharing the rewards and the challenges of business ownership.

Marketing Plan and Strategy

This section of the business plan is a description of how you propose to communicate your business to your market. It is important to research the various options carefully, as many marketing opportunities are expensive in money and time. Marketing tasks include Web site building or sourcing; social networking; and creating business cards, brochures, blogs, newsletters, and other printed materials. How will you advertise beyond the basics of printed material and your Web site? Will you collaborate with another service provider or practitioner to save on costs? Answering these questions will help you develop this section and give you specific details and ideas on building your marketing plan (Figure 7–5).

Marketing Vehicles			
Vehicle type	**Cost per year**	**Cost per month**	**Frequency**
Professional support:			
• Graphics/design			
• Social media			
• Advertising			
• Online search engine(s)			
Social networking			
Brochures/business cards			
Signs			
Multimedia advertising:			
• Radio			
• TV			
• Print			
• Online newsletter(s)			
Phonebook			
Direct mail			
Business development			
• Trade shows/business expos			
• Organizations			
• Memberships			

© Milady, a part of Cengage Learning.

Figure 7–5 A marketing vehicle form.

Public Relations

Public relations and positive exposure are critical for estheticians. Face-to-face networking is important in the skin care business, as people need to meet you directly. You do this by speaking to women's groups and helping on committees for service clubs. These are both great options for raising your profile in your community. Get involved.

Obtaining New Markets from Specific Demographics in Your Area

Including a note about how you could add new market opportunities to your plan can be effective. Describe how you would segment geographical factors and demographics for product and services. Using numbers, here is an example: If you were located near a college or university of 20,000 students between the ages of 18 and 26, it would be a good idea to market special treatments for acne to students, and offer a product gift as part of their first visit. You can use this worksheet to strategize your marketing plan to determine types, costs, and frequency of specific marketing vehicles.

Building your business plan will help set up a budget for your marketing needs. The old saying that "word-of-mouth is the best advertising" is true providing that the *word* is positive. You still need clients coming in to start the process, and you need new ones to continually build and increase your business.

Using Social Networking

Today's online marketing opportunities are endless and can provide a vast array of challenges as well. It is important that you use them wisely. As we know, there are message boards, Web sites with spa reviews, and social networking sites with open commentary where dialogue is exchanged. The comments may not be positive or true. Most of us are not able to spend countless hours tweeting or posting on Facebook. If you are, make sure that you avoid boxing yourself into a corner by badmouthing a competitor or responding to endless online chatter on line. It can degrade the level of professionalism of your business. Look at these opportunities as a chance to improve your image and to create awareness of your business. If your efforts do not achieve these goals, do not expect that they will help your practice. Do not ever put down another business or person online. It will be there forever.

A Poor Review

If you receive a poor review by a disgruntled "professional miserable," or from someone else, respond immediately for the entire world to see. Confronting this head on is the best remedy. That way, whoever is looking at the review will see that you are on top of your business. Furthermore, if you offer to give this person a free service or product, it will place you head and shoulders above the naysayer and demonstrate your extreme professionalism. Use the media to shine the light brightly on your business and practice. Have your own clients write your reviews. Contact editors of journals, industry magazines, and trade reviews to pitch editorials about your business. Write articles and give interviews to ethical companies interested in learning about your spa, salon, skin care center, or clinic. Offer to give a complimentary service or product to industry writers and affiliates. It is always advantageous to ask yourself this risk management question, "What will the exposure in this marketing tactic cost my business?"

If you can generally answer very little cost, with potential for high gain, it will guide your decisions on which techniques to employ and how much time to devote to the task.

Competition

Knowing who your competitors are is important. Make sure that you have a clear marketing message that is yours alone, and always be a professional competitor. Be fair when discussing competitors. You never know what the future may bring. A competitor may someday be a friend, a partner, or... your boss. Put a section in the business plan to do a **SWOT** analysis of your competition. This acronym stands for strengths, weaknesses, opportunities, and threats. It requires that you analyze each competitor, in each category, to determine what you would like to know about the competition and what you need to know in order to compete with them. To get really serious about SWOT-ing your competition, ask a college intern studying business to visit some of the local spas and salons and "mystery shop" for you. Have the student make an appointment, go in for a service, or purchase a product from the competitor just to see how the business treats their clients. You will obtain invaluable information, much beyond the actual dollars spent on a product or service. Keep in mind that the notes that you keep about your competitors may be viewed by friends, colleagues, and future employees of the business (some employees leave to go work for the competition; this also includes lenders, accountants, attorneys, etc., who may be friends). Always make them as positive as possible (Table 7–2).

SWOT
Is a business tool to use for analyzing one's competition. Often termed "SWOT" your business.

Operations

This section should provide a general overview of issues that are important to the success of running your business (such as the benefit of a location), illustrate your competitive edge (such as walk-in traffic at your storefront), and discuss how to mitigate issues.

Financials

The financials represent the basis of your business. Some experts will tell you that without financials in place, you should technically not be in business. We cannot make any decisions to purchase products and devices, market our business, hire employees, improve upon a Web site, or perform any other task. In short, without financial documents and statements we have no idea where we are, what we can do once we "get there," and, most importantly, where we go in the future.

projected income statement
A financial document that projects financial performance over a specified time frame.

Table 7–2 SWOT Your Competition

Name of SPA, Salon, Medical Facility, Skin Care Center	Strengths	Weaknesses	Opportunities	Threats
Competitor 1	Spa is new, looks fresh and inviting	On dead-end street, off the main path for foot traffic	Work together to refer clients back and forth	Clients like to try new venues
Competitor 2	Has medical focus offering injectables and laser services	Not very friendly	Partner and share clients, as they do not offer facials	Could hire more friendly staff, and become more of a threat
Competitor 3	Very good esthetician, well known, long time in community	Older facility, looks dated	Share an event or coop adverts	Could make space more upscale and look fresher, which may pull some clients in their direction
Competitor 4	Independent, one-person practice	Can only see so many clients a day	Connect and see if she may be willing to refer her overload to us (this does happen)	May add another practitioner
Competitor 5	Has many clients as offers motile service options and products	Has a mixture of services and product, no clear direction; very confusing as to what they do	May offer different services and products	May streamline practice and become more organized

© Milady, a part of Cengage Learning.

projected net income cash flow
A financial document that projects the amount of cash generated by a business during a specific time period.

profit and loss statement
A financial document that summarizes the revenues, cost and expenses incurred during a specific time frame.

balance sheet
A summary of a businesses assets, liabilities and the owner's equity.

Each document in the business plan serves as a directive for putting the pieces of your business story together. It systematically allows you the freedom to make decisions and determine how your business is working.

Include these financial documents in your business plan: a **projected income statement**, **projected net income cash flow**, **profit and loss statement**, and **balance sheet**. If you are starting a new enterprise, provide start-up costs, and create a source and use of funds document (Table 7–3), (Table 7–4), (Table 7–5), (Table 7–6).

Figure 7–6 is a sample business plan. It provides you with a context to develop your own or gives you ideas on how to adjust an existing one. The figures described in the report, the estimate costs, and all other materials are to be used for educational purposes and make no claim to profits/earnings or sales.

Table 7-3 Projected Income

Projected Income	Jan	Feb	Mar	Apr	May	Jun	Jul	Aug	Sep	Oct	Nov	Dec	Projected YTD
Treatments													
Average Price per Treatment	$ 130	$ 130	$ 130	$ 130	$ 130	$ 130	$ 130	$ 130	$ 130	$ 130	$ 130	$ 130	
Average # of Treatments	55 / 7,150	55 / 7,150	55 / 7,150	55 / 7,150	60 / 7,800	60 / 7,800	60 / 7,800	60 / 7,800	60 / 7,800	75 / 9,750	75 / 9,750	75 / 9,750	96,850
Products													
Average Price per Product	$ 40	$ 40	$ 40	$ 40	$ 40	$ 40	$ 40	$ 40	$ 40	$ 40	$ 40	$ 40	
Average # of Products Sold	25 / 1,000	25 / 1,000	25 / 1,000	30 / 1,200	20 / 800	35 / 1,400	35 / 1,400	25 / 1,000	20 / 800	30 / 1,200	20 / 800	40 / 1,600	13,200
Discounts Given	$ (100)	$ (100)	$ (150)	$ (200)	$ (250)	$ (200)	$ (200)	$ (250)	$ (250)	$ (300)	$ (250)	$ (250)	$ (2,500)
Returns & Allowances													
Average Price per Product	$ 50	$ 50	$ 50	$ 50	$ 50	$ 50	$ 50	$ 50	$ 50	$ 50	$ 50	$ 50	
Average # of Products Returned	2 / (100)	1 / (50)	3 / (150)	3 / (150)	2 / (100)	2 / (100)	2 / (100)	3 / (150)	2 / (100)	3 / (150)	2 / (100)	2 / (100)	(1,350)
Total Net Income	$7,950	$8,000	$7,850	$8,000	$8,250	$8,900	$8,900	$8,400	$8,250	$10,500	$10,200	$11,000	$106,200

Terrance Luke, Controller.

Table 7–4 Projected Net Income (Loss) and Cash Flow

	Jan	Feb	Mar	Apr	May	Jun	Jul	Aug	Sep	Oct	Nov	Dec	Projected YTD
Income													
Treatments	$7,150	$7,150	$7,150	$7,150	$7,800	$7,800	$7,800	$7,800	$7,800	$9,750	$9,750	$9,750	96,850
Products	1,000	1,000	1,000	1,200	800	1,400	1,400	1,000	800	1,200	800	1,600	13,200
Discounts Given	(100)	(100)	(150)	(200)	(250)	(200)	(200)	(250)	(250)	(300)	(250)	(250)	(2,500)
Returns and Allowances	(100)	(50)	(150)	(150)	(100)	(100)	(100)	(150)	(100)	(150)	(100)	(100)	(1,350)
Total Income	7,950	8,000	7,850	8,000	8,250	8,900	8,900	8,400	8,250	10,500	10,200	11,000	106,200
Cost of Goods Sold													
Treatments	715	715	715	715	780	780	780	780	780	975	975	975	9,685
Products	500	500	500	600	400	700	700	500	400	600	400	800	6,600
Total COGS	1,215	1,215	1,215	1,315	1,180	1,480	1,480	1,280	1,180	1,575	1,375	1,775	16,285
Gross Profits	6,735	6,785	6,635	6,685	7,070	7,420	7,420	7,120	7,070	8,925	8,825	9,225	89,915
Expenses													
Advertising and Marketing	250	250	250	250	250	250	250	250	250	250	250	250	3,000
Bank Fees	25	25	25	25	25	25	25	25	25	25	25	25	300
Business Licenses and Permits	40	40	40	40	40	40	40	40	40	40	40	40	480
Business Taxes	150	150	150	150	150	150	150	150	150	150	150	150	1,800
Credit Card Fees	163	163	163	167	172	184	184	176	172	219	211	227	2,201
Depreciation Expense	400	400	400	400	400	400	400	400	400	400	400	400	4,800
Education/Training	100	100	100	100	100	100	100	100	100	100	100	100	1,200
Finance Charges	-	-	-	-	-	-	-	-	-	-	-	-	-
Insurance	125	125	125	125	125	125	125	125	125	125	125	125	1,500
Internet Access/WEB Site Host	75	75	75	75	75	75	75	75	75	75	75	75	900
Legal and Accounting	100	100	100	100	100	100	100	100	100	100	100	100	1,200
Magazine Subscriptions	10	10	10	10	10	10	10	10	10	10	10	10	120

Terrance Luke, Controller.

													Total
Meals & Entertainment	50	50	50	50	50	50	50	50	50	50	50	50	600
Miscellaneous Expenses	25	25	25	25	25	25	25	25	25	25	25	25	300
Office Supplies	50	50	50	50	50	50	50	50	50	50	50	50	600
Wages	3,333	3,333	3,333	3,333	3,333	3,333	3,333	3,333	3,333	3,333	3,333	3,333	39,996
Payroll Taxes	333	333	333	333	333	333	333	333	333	333	333	333	4,000
Rent	1,100	1,100	1,100	1,100	1,100	1,100	1,100	1,100	1,100	1,100	1,100	1,100	13,200
Salon Supplies, Linen, Laundry	150	150	150	150	150	150	150	150	150	150	150	150	1,800
Telephone	50	50	50	50	50	50	50	50	50	50	50	50	600
Travel	50	50	50	50	50	50	50	50	50	50	50	50	600
Utilities	75	75	75	75	75	75	75	75	75	75	75	75	900
Total Operating Expenses	6,654	6,654	6,654	6,658	6,663	6,675	6,675	6,667	6,663	6,710	6,702	6,718	80,097
Operating Profit	81	131	(19)	27	407	745	745	453	407	2,215	2,123	2,507	9,818
Interest Income (Expense)	(50)	(50)	(50)	(50)	(50)	(50)	(50)	(50)	(50)	(50)	(50)	(50)	(600)
Net Profit Before Income Tax	31	81	(69)	(23)	357	695	695	403	357	2,165	2,073	2,457	9,218
Income Tax (estimated at 20%)	6	16			71	139	139	81	71	433	415	491	1,840
Net Profit After Income Tax	$ 25	$ 65	$ (69)	$ (23)	$ 285	$ 556	$ 556	$ 322	$ 285	$ 1,732	$ 1,658	$ 1,965	$ 7,356
Add Back Noncash Items													
Depreciation Expense	400	400	400	400	400	400	400	400	400	400	400	400	4,800
Projected Cash Flow	$ 425	$ 465	$ 331	$ 377	$ 685	$ 956	$ 956	$ 722	$ 685	$ 2,132	$ 2,058	$ 2,365	$ 12,156

271

Table 7-5 Serious Skin Care Profit and Loss Statement Jul-15

Income	
Treatments	$ 7,800
Products	$ 1,400
Discounts Given	$ (200)
Returns and Allowances	$ (100)
Total Income	8,900
Cost of Goods Sold	
Treatments	780
Products	700
Total COGS	1,480
Gross Profits	7,420
Expenses	
Advertising and Marketing	250
Bank Fees	25
Business Licenses and Permits	40
Business Taxes	150
Credit Card Fees	184
Depreciation Expense	400
Education/Training	100
Finance Charges	-
Insurance	125
Internet Access/Web Site Host	75
Legal and Accounting	100
Magazine Subscriptions	10
Meals & Entertainment	50
Miscellaneous Expenses	25
Office Supplies	50
Wages	3,333
Payroll Taxes	333
Rent	1,100
Salon Supplies, Linen, Laundry	150
Telephone	50
Travel	50
Utilities	75
Total Operating Expenses	6,675
Operating Profit	745
Interest Income (Expense)	(50)
Net Profit Before Income Tax	695
Income Tax (estimated at 20%)	139
Net Profit After Income Tax	$ 556

Terrance Luke, Controller.

Table 7–6 Serious Skin Care Balance Sheet As of July 31, 2015

Assets

Current Assets

Checking Account	$ 14,000
Savings Account	4,500
Accounts Receivable	800
Allowance for Bad Debt	(100)
Inventory	8,500
Total Current Assets	27,700

Fixed Assets

Furniture & Fixtures	5,000
Spa Equipment	20,000
Computer Equipment	3,500
Software	500
Leasehold Improvements	1,000
Accumulated Depreciation	(2,900)
Total Fixed Assets	27,100

Other Assets

Note Receivable	500
Total Other Assets	500
Total Assets	$ 55,300

Liabilities & Equity

Current Liabilities

Account Payable	$ 8,000
Payroll Tax Payable	207
Sales Tax Payable	200
Customer Deposits	500
Total Current Liabilities	8,907

Long Term Liabilities

Bank Loan	25,000
Total Long-Term Liabilities	25,000

Equity

Capital Stock	15,000
Retained Earnings	5,000
Year-to-Date Net Income	1,393
Total Equity	21,393
Total Liabilities and Equity	$ 55,300

Terrance Luke, Controller.

Business Plan for Serious Skin Care
Suzanne Martin and Merilee Morgan

Executive Summary
Serious Skin Care

Serious Skin Care is a skin care center that offers the latest cutting-edge technology and products for clients ranging from ages 14 to 70. It is located in Rose City, Oregon, where it targets clients from Portland, Cannon Beach, Lincoln City, and Seaside, Oregon. The owners, Suzanne Martin and Merilee Morgan, are both long-term licensed estheticians and licensed instructors with a large client base and a history in the region. They offer services for age management, acne, and sensitive/reactive skin types.

Mission/Vision

Serious Skin Care strives to provide excellence in comprehensive and compassionate, science-based skin care treatments, products, and client education to clients, the public, and students.

Serious Skin Care plans to expand and liaise with the local university. The university will develop a training center for esthetic professionals, which will offer services, products, and training for undergraduate esthetic students in the Pacific Northwest.

Products and Services

The business offers microdermabrasion, LED, microcurrent, oxygen therapy, chemical peels, and European facials. Serious Skin Care uses and retails a private label product line called Premiere Skin Care, formulated for the business by Private Label Manufacturing Inc. located in Bright City, Illinois. It contains cell and tissue support ingredients, antioxidants, and environmental protection. Private Label Manufacturing, Inc. is ISO certified, FDA registered and OTC licensed.

Competition

The general competition for Serious Skin Care is plentiful; however, there are no direct competitors. There are salons and spas on most corners of the downtown area, but none of them feature the more comprehensive services or higher-end products that our clientele is accustomed to using. This creates multiple opportunities for Serious Skin Care and for the future of our training enterprise as well. We will offer cutting-edge technology for training and will host e-learning classes as an outreach program to colleagues and learning institutions throughout the United States and the world.

Marketing Strategy

Serious Skin Care has a successful marketing plan, which includes an interactive Web site with questionnaires on skin types and conditions, an appointment reservation feature, a product-purchasing program, and a weekly one-minute podcast describing our latest specials. We plan to continue to network in strategic partnerships, such as local women's groups and services organizations, and to participate in fund-raising for local children's programs. We support cooperative

Figure 7–6 A sample business plan.

advertising annually and seasonally with local merchants by purchasing space on the Rose City Chamber of Commerce Web site. We plan to use social networking to build referral resources and networking connections with esthetic schools out of the area. We plan to team-teach classes with colleagues on various topics and will include advanced programs for professionals. We will offer an e-mail newsletter to clients, and students.

Operations

Serious Skin Care leases a space near the university that is a storefront location, which is excellent for foot traffic. Additionally, we will lease a space from the university for our esthetics training center and will use the store front as a real-life educational experience for students to transition to the marketplace.

Financials

The financial strategy of Serious Skin Care and the esthetics-training center will be to use reinvestment of income for growth during the initial setup phase of the training center. The training center will reach profitability within two years of operation. The annual projections for current year are $500,000; for year two, $600,000; and for year three, $750,000.

Source and Use of Funds

The business is currently seeking $150,000 in investment financing to expand and develop the training center. The funds will be used to acquire devices, hire new staff, and increase marketing plans.

Industry Analysis Information

The skin care industry is a multibillion-dollar industry and continues to grow annually by 6 to 8 percent. Spa goers and skin care supporters continue to spend money on treatments and products even during a downturned economy, as people have the desire to look and feel their best. Treatment and services have become shorter/abbreviated, making them more affordable, and salon and spa owners have purchased less expensive products. Some have gone to private label products to increase profitability.

Marketing Conditions

- Market size: Population 153,987, median age 33, average housed hold income $62,000
- Trends: There is a movement toward smaller communities from larger cities where services were plentiful. The demand for personal product and services is increasing, and the income base supports that notion. Additionally, the average age of these individuals moving to the community indicates that they will request product and services for many years to come.
- Target market: 30 to 65, 65 percent female, 30 percent male; with 5 percent teen clientele for acne services and products.

Rose City, Oregon, is an affluent community with a university and a technology sector that heavily supports the community. Trends have shown the population to be increasing by 8 percent annually. The average homebuyer spends $500,000 on real estate.

© Milady, a part of Cengage Learning.

Figure 7–6 Continued

Avoidance
A technique of risk management that involves taking steps to remove a risk completely, or choose an alternate route in business to reduce exposure to risks. One example would be eliminating a device that is not working consistently.

Reduction
A risk management technique that takes measures the reduce the potential of loss. An example might be removing a marketing piece that may make a false claim.

Retention
A risk management technique where the owner of a business assumes all of the risk rather than seeking outside help. This might be where a spa owner takes on the responsibility to replace a product or device if something goes wrong.

Transfer
A risk management technique where a business owner may transfer all if the risk to another party such as in purchasing an insurance policy.

RISK MANAGEMENT

According to www.entrepreneuer.com, risk management is: "Decisions to accept exposure or reduce vulnerabilities by either mitigating the risks or applying cost effective controls."

Accepted conventional views place risk management in four basic categories:

Avoidance: eliminating all potential risks

Reduction: reducing risks by employing measures that minimize potential risks

Retention: totally accepting risks

Transfer: shifting the risks to another body, such as by purchasing insurance and/or making contractual agreements, which ultimately makes other parties share in the risk.

MINIMIZE RISKS

We know that skin care and beauty professionals are truly a special group of people. Many have angel wings. Estheticians are naturally focused on and motivated by helping people. We tend to be visually oriented, tactile (*we touch people…* very few other professions do), sensitive, compassionate, empathetic, and intelligent multitaskers. We generally care about the health and well-being of others. Broadly speaking, we are still learning about the care and protection of ourselves, namely our exposure risks as practitioners and business owners.

When just a few of us were practicing, the rules seemed clear. One went to school, became licensed, obtained a job, and the employer often took care of the business details. If one opened a salon or skin care center, he or she followed the advice of well-meaning friends, family members, and maybe a banker if there was a need for a loan, and an insurance agent wrote a policy to insure the building or equipment. Back then, it was unheard of for licensees to have an accountant, a lawyer, a public relations/marketing professional, 5 to 10 manufacturers' sales representatives (most had one or two at the most), or other professionals to rely on regularly for support and advice. Our society was not as litigious then, and in general, one could earn a great living if you went to work every day and took good care of your clients.

As a general practice, we diligently complied with the essentials in business practices, not really knowing all of the ramifications of being underinsured and overexposed to unknown risks. The term "risk management" was not well known or understood.

Today, a myriad of issues have changed the business environment of estheticians, skin care specialists, or beauty professionals. With the

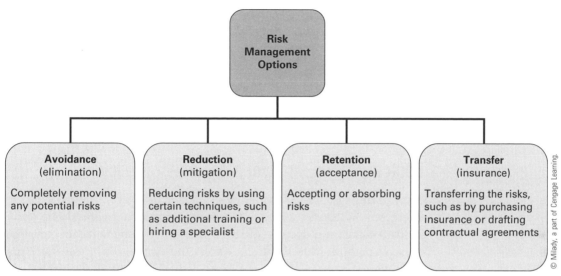

Figure 7–7 Risk management.

globalization in trade of goods and services, we are now all business people. Like it or not, we are in charge of our work–lifestyle pursuits and of managing our own risks, whether we are an employee or business owner. In this next section, we will look at the recommendations of risk management professionals for learning to reduce the likelihood of ending up in litigation, or for protecting our investment if we do how (Figure 7–7).

Obtain Professional and General Liability Insurance

Insurance professionals say that it may not be enough for an independent contractor to have **professional liability insurance** in the event that one is named individually in a claim. According to Samantha Tradelius of Strickler Insurance, in San Francisco, California, "If you are working for a salon as an independent contractor, leave the wax machine on, and a fire ensues, the salon owner's **general liability insurance** will cover the recovery expenses. However, the owner could ask you for expenses; these would be out of pocket if you do not have adequate coverage." Tradelius further states, "In addition to having professional liability insurance as an independent contractor, it is wise to have general liability insurance as well."

Documentation and Conventional Charting Methods

It is important to document any deviations from the normal protocol of a treatment or service. Moreover, **papering your file**, which means to

professional liability insurance
Insurance that protects a professional in business from litigation caused by charges of professional negligence or failure to perform professional duties.

general liability insurance
Comprehensive insurance that covers a business from unforeseen accidents and events with products and services.

papering your file
Clearly documenting in clients' files all visits and events.

include as much documentation as possible, is another recommendation that Samantha Tradelius of Strickler Insurance requires of her estheticians and skin therapist clients. Tradelius explains, "If a claim does occur against you, you can paint a picture for your defense with your documentation. Without it, you may be proven negligent." When making a claim, it is also necessary to show that you are following what is known as a **standard of care**. This means that you are following reasonable standard protocols, which may make a difference in whether a claim is paid.

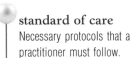

standard of care
Necessary protocols that a practitioner must follow.

Look at Your Employer's Insurance Policy

Katie Armitage, president of Associated Skin Care Professionals, in Evergreen, Colorado, states, "Many skin care professionals who work in spas, salons, and doctors' offices mistakenly believe that their employer's coverage protects them. However, the employer's policy may not cover you if you are individually named in a claim. It is unlikely to cover your court costs, legal expenses, and settlement fees. Review the employer's policy carefully and read the fine print, otherwise you are at risk." Armitage adds, "Employers often assume that their staff are protected because they don't fully understand their own insurance policy. One of our own staff members owned a small day spa and made this mistake. When she came to work for us and learned more about insurance, she dug deeper and discovered her staff were *not* covered. An employer might also forget a payment or fail to renew their policy, leaving staff at risk. Most often, an employer's policy will not cover you if you work in locations outside the business premises or offer services out of your home. Some treatments or techniques that you provide may not be covered by the employer's policy. If something goes wrong and you find out too late that your employer's insurance doesn't cover you, guess who's responsible for those costs? You are."

Add a Client Waiver Statement

Often our clients become like family members or friends. We tend to become *laissez-faire* in some of these instances. If you go ahead and perform a treatment or service, the client may not see the referral that you are making as important or as necessary. They see us as the expert. They believe that if we really thought something was wrong, we would know for sure what it is. It may not occur to them that many skin issues are below the surface entirely, and that in some cases, applying a service or treatment may even mask a lesion. Or lesions may recede for a time, such as in **actinic keratosis**, or others. You need to reschedule the treatment until a dermatologist or a qualified health care

actinic keratosis
Lesions created by UV exposure that are often dry and flaky; can be precancerous.

professional has seen the client and make sure that you have confirmation of that visit to place in his or her file or chart.

Good Risk Management Measures

- Do not publicize or tell a client that you have professional and/or general liability insurance. This gives unprincipled, scheming-types *free rein* to your insurance capital. Experts say it does not matter how well you may know an individual, it is best not to share your insurance coverage or any business information that may potentially be a risk management issue.
- While doing business out of the United States, make sure that you have systems in place to safeguard your products, equipment, and transactions. You need to have a monitoring body, which is responsible for keeping your products and services safe, environmentally sound, reliable, efficient, and cost-effective.
- Make sure that your equipment is in good repair. Inspect it as a routine practice. If a device is not working properly, get it in for repair as soon as possible. Also, look for unexpected risk management issues, or sleepers, that can become a problem, such as the treatment bed or a chair on wheels. Remember that these items have brake features.
- Obtain and use protocol home care compliance documents. This means that you have done your part to make sure that your clients are using their home care products correctly. This becomes especially important if the client is preparing for a surgical procedure. Always put a signed copy in the client's chart.
- Attend continuing educational events and workshops. As skin care professionals, it is our responsibility to make sure that we remain qualified to use the equipment, peels, and/or other devices that we apply to a client. For example, do not assume that a peel that you have used for years has not been through some changes. Ask for updates on MSDS sheets as well.

OWNER RISK MANAGEMENT CONSIDERATIONS

Along with the countless details that an owner of spa, clinic, salon, or other skin care facility has to manage, it is necessary to put in place a very proactive and transparent risk management program that may involve multiple layers. Here are a few unconventional risk management techniques for the forward-thinking entrepreneurial business owner.

Remain Detached

This sounds like something out of a new age catalogue; however, we have all made emotional decisions about our businesses because we somehow believe it is our "baby." But sometimes a business needs to grow up! Get outside help if you find that you are not objective about your business. Local, small-business development centers often offer this support for free, and can offer advice on how to minimize risks on everything from financial matters to having employees sign non-compete agreements. The more impartial we can be about our business, the more precise our decisions will be in providing for its longevity.

Trust Your "Gut-Level" Feelings

We often can look back at a circumstance or incident that created a business or personnel problem, and recall something that just did not feel right. It is important to trust our intuition. For many, intuition, or that "sixth-sense," offers a direct link to risk management by keeping us "awake," thus diverting a mishap.

Bring in a Qualified Mediator

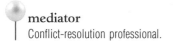

mediator
Conflict-resolution professional.

Sometimes we just "hit the wall" with someone, and our plight in conflict resolution drifts away. Maybe the situation has become too hurtful or depressing to deal with effectively. These are both good reasons to hire a **mediator** to help resolve a dispute. Sometimes it can be a lengthy proposition, but it might be money well spent in the long run. Through the process, you may discover unhealthy patterns repeating within your operations that are crying for a "call to action." It can be difficult to look at our own shortcomings, but it is necessary.

Purchase Liability Insurance for Your Equipment

You may find that while your waxing services, microdermabrasion, and chemical peels are covered, permanent cosmetic applications or electrolysis may not be. Check with your state laws, rules, and regulations in order to remain compliant and official. Due diligence goes a long way to avoid expensive course corrections.

Risk Management for Product and Equipment Manufacturers

If you own or work for a skin care manufacturing company, here are some key suggestions as an overview to spa/salon product and equipment manufacturers. Many of these ideas could be carried over to anyone in business where products and equipment are being developed.

- **Product labels and instructions for use.** These should be periodically reviewed by legal counsel to ensure accuracy, FDA compliance, and ease of understanding (for the consumers).
- **Insurance from suppliers.** Obtain evidence of product liability insurance from all suppliers. David Suzuki, president of Bio-Therapeutic, Inc. states, "Evidence of product liability is standard practice for reputable manufacturers. Furthermore, you should inquire about **ISO (International Organization for Standardization)** and **CSA (Canadian Standard Association)** certifications. These prestigious certifications ensure you are dealing with a company who takes safety, consistency, and quality seriously."
- **Independent testing.** Quality control is a critical issue for all manufacturers and distributors. Where possible, periodic independent testing/certification is a great idea.
- **Batch number.** Charles Stevens, program division manager for Marine Agency Corporation, Maplewood, NJ, states that batch numbering products according to production line and date is important, and that the batch numbers should be tied to sales information in order to facilitate an expedient recall if necessary

ISO (International Organization for Standardization)
Organization that develops standards for businesses and industries worldwide.

independent testing
Testing performed by a third party or someone other than the developer of a product.

TYPES OF INSURANCE COVERAGE

- **General liability** includes product liability coverage, which covers lawsuits arising out of the operations of a business
- **Property coverage** includes buildings (if owned) and contents, including furnishings/fixtures, supplies, and inventory
- **Business interruption and extra expense coverage** covers loss of income following a covered loss (like a fire)
- **Workers' compensation** covers on-the-job injuries and disease

property coverage
Insurance that protects the physical property and equipment of a business against loss from theft, fire, or other perils.

Worker's compensation
System of insurance that reimburses an employer for damages that must be paid to an employee for injury occurring in the course of employment.

Hidden Risk Management Issues

There can be unique or hidden risk management issues that rarely come up, such as product recalls from a company in your primary product line. Or maybe you have an employee who has also been a long-term friend; she experiences an unfavorable encounter with someone within your business and decides to press charges unexpectedly. It is best to make sure that you have the most comprehensive policy possible. Here are a few situations for which you want to be prepared should you need help:

- Product recalls can be very expensive and are not automatically covered under a general liability/product liability policy. Separate coverage may be available.
- Employment practice suits (sexual harassment, wrongful termination, hostile work environment, etc.) usually come without warning. Defending a single suit (even if groundless) can cost $25,000 or more in legal fees. Separate coverage called **employment practices liability insurance (EPL or EPLI)** is available to protect employers from employees' claims.
- A crisis management and disaster recovery plan should be included in your overall risk management plans. Businesses should plan ahead for all possible contingencies, including everything from incidents of workplace violence, product recalls, and temporary locations (and emergency supplies/inventory) following a property loss.

employment practices liability insurance (EPL or EPLI)

EPL or EPLI is a type of insurance that provides protection for an employer against claims made by employees, former employees or potential employees.

RISK MANAGEMENT IN MARKETING

Janet D'Angelo, president of J. Angel Communications, a marketing and public relations company based in Scituate, MA, is the author of *Spa Business Strategies: A Plan for Success* (Milady Publishing). D'Angelo has many useful tips for new and existing businesses engaging in the practice of marketing and advertising. She states, "When it comes to marketing, creating a name and logo is the first order of business in branding a salon or spa's identity. This is a task that most spa owners take great pride in, but it is important for small business owners to understand the legalities involved. This generally includes registering your business name at both the state and local levels. You should also check with the U.S. Patent and Trademark office to be sure you are not infringing upon the trademark rights of another business. Unwittingly, copying the design or name of another business can get you into trouble even if that other business has not registered a trademark. All of this can be confusing to the new business owner, so it is always best to seek expert legal advice in these matters."

D'Angelo has more advice for spa owners, "Spa owners should also be aware of any restrictions or requirements when it comes to advertising name brand products and patented techniques. Most manufacturers and developers are eager to showcase their products and are often happy to support you in your efforts; however, when it comes to representing their wares they may require the use of certain trademark symbols and/or language. Marketing professionals take extra care to research these facts before placing them in media outlets. If you are creating your own advertising materials or relying on media personnel to create a design, be sure to investigate these important items yourself. While media representatives are often happy to assist you in creating an ad, the ultimate responsibility for content is yours."

 ## SEEK GOOD COUNSEL

It is important to have a diverse and comprehensive support team of other professionals. These should be people with whom you can have a confidential discussion. They should be current on rules and regulations, laws, procedures, and education. Some topics are better discussed with a paid professional, over the phone or in their office, rather than in a last-minute panic with a friend.

Insurance is one of these topics. Policies can be confusing to review on your own, so it's always a good idea to have a qualified insurance agent/broker or attorney assist you. Make sure that you have the best resources in front of you for conversations involving a potential liability. Debbie Higdon of Associated Skin Care Professionals in Evergreen, CO, serves in risk management and says, "I'm often the first person a skin care professional talks with if a claim is made, and I can hear the anxiety in their voice, even if they don't believe the claim has merit. Having someone to turn to is so important to them. They are always so relieved to have the matter settled."

There is nothing like having a calm, well-trained professional at the other end of the phone when you need advice.

 ## LOOK WITHIN

Having an emotional safety net in place for support is invaluable with the busy lives that we lead today. It is imperative that we have people around us who care for and support us as individuals. If you feel at risk personally, it is vital to enlist the help of a good therapist or mental health specialist to work through difficult issues. Risk management issues can crop up for people who have experienced a loss of confidence. Perhaps a domestic issue, or another personal problem, may be affecting the way we are functioning on the job, thus lowering our ability to concentrate or perform well. Knowing yourself and when to reach for help is good business.

Looking at the Big Picture

Every skin care professional knows that the pulse of his or her practice revolves around the caring of their clients. We develop relationships with clients and to our work, which supports us on many levels. It is rare that we incur problems; however, we must anticipate unforeseen events by being stewards not only to ourselves, but to our profession. Once risk management systems are in place and are reevaluated on a continual basis, it becomes more an issue of practice management.

SUMMING IT UP

Working in or owning a salon, spa, skin care center, or esthetic medical clinic can be an extremely rewarding business pursuit, from every angle. It is very exciting to be at the helm of running a business or to be support anywhere along the line; it is also vital to make sure that you have a well thought-out plan to thrive and exceed in your endeavor year after year. As part of the business culture, you must take good care of yourself, your coworkers, staff members, and clients while employing good business practices. Issues do arise, and you want to be able to mitigate the challenges as best as you can. Having a business plan will help you do just that, as it will provide you with the necessary road map to success. Here are a few details to keep in mind while building your business plan:

- **Use images, graphics, bullet points, white space, and numbers for impact makers.** Give the reader some diversity in the text (this includes staff members, employers, yourself, lenders, attorneys, and accountants) by making it clear, easy to read, and engaging. Review and rework the plan regularly.
- **Keep it short**. A business plan need only be approximately 20 pages. Some sections will be used more frequently than others. Keep in mind that if you are obtaining financial support from a bank or lending institution, you will need to be concise and be able to prove that there is a market for your services.
- **Make sure that the financials are realistic.** It is important to set forth reasonable goals in your plan, not only to obtain financial backing, but for your income and the sustainability of the business. It is best to explore all of the financial configurations prior to meeting with a lender.
- **Watch a tendency to self-promote**. This can be confusing. On one hand, we need to present ourselves as confident and assertive. On the other, we must be aware that lenders will suspect us of

embellishment if during important meetings we continually discuss how wonderful we are and how our services and products are the best ones on the market.

- **Look at risk management from all angles.** Make sure to have the professional liability insurance that you need. Go beyond what you might be able to imagine. Find an insurance representative that you can relate to and speak frankly with. You will need to trust his or her willingness to help you with your practice. The agent will help you navigate the probability of and potential exposure to issues that you may not even want to think about, but must.

ESTHETICIAN **PROFILE**

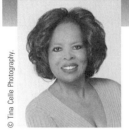

© Tina Celle Photography.

Pamela Springer, LA
Owner, Global Skin Solutions

Product Developer, Author, and Speaker

I am Pamela R. Springer, founder of The Skin & Makeup Institute of Arizona and the Academy of Advanced Aesthetics and Permanent Cosmetics. I am the product developer of Global Skin Solutions, a corrective skin care line for Global skin tones 3 to 6 and author of *Natural Radiance, A Guide for Ethnic Skin Care*.

I am originally from Boston, MA. My journey, as an adult, began in Northern California's Bay area in 1973. My entrepreneurial spirit became evident after I moved to Los Angeles in 1975 to discover my purpose. As a plus-size woman, I modeled for fashion magazines, and eventually became an image consultant for this market. Because it was such an untapped market, I built a successful brand as Pamela Springer, The Image Maker, appearing on national talk shows, and hosting my own television show, *Full Dimensions* on the Fashion Channel, which is now QVC. I began producing fashion shows in the Southwest and Western regions of the United States for the plus-size departments of major retail stores (Nordstrom, Bullocks, Saks Fifth Ave, Macys and the now defunct Robinson's, May Company and Broadway).

I established a production company called Rich-In-Body Productions, which allowed me to create special events for major shopping centers throughout Northern and Southern California. Unfortunately, after almost 20 years of building a successful brand, I lost my business due to the recession in 1993. In October 1994, I packed what was necessary and moved to Scottsdale, Arizona.

Training

I enrolled in Carsten Aveda Institute, and received my aesthetics license in1995.

Because of my interest in the clinical areas of aesthetics, immediately after getting out of school, I interned for six months with a plastic surgeon. In 1996, I was given the opportunity to intern with a dermatologist who specialized in ethnic skin. At that time, she was an assistant professor of dermatology at the Charles Drew Medical School in Los Angeles. This school is one of the few black medical schools in the United States. Her in-depth training and mentoring allowed me to provide services and education for another untapped market, ethnic skins. I wanted to have my own business, so I leased a small room at a hair salon in Scottsdale. After four years, I opened a skin care center employing two aestheticians, a natural nail tech, and a massage therapist.

Because of the success of using Jessner's solutions on ethnic skin, Doctor's Dermatologic Formula (DDF) hired me as an educator to train aestheticians in peeling techniques for ethnic skins at aesthetic trade shows. This led me to launch The Skin & Makeup Institute of Arizona in 2000, which is a facility that trains aestheticians on advanced treatments using peeling agents and offers a program called "Practice of Aesthetics in a Medical Office." In 2002, the Institute became licensed by Arizona State Board of Cosmetology.

Practice Demographic

I treat all ages and skin types in clinical treatments for pigmentation anomalies, acne, and aging skins. I specialize in the corrective treatments for skin types 3 to 6.

Services/Treatments Offered

Global Skin Solutions's tagline is "We believe every skin deserves to be flawless!" I take this statement to heart and passionately deliver results for a market that has been overlooked. There are many myths about pigmented skins that limit clinicians from understanding how to "tweak" certain treatments to get optimum results. With a tweaked treatment intervention, clinicians have the ability to uncover the ethnic skin's natural radiance.

Personal Philosophy

I have enjoyed the challenges and rewards of specializing in skin types 3 to 6 for approximately 15 years. My work has given me the opportunity to travel, educate, and have my voice heard. I write articles for industry magazines, appear on local radio and television stations, and have numerous speaking opportunities for a variety of organizations. I have enjoyed the opportunity to develop a corrective product line for this special market.

Launching Global Skin Solutions has allowed me to establish a voice in the skin care community. The enthusiasm and openness of skin care professionals across the country have afforded me the opportunity to slowly recover from this economy. The institute that I founded

over 11 years ago has been at its all-time high since 2009. Our student spa services have increased for both our day and evening hours. In 2011, the institute also received the honor of being named number one in *New Beauty* magazine's Five-Star Beauty Destination program, which recognizes the country's most elegant and extraordinary beauty destinations.

Additional Contributions to the Industry

Our "Don't Be Afraid of the Dark" series is a forum used to educate the general population of skin care professionals. We conduct workshops, presentations, speaking engagements, webinars, and write articles. The Academy of Advanced Aesthetics and Permanent Makeup (AAAPC), a subsidiary of the institute, is licensed by the postsecondary licensing board and conducts ongoing advanced classes and programs for clinical technicians in advanced protocols for chemical peels, microdermabrasion, dermaplaning, skin needling, laser training, and LED, and offers training in certifying permanent makeup technicians.

I am or have been involved with the following industry-related organizations:

- National Aesthetic Spa Network (NASN)—Arizona director
- Associated Skin Care Professionals—member
- American Association of Cosmetology Schools—member
- Board of Trustees for the Arizona Theatre Company—secretary and former board member
- Greenway Medical & Professional Association—former president
- Black Board of Directors Project—member
- American Heart Association—former board member
- Arizona State Board of Cosmetology—former member (appointed by former Arizona Governor Janet Napolitano; I was the first aesthetician to receive this honor)

My writing encompasses beauty advice columns for national women's publications, and serving as a contributing author for the industry magazines *Les Nouvelles Esthetiques, Beauty Link,* and *Skin Deep.*

ESTHETICIAN **PROFILE**

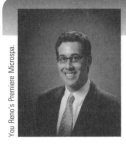

You Reno's Premiere Microspa.

Alex Leeder, LE
Owner, You Micro Spa

Reno, Nevada

Born in New Jersey, and I later moved to Reno, Nevada, where I attended high school and college. During college, I worked with various cosmetic lines retailing skin care and makeup and learned to love the innovation and ingredient technologies that skin care offered. I took my time completing my college studies, first at the University of Nevada, Reno; then at San Francisco State University; University of Massachusetts at Amherst; and finally Humboldt State University in Northern California. Each year (and at each location!), I worked as a makeup artist for Sonya Pugh with Sebastian Cosmetics of Manhattan Beach, CA. I also worked with Premiere Collection Cosmetics (owned by Colleen Moon), and in retail for Sue Santsche at Personal Choice Skin Care Center & Spa in Eureka, CA. These three women were my early mentors and defined my philosophy of client care and service.

Training
My initial training prompted my attendance at Northern Nevada Beauty Academy, a local beauty school, and my graduation from the Paris Beauty College where I learned the traditional French facial.

I worked as a licensed aesthetician with Kimberly Kolar, MD, who further solidified my skills in protecting and maintaining the health of the skin. I was the founding manager of Aesthetic Services at Skin Cancer & Dermatology Institute in Carson City and Reno. I was responsible for managing cosmetic dermatology patient services and dermatopathology records and provided chemexfoliation facials and skin cancer surgery-assist to Dr. Kolar. I served as the editor of Skin Sense, a series of featured articles in the *Nevada Appeal,* a Carson City, Nevada, newspaper.

I continued studying postgraduate master aesthetics with Douglas Preston, and was personally tutored in Hungarian cleansing techniques by Eva Claiborne of Euro-Skin. Each of these mentors enabled me to take the leap into my private practice.

Services Offered
I maintain dual licensing in California and Nevada and continue to enjoy my own skin care practice and private label skin care line servicing clients from the greater Truckee Meadows. My very first clients, Phyllis Williams, Florence Suenaga, Martha Berger, Diane Schnaser, Laurie Newmark, Juanita Ydiando, and Michele McGarraugh, continue to enjoy superior skin care after 14 years of regular facial care. Each has been a valuable client and our relationships have strengthened over time, and with my improved skills and experience.

My signature skin care techniques are a blend of Western therapies with Eastern philosophies. I am a Reiki master specializing in the traditional French facial with a Hungarian cleanse. I earned my IDI postgraduate diploma and am certified in Face Mapping, Successful Acne Care and European skin care techniques, and in Chinese acupressure. I have trained with Narendra Mehta in Indian Champissage, which is a massage of the head, shoulders, and neck. I am also certified in the thermal healing of LaStone, an incredibly relaxing treatment using heated and cooled stones to increase circulation and balance body energy.

Client Demographics
The current demographics for my skin care center skew 70 percent female and 30 percent male; ages range from 8 to 94, with most clients between 40 and 70 years of age. Most clients want to minimize signs of premature aging and reduce the likelihood of "break outs." I specialize in expert eyebrow design for men and women (the age range is 20 to 50); 20 percent of my income is derived from this waxing service. Over the past four years, I developed a complete and relaxing body treatment service called the "Wake Up Refreshed!"

(90 min/$125), and this service now accounts for 40 percent of my total annual income.

Contributions to the Esthetics Industry and Beyond

I serve as vice chair on the Nevada State Board of Cosmetology, having received my commission from Governor Kenny Guinn and my reappointment from Governor Jim Gibbons. I am a nationally recognized, award-winning spa business manager certified by the International Dermal Institute and Dermalogica, a world choice professional skin care product. I also worked as a multidisciplinary arts agency director and am an honorary board trustee of the Sierra Arts Foundation. I developed AMS, Artists' Management Services, and offer expert technical support to local artists, businesses, nonprofits, and regional arts organizations, as well as HOPE (Helping Other People Everyday), certified mediation confidential facilitation.

Products and Positioning Products in Your Business

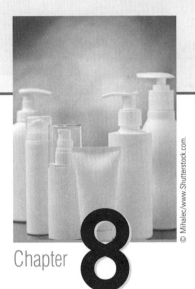

Chapter **8**

> "It is imperative that we educate our clients and send them home with the appropriate products and home care technology if we truly expect to meet our objective and satisfy our customers."
>
> *—David Suzuki, President, Bio-Therapeutic*

Chapter Capture

After completing this chapter, you will be able to:

- Choose professional products for your practice.
- Decide on a single product line.
- Work with multiple product lines.
- Conduct business with private-label products.
- Buy and sell generic private-label products.
- Work with physician-exclusive products.

PRODUCT SELECTION AND APPLICATIONS

Products are the foundation of our business. A wise old esthetician once said, "If you do not have products to sell, you do not have an esthetics practice." Practitioners need to anchor their business with excellent products that support the services that they provide. We can do a beautiful job on a treatment only to find that the client goes home to use products with waxes and comedogenic ingredients that diminish our efforts, and wastes the money and time that they spent with us. We need to educate them on why we have recommended specific products to them, and to determine their willingness to be compliant in using them. Whether we imbed the cost of the product into our treatment series prices, or sell them out right, clients must follow our protocols and use skin-type- and condition-appropriate home care in order to achieve the results that we know are possible. Clients must be compliant (Figure 8–1).

Compliance and the Esthetician

Compliance also means that we must follow our own protocols and standards as estheticians. As we know, offering tanning services and then selling the client a high-level AHA product is counterproductive and dangerous for the client. Better to spend that time educating the client on the benefits of not using tanning devices and offering a product with SPF, antioxidants, cell protectants, and antiglycation benefits.

Another important aspect of compliance, which enters into the realm of ethics, is not to recommend a product simply because we

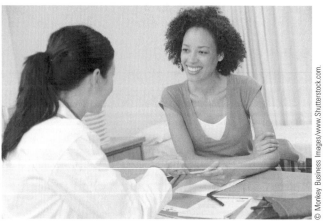

Figure 8–1 Clinical esthetician going over protocols.

GUEST SPOT

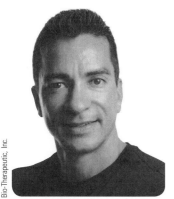

Bio-Therapeutic, Inc.

DAVID SUZUKI, PRESIDENT OF BIO-THERAPEUTIC, INC.

As skin therapists, our objective is clear: to create and maintain beautiful skin. We achieve this through our services, the use of well-designed technology, and our knowledge, experience, and intuition. However, our job is not finished the moment our clients are out of our sight. On the contrary, this is where the work begins. Even the most diligent clients typically have only one facial every four weeks. That means that they are treating their own skin nearly 100 times in between every one of our professional services. So it is imperative that we educate our clients and send them home with the appropriate products and home care technology if we truly expect to meet our objective and satisfy our customers.

Our clients are inundated with information on skin care products, and it is hard to avoid ending up with a collection of miscellaneous products, brands, and concepts. As with vitamins, we know just enough to understand that they are good for us and that we should take them, and as a result, we collect them—literally. It is also our job to make our clients understand that beautiful skin is a lifestyle that must be attended to every day! Remember that we are their coach, not miracle workers.

---

have it on the shelf. Rather, we must offer our clients the right choice or wait for a more appropriate product to arrive. In the end, products that we should not have recommended in the first place often end up as returns, so we have gained nothing and may even have lost a little credibility. As diligent as we are, however, on occasion, we might run out of a product. We can always give out samples to hold clients over until our order arrives. Many of us have found that it is important to have a safety net of an emergency stock of our best-selling products kept in a location separate from our "live merchandise." Do not dip into these emergency supplies except to take inventory and rotate stock to keep ahead of expiration dates. Some estheticians have cultivated good referral relationships with other estheticians in their community and can help each other out in a bind by selling products to each other either at cost or at retail and then selling them to their clients. While we would not want to make a habit out of doing this—as you may lose your business to them—it may work in some circumstances.

When you have a long-term client and client retention and satisfaction are at the top of your priority list, the decision to provide a product is simple. Knowing that you have built trust with clients, and spent time and energy telling them why they need this product in the first place, it is always best to provide the best for them at every opportunity.

Anticipate Retail Needs

In the big picture however, it is best to stay ahead of low stock issues by diligently keeping track of inventory and ordering ahead. Keep in mind that manufacturers may cause delays and make changes to products. They may be waiting for an exotic ingredient, be forced to recall a product, or, as in many cases today, discontinue a product that has been a low performer for them (even though it may have been your best seller).

Clients, Product Selection, and Home Care Compliance

Client selection is as important as product selection. You want clients to be compliant, and it is important to assess their compliance level when you take them on. Do they follow instructions? Are they using protocols now with their home care or do they omit the nighttime regimen on a regular basis? Find out. We can perform a fantastic service for our client, and find it squandered when they pick up and use a product that counteracts the effects of our session. The message here is that you must know your client. We all have examples of clients who used products recommended by a well-meaning friend that turned out to be the culprit in acne outbreaks. Other products impair barrier functions (such as a pH that is too high or too low), causing a caustic reaction and further irritation, which exacerbate the very condition we are working to remedy. Many of us have had clients who have been on a great peel series, and then through self-referral, pick up an OTC peeling product that they believe will accelerate the work you are doing, only to find that they must postpone the next peel in the series due to irritation and sensitivity. The trust that is required in our relationship with our clients works both ways. They must trust us and follow our recommendations, and we need to make realistic, plausible plans for them to follow. The truth is that client and product selection, along with product use, matter.

PROFESSIONAL PRODUCTS

As one of the most exciting business ventures on the planet, esthetics continues to produce and delight us not only with advancements in technology annually, monthly, weekly, and nearly daily, but also by giving us various options for products and product ingredient technology (Figure 8–2).

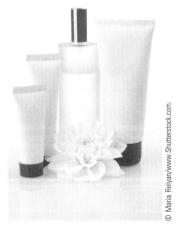

Figure 8–2 Professional products.

© Maria Relyan/www.Shutterstock.com.

There is not an esthetician among us who is not eager to see the newest products on the market. We know exactly what the electronics and computer industries experience when new products are revealed to the consumer. It becomes the topic of conversation among users, and creates a strong desire to buy the product. As skin care professionals, we deal with technology in our work, as well as beauty, fitness, and well-being. All these aspects are layered in the tightly woven, sometimes misunderstood industry of skin care. We continue to be an emerging industry, with opportunities for growth; there seem to no end to the innovation. It is exciting indeed. It is a powerful position to be in an industry that is advancing technologically and that has enjoyed a solid, strong past. If history is the best predictor of what is to come, our future is bright. Even during lean economic periods, skin care products will continue to dominate the market share of personal care products, as we now have a multibillion dollar, global industry.

There are many options for offering products. It is necessary to know your market, select a quality product line, and make certain that your line fits your needs. We next will explore the benefits, challenges, and solutions involved in the various options in product selection.

THE SINGLE PRODUCT LINE

Carrying a single product line has been a protocol for many estheticians over time. For some, it serves as only a starting point. There are advantages and challenges in carrying one product line. These are explored below (Figure 8–3).

The Benefits of Offering a Single Product Line

For a spa, salon, skin care center, or clinic to offer a single line is often the best option. This is particularly true if there is a specific line that covers the needs of the client base and the business's need to consolidate information and keep a tight control on training and inventory. Furthermore, it can be the best option if the business has selected a high-profile line with a presence in the marketplace via advertising, and a generous sampling program. It can also be helpful during the expansion of a newer business, where trainers are available for routine in-service training of the staff, or offer regular online courses. A single product line may be the best option when staff members are enthusiastic and eager to learn, younger, yet new to the business—or when the business is run by a sole esthetician.

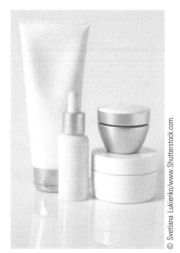

Figure 8–3 A single product line.

© Svetlana Lukienko/www.Shutterstock.com.

The Challenges in Carrying a Single Line

Clients and personnel may become bored with a one-choice option. If a client has allergies to the line that you carry, it may preclude them from making purchases and later fuel a decision to look elsewhere for products and services. Also, many veteran estheticians have the perception that one line cannot do it all. If you have talented and seasoned esthetic personnel, with experience and knowledge of ingredients, delivery systems and exposure to multiple product lines, they may have some buried secrets worth pulling up for discussion.

If a product company is happy with its product line up and has not made changes for decades, it may look as though the company is dated or not on the cutting-edge of technology. If a product line has been oversold in your neighborhood, it may not be the best line for you if you are not a "me too" type of salon, spa, skin care center, or medical-spa. Many businesses will try to steal clients from a good solid business by copying what has been successful. Watch for a product company that saturates an area with its brand.

Ways to Successfully Carry a Single Product Line

Adding an additional line may provide the diversity that you need without removing the focus from your primary line. A second line might be one that does not compete with the primary line. For example, it could be a specific, targeted line that is strictly organic or "green" in nature or a smaller age-management line with stronger performance ingredients than the primary line. Naturally, you would want to select a line that aligns with your mission/vision statements and philosophical beliefs and value system. There are many great lines available to support your core positions.

If you are not interested in carrying a small supplemental line and wish to create excitement for a primary single line, merchandise often and create multiple vignettes throughout your space. In a boutique-style display, place products for body, eye care, or age management together. Place antioxidants and environmental protection products in the middle of every display. Make a strong statement by using shelf talkers and images of people next to each cluster of products. Work with vendors on obtaining marketing materials that you can change often to keep movement and action in the product line.

MULTIPLE PRODUCT LINES

Carrying multiple product lines is often the cumulative effect of a practitioner having been in practice for some time. Esthetic professionals may start with one line and then add another when they find that they need something new or want to round out options for their clients. There are benefits and challenges in carrying multiple product lines (Figure 8–4).

The Benefits of Offering Multiple Product Lines

Many of us have successfully risen to the challenge of carrying multiple lines. However, it requires diligence, knowledge of products on the market, awareness of your target market profiles (acne, age-management, men), and a great enthusiasm for buying and selling.

One of the greatest benefits of offering multiple options is that you always have a product for your clients and a direction in which to move them. Whether they are working in makeup, hair, clothing, or home décor, great stylists and designers know they need to coach their clients toward the best that they can be. As we know, clients today become very restless, particularly those without skin conditions that prohibit sampling a variety of products. They love receiving the many benefits that a wonderful esthetician brings to their life, including sampling something new. Our clients are exposed to many options while online or out shopping, or in the recommendations they receive from well-meaning friends and colleagues. If they see us as a cutting-edge skin health coach, they are likely to be faithful to us. Many clients want to retain the skin health that they have, but more want to see continual improvements as well.

Another benefit of carrying multiple lines is that it demonstrates that you are well versed in what is available in the market. It shows that you are current and savvy about trends. There is a presumption that you follow continuing educational programs too. By demonstrating the various products available in your salon, spa, or skin care center, you show that you believe in the use of products. It is also advisable to offer makeup to clients too. If clients go back to work after a service (which most do), it is a good business practice to select the product that they put on their freshly treated skin, whether you apply it for them or not. Mineral powders are the best posttreatment or service choices. Make certain that you choose professional products that contain ingredients that are healthy for the skin (Figure 8–5).

The Challenges in Carrying Multiple Product Lines

Inventory becomes of paramount importance whether you are a solo provider or a team of many. You do not want too much product taking

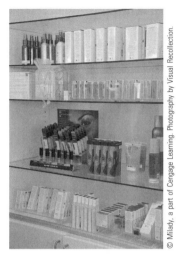

Figure 8–4 Multiple product lines.

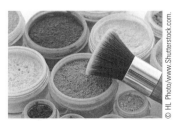

Figure 8–5 Mineral makeup.

up the real estate on the shelf; however, if you are routinely out of a favorite product, clients may become frustrated waiting for it to arrive. In the new economy, we have all been subject to fewer supplies on the shelf and fluctuations in demand. If there has ever been a time where patience has been practiced equally by practitioners, product companies, and clients, it is now.

Another challenge in carrying multiple lines is that you must stay on top of all of the product indications and ingredients. This can be a full-time job. Ingredients can vary slightly: one supplier may use an ingredient for a humectant, for example, and another uses it as a binder. Ingredients may serve different functions depending upon what the supplier chooses and needs in order to build the formula. Clients want to know that we are committed to providing information about what the product contains, what the product benefits are, and that the formula is the best choice for their skin.

Challenges in Training with Multiple Product Lines

Training other staff members on multiple product lines can be demanding. If your team includes multiple estheticians, a receptionist, or a medical assistant and a nurse, you will need to train them on the products so that you can provide a united front when it comes to conveying information to the client or patient.

Ways to Successfully Manage Multiple Product Lines

Work with companies that supply you with good, solid information about their products. It will save you time if they can provide quick selling tips. This does not need to be an exhaustive or extensive list: five to seven bullet points that are intelligently and strategically drafted are easy to memorize, train from, and share with the client. Sharing product ingredient benefits is a good idea as long as it does not take up too much time and/or is so complex that you to lose the client in the translation. Even the most well-informed skin care aficionado, who travels the world, will have limitations on what he or she wants to know when listening to a product orientation. Allow clients to ask questions along the way—this helps engage them and helps you focus your presentation.

As a confidence builder for the new client, have an idea of what you might recommend. While you greet the client and are handing him or her the intake form, begin to think about which product line is the best for the client's needs. Further, while you are going through your consultation and skin analysis, your assessment develops the plan for the product you will choose for your client.

Inventory and Training

As a solo practitioner, you will have a good idea of what products you are running low on. Even still, take 15 to 20 minutes every day to do a quick count on fast-selling products. Keep a running list of what needs to be reordered. If you have staff members, assign them each a line or two to monitor. Have them apply low stock items to the reorder list or place the orders (Figure 8–6).

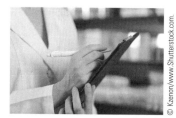

Figure 8–6 An esthetician taking inventory.

Initial or continual product training for you or your staff can be easy and fun if it is a weekly routine and lasts no more than 15 to 20 minutes per session. If you are a sole practitioner, make time every day to look at materials provided by your suppliers, vendors, and sale representatives. Allow quick meetings with them when they come to town. This is a great opportunity for you, as they can bring marketing, display ideas, and a fresh perspective to you and your space. They also know what everyone else is doing, so it is good to listen to what they have to offer. If you are dealing with a supplier who you do not like, or you dread meetings with your reps, look around. There are plenty of good, talented people to support your business. Chances are, if you are not happy with the service that a company provides, it will affect your performance in selling the product. This does not help either of you; it is best to be happy with your product lines and your account representatives. As we all know, there are fabulous and brilliant account managers and sale representatives just waiting to help us out. Many provide training on-line (Figure 8–7).

To train staff, ask each member of your team to present a 5- to 10-minute info session on a new product in a line or on a special ingredients change. This makes the staff and ownership accountable for moving products out the door.

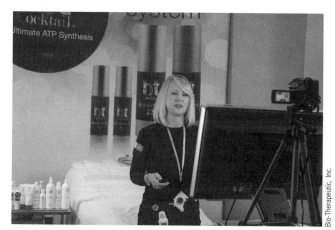

Figure 8–7 On-line training.

DID YOU **KNOW** (?)

Many comprehensive lines have back bar products, which are used for treatments. More recently, we see these larger sizes also sold for retail. There has been a movement in this direction for many years in the United States. Many estheticians want their clients to have the same benefits that they have, and will sell the back bar to the client. This does not diminish the value of the professional product, as clients feel that they are part of a private club, and will think that the esthetician is forward thinking for offering this option. Clients have a way of obtaining these products, so it may as well come from you. You can make up the difference in profit by adjusting the larger volume prices accordingly, or offering a percentage off for the larger sizes (manufactures generally give professionals value cost pricing). If you decide to do this, you will find that you can minimize the need to stock both retail and back bar, as you will only need one set for both applications. This saves time, costs, and shelf space and keeps the client happy.

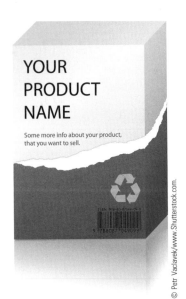

Figure 8–8 Private-label products.

© Petr Vaclavek/www.Shutterstock.com.

PRIVATE-LABEL PRODUCTS

Private-label products are favored by salons, spas, and medical settings for the exclusive image that can be created by having one's brand thread all the way through the business. Below, we will look at the benefits, challenges, and solutions involved in private-label branding (Figure 8–8).

The Benefits of Offering Private-Label Products

The opportunity to create a private label for your own product line has never been easier, more cost-effective, and more fun. To see your name or salon, spa, or skin care center's name on the label of a product is rewarding and can be the realization of a dream. Private labeling also brings the full circle to your clients as they perceive that you have done your homework, believe in your business, and are willing to share with the world that you are endorsing your name to your special brand.

Private labeling is also a way to streamline your target market. Clients are attracted to a private-label offering when they like what they see about a business. They assume that the products are an extension of a practice's mission/vision and personal philosophy. There is nothing more congruent than making a statement that is supported all the way through your marketing materials, Web site presence, service/ treatment plans, and home care protocols (this was discussed in Chapter 7, in the business and marketing section).

One benefit of a private-label product line is that it appears that you have an accomplished practice and are successful enough to afford your own line. The perception is that you have done massive research, understand cosmetic chemistry, have spent a fair amount of money on your products, and may even have a laboratory somewhere. Some of these perceptions may be true. Other benefits are that you can have a markup that is uncontested in the marketplace, and that there is not another product with your name, logo, coloration, or style in your community (it is important to research this before you decide to create a private label). Many large vendors have used private-label product companies and have been extremely successful at every turn, albeit they have had to deal with the challenges that come up in doing business of any type.

The Challenges in Offering Your Own Private-Label Line

One challenge of having a private label line can be that the company uses the same packaging for all clients. Your products will have your artwork, but the bottles, tubes, and pumps may be the same as many other private-label products. This reveals a common supplier. Some clients may not care or may not travel to other locations where they would see the same bottle on another practitioner's or provider's shelf. However, for discerning clients, this may pose the question, "Are those my products... the products that I get at Super Special Skin Care Clinic?" One must be ready to answer these types of questions. They will come up.

Another issue that may arise is that if the product manufacturer lists its name on the back of the packaging, a client may research that supplier and recognize that you are competing with the manufacturer and may be charging more for your product than the manufacturer or another practitioner is charging. This gets everybody in trouble.

Ways to Successfully Carry Your Own Private-Label Product Line

Make certain that your manufacturer can supply you with alternate packaging, or be prepared to pay for packaging from someone besides your manufacturer. If the private-label manufacturer is doing the printing/artwork for your packaging, check to make sure it is willing to put "Manufactured for [your name]" on the packaging details. You do not want to be competing with the manufacturer, or with any other company, for that matter, when you are building your brand.

This makes for a cleaner demarcation, is less confusing, and will not lower the integrity of the work that you are both providing for your client on both sides of the aisle.

If you are not concerned about the manufacturer's name printed on the label, and instead feel that it adds credibility to your line, make sure that your prices are in alignment with others who offer the same products with their names on the label. This reduces the motivation for clients to order online from the manufacturer or from another business.

GENERIC PRIVATE-LABEL PRODUCTS

Private labeling a generic brand is a great way to purchase a line that is competitive in the market and that may have specific ingredients that you enjoy. You may even be able to offer a generic product at a lower cost, as you may be looking for volume in this case. You may see these product types in health food stores, with one label for in-store point of purchase, and upon further investigation, find that they have another label available for professionals. They may use the same ingredients, preservative systems, and packaging, but have a different name for the professional application. These are great products and have a market share of their own. You might select a smaller run for a few specialty items or to have as a second product-line offering. They do not typically have label options or provide client specific artwork applications. Below, we will look at the benefits, challenges, and solutions involved in offering generic private-label products (Figure 8–9).

The Benefits of Offering a Generic Private-Label Line

One benefit to offering a generic private-label line is that they are often less expensive than other brands. They appeal to value-focused consumers, who have done their homework on ingredients, the company, and their needs and trust the esthetician offering the product. Sometimes these companies provide larger vendors with specific products, such as specialty masques, gels and cream bases, and sunscreen products.

The package profiles are simple. They do not take up space, so they are easy to merchandise in the spa, salon, or skin care center. They typically travel well. Many clients like the simplicity of a simple jar or bottle to take to the gym or on business trips.

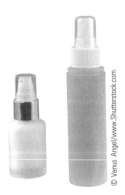

Figure 8–9 Generic products.

© Venus Angel/www.Shutterstock.com.

Challenges in Offering a Generic Private-Label Line

One challenge is that the packaging is often minimal, and not negotiable. Even though the product may contain excellent ingredients and perform beautifully, there will be a certain population of clients for whom packaging does make a difference. They will not be interested in trying a product with value-focused packaging.

Competitors may carry the brand; this happens with very mainstream lines as well. These companies may be smaller and may run short of products, and you may be out of the product for some time if you do not stock up. Shortages can plague vendor and suppliers of all sizes.

Ways to Successfully Offer a Generic, Private-Label Product Line

As with all purchasing decisions, you should determine your rate of sale on products. At a minimum, keep a two-month supply of products on hand for a smaller business, and a three- to four-month supply for larger businesses (some recommend a six-month supply). Suppliers may face changes in their product run; a shortage of ingredients; and manufacturing issues, such as with bottles, labels, and behind-the-scene challenges. Make sure that the generic private label line that you introduce matches the style, profile, and sensibility of your business. You do not want a product that sits on the shelf because it does not match anything else that you do. If you are in love with a generic product line, and it does not look good on a shelf, put one piece in a special point-of-sale (POS) position—perhaps near the checkout for an impulse buy—price it well, and offer a 20-second tutorial on the product. It may fly out the door.

 ## PHYSICIAN-EXCLUSIVE PRODUCTS

There have been several medical-focused and medical-grade product lines in the market for at least 20 years. Some of these products have found their way into the mainstream through online product discount houses and other Web-based marketing vehicles. These are often the most active and beneficial products for certain indications and conditions that we have on the market today. The companies that have developed these often hybrid products enjoy annual growth; and age- and acne-management patients and clients will continue to seek them (Figure 8–10).

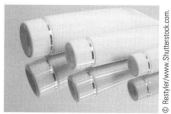

Figure 8–10 Physician-exclusive products.

Physician-Exclusive Skin Care Products

There is a perception that the products used in skin care treatments and services offered in a plastic surgery center, dermatology office, medi-spa, family practice, or other medical facility are more aggressive, active, and possibly more effective than those found in a spa or salon setting. In some cases, this may be true; however, if the efficacy of a product creates some undesirable side effects, client satisfaction may suffer. If a client uses a very aggressive home care program to reduce hyperpigmentation, for example, but develops a chronic secondary condition—such as erythema or a heightened sensitivity—due to the use of the product, it will no longer seem effective to that client. Therefore, as when physicians recommend a surgical procedure or the use of soft-tissue fillers, it is necessary to look at the reality of what the patient is requesting, and determine whether the request will be fulfilled by the procedure. If it is determined that the procedure will satisfy the client's request, then a great deal of patient education must follow to ensure that each step in the process is necessary. It is made clear to the patient that he or she must follow the protocol set by the medical team for a good outcome.

This is also true for estheticians when recommending more active, medical-grade products. We must provide additional education on the use and side effects of products that contain more active ingredients. When the products are of a medical grade, and contain pharmaceuticals as defined by the FDA (which are those that claim to treat conditions and have an effect on the structure and functions of the skin), we need a prescription for them.

Keep in mind, our ultimate objective in any setting is to care for the patient or client and provide compassionate, results-oriented skin care and experiences with ongoing excellence in service. Next, we will look at the benefits, challenges, and solutions involved in offering medical grade products.

The Benefits of Offering Medical-Grade Skin Care Products in a Medical Facility

As we know, offering medical skin care products in your practice spares your patients and clients the trouble of going to another facility, store, or esthetician. It is well known that in our multibillion-dollar business, that consumers are buying personal care products from a variety of sources. They might as well be buying them from you, their trusted esthetic professional. It is common practice for a client to spend between $200 and $400 on home care products every two to four months. As we know, it is a maintenance business. The average annual expenditure on personal care products in the United States is $1,220 per household. Why shouldn't they spend this money, with us?

Patient Education and Product Knowledge

In addition to medical support, the patient will have their skin care needs met by a well-appointed esthetician, nurse, PA or physician who is trained in patient education and product knowledge. This foundational training supplies us with most of the necessary skills to educate patients on the benefits of using skin care. Most skin care professionals tend to be excellent continuing education students themselves, and are often exceptional teachers, so having an esthetician on staff in a medical office is highly desirable.

Training the staff in a medical office

The in-service training offered by sales representatives is typically excellent. Training happens routinely, as reps often provide other specialty products such as soft-tissue fillers, neurotoxins, instruments, and/or devices. They are also diligent about managing their accounts.

The Challenges in Offering Medical-Strength Skin Care Products in a Medical Facility

Medical-strength skin care products that are administered in a medical setting can be stronger, and more aggressive. The client may not have been listening to the instructions for use during the consult, may have left the written instructions in the car (sometimes there will be a variety of reasons for misunderstanding important information). Or, was not properly introduced to the differences in active ingredients between OTC products and higher-level concentrations. This can result in irritated skin and emergency visits to other health care professionals or well-meaning friends or family members: this can be both frightening for the patient and not good for the office's reputation.

Many medical providers do not have an interest in skin care products. If some team members are negative or indifferent about the office providing skin care products in a medical office, patients notice this will go where they feel justified in spending their money.

Ways to Successfully Offer Medical-Strength Skin Care Products in a Medical Facility

Make sure that there is plenty of time to go over the protocol for the product with the patient. It may be that the client starts with a low-level product, and then gradually moves to a product with a higher concentration once his or her skin has had a chance to adapt and acclimate to the active ingredients or pharmaceutical. With pharmaceuticals, it is also necessary to reduce exposure to risk by having the appropriate medical personnel working with the patient.

If you have members on the staff who do not support the sale of products, it creates a challenge in building your business. It may be that these employees do not know enough about what the products can supply for the patient, have not looked at the financials, or are just not interested. If the problem is a lack of education, you may be able to change an employee's perspective simply by sharing the antioxidant benefits in a sunscreen, for example. Looking at a good month of product sales and the cash flow that has been provided by the profit center may inspire a product cynic to take a more positive approach toward products.

SUMMING IT UP

It is important for you to stay on top of your purchasing decisions and sell products to not only avoid expiration date issues, but to keep your business healthy. There are multiple options in products for salon, spa, and skin care center businesses: it is truly a matter of which plan works best for your business. Many product companies will share their records of success with suppliers and vendors. Request to see them. You can ask the vendor if they have satisfied clients that you may call to provide a testimony. It is also important to evaluate your vendor's point of contact or representative as well as the product. Ask yourself a few questions when evaluating or reevaluating along the way:

- Do they get back to me in a timely manner?
- Are they respectful of my business and my questions?
- Do they have options for me if a product is out of stock?
- Do they have someone whom I can contact if my account manager is out of the office?
- Are they forthcoming with product information and education, and do they have a Web presence? Do they make trade show appearances?
- Do they offer continuing education (is there an online alternative)?
- Do they care about me and our practice?
- Are they solvent?
- Are they current? Do they have new products coming out regularly?
- Will they trade out a product if it is just not moving for me after attempts, training, and applying selling techniques?

It is often best to work with someone who you feel is looking out for you and your business. You are looking for a partnership and real people who will support your success.

ESTHETICIAN **PROFILE**

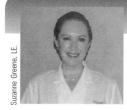

Suzanne Greene, LE.

Suzanne Greene, LE

Account Executive and Educator for Murad

I am a Seattle native. I have always been passionate about the beauty industry. I took that passion to the next level and became licensed in esthetics and manicuring in 1982. I then went on to work in the cosmetic industry, where I was fortunate enough to work for Nordstrom and Chanel Beauté for the majority of my sales career. While at Nordstrom, I was awarded the prestigious Pacesetter (now called All Star) annually, and developed a clientele equal to many of the larger lines that were in our department. I truly felt connected to each customer and made many friends while working for Chanel. This experience provided a strong background in sales and in business. I learned early in my career how important it was to become an advisor, to be consistent with customers and clients, and to follow up with the client. These three important steps help make not only sales goals, but keep the client very loyal.

In 2005, I decided to get back into the professional esthetics world by working for Murad as an account executive and working closely with estheticians to help them build their practices. With my background in sales and being licensed, it has been an amazing journey. It has set up a lifelong career that never gets old. With the constant changes in the industry, it continues to stay fresh. There is always something new to learn and then share with our devoted clients. This allows us to grow and develop our careers as well.

Training

I attended Bellevue Beauty School, where I learned the basics. I went on to get additional training through working with Dr. Murad. Meeting Dr. Murad and working under his philosophy has been an incredible journey and has changed my life in so many ways. I have been able to meet amazing people due to the extensive travel that my job provides.

I routinely continue my education by participating in multiple training programs on skin physiology, ingredients, sales updates and applications, merchandising and display, account management, and various business classes. We also have routine meetings with Murad that provide educational opportunities as well.

Practice Demographic

I deal with all skin types, conditions, and ages and am fortunate to work with a line that provides care for all. I work with students and professionals, in both esthetic and medical settings. The demographic is varied, as I work with schools, spas, salons, skin care centers, medi-spas, plastic surgery and dermatology offices, and wellness centers.

Services/Treatments Offered

The services I provide are based on the individual needs of each of my accounts. I am able to treat the first signs of aging all the way to hormonal aging: this enables me to assist all skin concerns. As an account executive, I offer a detailed, comprehensive skin care plan to clients, which involves assessing their needs to determine what type of product knowledge they will require in their place of business, training requirements, and ultimately support their implementation of the plan for their customers and clients. We manage their accounts closely to make certain that their needs are not only met, but exceeded.

Personal Philosophy

The personal contact that I have with people and the outstanding customer service that I provide is where my passion is. It is very rewarding to help an esthetician start with a line, progress through the learning process, create a stable, thriving business, and then become one of my top accounts.

In these ever-changing times, I believe if that if you care enough and give the best service possible, you can make it through any changes that come along your path. Some days can be more challenging than we would like them to be, but if we stay focused and keep moving, we can conquer setbacks, life changes, and fear. Our work with clients can also provide a great deal of strength and hope to our days as well.

Additional Contributions to the Industry

Sales is not my only passion. I have found that becoming an educator and being involved in education is also a passion and gives me a way to touch estheticians' lives in a totally different way. It is great to see the expressions on the faces of estheticians when they are learning about new and exciting changes with Murad, as we are constantly evolving and expanding our product line to include the latest ingredients in skin care. The excitement that I have found in teaching others is something I never thought I would enjoy; however, it has been a very positive development for me. I learn so much myself from every teaching experience, and that in itself is a reward. That is what is so amazing about our industry ... you can do anything and go everywhere.

Concluding Thoughts

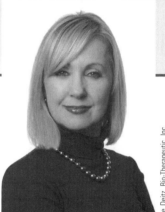

Sallie Deitz, Bio-Therapeutic, Inc.

The career choice to serve as an esthetician in any environment today is rewarding and offers great diversity, which is not available in most industries. We are fortunate to have options for growth and change and yet belong to a profession that has a strong history routed in ancient times. Esthetics and the interest in beauty are well understood, documented, and have survived and thrived for thousands of years.

Technology and training for estheticians and skin care professionals is limited only by our thoughts and perceptions. As highly respected professionals, we are sought out for our knowledge, compassion, adaptability, intelligence, talent, and skills. There are many professions that an esthetician or skin care professional can transfer into because of the cross-training and education that esthetics provides. In many ways, we are just getting started, and yet when you look at our collective résumé, it is impressive. We know that we must follow our state regulations and work within of the scope of practice; this is easy to do, as it provides the necessary boundary to stay focused on what we are licensed to do. Many estheticians are expanding their horizons to include master's programs in both technical realms and academic programs as well as completing doctoral programs and business entrepreneurship programs. If you can conceive of the perfect livelihood, you can create it in the world of esthetics and continue to reinvent yourself indefinitely.

Many blessings!
Sallie Deitz, LE

Glossary

A

accelerated hydrogen peroxide (AHP) Disinfectant based on stabilized hydrogen peroxide that needs to be changed only every 14 days. It is nontoxic to the skin and the environment.

actinic keratosis Lesions created by UV exposure that are often dry and flaky; can be precancerous.

andragogy Theory developed by Malcolm Knowles, PhD, that focuses on relevant learning and teaching methods for adults.

artefill Permanent soft-tissue filler.

auricularis anterior Muscle in front of the ear that draws the ear forward.

autonomous Independent in origin, action, or function; self-governing.

avoidance A technique of risk management that involves taking steps to remove a risk completely, or choose an alternate route in business to reduce exposure to risks. One example would be eliminating a device that is not working consistently.

B

Beta hydroxy acid peel Exfoliating organic acid; salicylic acid; milder than some alpha hydroxy acids; excellent for oily skin.

biofilm Single type of microorganism or, in nature, an aggregate of living microorganisms, such as bacteria, fungi, and protozoa, which form a biofilm community and further attach to a moisture-rich surface environment and begin to reproduce.

blepharospasm Uncontrollable blinking.

blue light Light-emitting diode for use on clients with acne.

bodily-kinesthetic intelligence Excellence in physical movement; an individual who demonstrates this intelligence needs a "hands-on" approach to learning.

Botox® Botulinum toxin type A that, when injected into a muscle, restricts its movement.

brain plasticity The idea that the human brain is wired to learn; also known as neuroplasticity.

buccinator Thin, flat muscle of the cheek between the upper and lower jaw that compresses the cheeks and expels air between the lips.

C

Candida albicans Yeast that thrives in dark, moisture-rich environments.

cervical dystonia Neck muscles that contract abnormally, causing pain.

circadian rhythms Natural biological rhythms.

cimicidae Parasite commonly known as a bed bug.

Climex lectularius Parasite commonly known as a bed bug.

community-associated methicillin-resistant staphylococcus aureus (CA-MRSA) Type of staph infection that is highly contagious, resistant to antibiotics, and found in the community.

corrugators Facial muscles that draw eyebrows down and wrinkle the forehead vertically.

covalent bond A form of chemical bonding characterized by the sharing of pairs of electrons between atoms.

D

Depressor anguli oris Muscle found on the chin, also called the triangularis, which depress the corners of the mouth.

Depressor labii inferioris Muscle found in the chin, which depress the lower lip and allows movement from side to side.

dermatitis Any inflammatory condition of the skin; various forms of lesions, such as eczema, vesicles, or papules; the three main categories are atopic, contact, and seborrheic dermatitis.

dermatophytes Fungi that cause skin, nail, and hair infections.

distress Associated with generalized stress, which tends to be chronic; can pose health concerns and has a negative and cumulative effect.

Dysport™ Botulinum toxin type A that, when injected into a muscle, restricts its movement.

E

eczema Inflammatory, painful itching disease of the skin, acute or chronic in nature, with dry or moist lesions. This condition should be referred to a physician. Seborrheic dermatitis, mainly affecting oily areas, is a common form of eczema.

employment practices liability insurance (EPL or EPLI) EPL or EPLI is a type of insurance that provides protection for an employer against claims made by employees, former employees or potential employees.

ephelides Light-colored freckles.

erythema Redness caused by inflammation; a red lesion is erythemic.

eurstress Stress that culminates in a positive result is often short term. Eustress can enhance productivity, increase a sense of well-being, and supply the necessary motivation to complete goals in life.

executive summary The overview of a business in a business plan.

F

fibroblasts Cells that are responsible for making connective tissue such as collagen.

fight or flight response Brain-stimulated response to stress that prepares the body for trauma.

fissures Cracks in the skin that penetrate the dermis; examples include severely cracked and/or chapped hands or lips.

Fitzpatrick skin type Scale used to measure the skin type's ability to tolerate sun exposure.

flourishing Prospering, growing well, thriving, being successful and productive.

G

Gardner, Howard, PhD Harvard professor who developed the theory of multiple intelligences.

general liability insurance Comprehensive insurance that covers a business from unforeseen accidents and events with products and services.

glabellar lines Vertical and horizontal forehead lines found between the eyebrows and across the forehead.

Globalization A worldwide movement toward integrating cultures, communication, business, and trading

Glogau Photodamage Classification Categorization of wrinkle activity developed by Richard Glogau, MD.

granulomas Nodular lesion on the skin.

green light Light-emitting diode for use on clients with hyperpigmentation or to detoxify the skin.

H

heterologous Derived from a different species.

High-glycemic Higher levels of sugar substances being absorbed into the bloodstream.

home care compliance Clients or patients using products at home in a manner consistent with a plan created by an esthetician and physician.

hospital associated Methicillin-resistant staphylococcus aureus (HA-MRSA) Type of staph infection that is highly contagious, resistant to antibiotics, and originates in a hospital setting.

Hyaluronic acid Hydrating fluids found in the skin and around joints for lubrication; also a hydrophilic agent with water binding properties found in skin care products.

hyperpigmentation Overproduction of pigment.

hypopigmentation Absence of pigment that results in light or white splotches.

I

independent testing Testing performed by a third party or someone other than the developer of a product.

interpersonal intelligence Talent for dealing with people; higher than usual amount of compassion and emotional depth.

intertrigo Type of fungal infection found in the body folds of the skin in areas such as the underarms and in the groin.

intrapersonal intelligence Great self-knowledge and self-awareness.

ISO (International Organization for Standardization) Organization that develops standards for businesses and industries worldwide.

isotretinoin Medication used for advanced cases of acne and extreme cases of rosacea; (formerly known as Accutane).

K

keloid Thick scar resulting from excessive growth of fibrous tissue (collagen).

keratosis Abnormally thick buildup of cells.

kinesthetic Tendency to respond positively to physical movement.

Knowles, Malcolm, MD Known as "the father of adult education."

Kojic acid Type of tyrosinase inhibitor used to stabilize and reduce melanin production.

L

lentigines Technical term for freckles; small, yellow-colored to brown-colored spots on skin exposed to sunlight and air.

linguistic intelligence Facility with words and language.

logical-mathematical intelligence Exceptional ability with numbers and logic.

M

malleable Brain's ability to adjust according to new information and situations in the environment.

masseter Muscle that coordinates with the temporalis, medial pterygoid, and lateral pterygoid muscles to open and close the mouth and bring the jaw forward; sometimes referred to as the chewing muscle.

mediator Conflict-resolution professional.

melanocytes Cell that produces pigment granules/melanin in the basal layer of the epidermis.

mentalis Muscle found on the chin which raise and protrudes the lower lip as in drinking from a glass.

mind mapping A diagram or graphic developed to link ideas, tasks, and information to help organize thinking on a specific theme.

mission/vision statement Mission statement is the foundational premise on which a business operates; vision statement relates more to the application of plans.

multiple intelligences A theory created by renowned psychologist Howard Gardner, PhD, that delineates eight different types of intelligence that people possess.

musical intelligence Above-average ability in music; someone who responds to rhythm and sound.

N

naturalistic intelligence Strong ability to interact with the natural world.

necrosis Premature death of cells in living tissue.

O

OD (optical density) Measurement of how much light an object absorbs and how much of the light passes through the object.

off-label Product or device being used for purposes other than its intended use.

onychomycosis Type of nail infection.

orbicularis oculi Ring muscle of the eye socket that closes the eyelid.

P

papering your file Clearly documenting in clients' files all visits and events.

pathogenic Harmful microorganisms that can cause disease or infection in humans when they invade the body.

Pediculosis capitis Infestation of the hair and scalp by head lice.

periorbital region Area around the eye; peri-orbital bone.

postinflammatory hyperpigmentation Dark melanin splotches caused by trauma to the skin that can result from acne pimples and papules.

Professional Beauty Association (PBA) Association that serves to advance the professional beauty industry by providing its members with business tools, government advocacy, education, and networking to ensure their success.

professional liability insurance Insurance that protects a professional in business from litigation caused by charges of professional negligence or failure to perform professional duties.

property coverage Insurance that protects the physical property and equipment of a business against loss from theft, fire, or other perils.

psychoneuroimmunology Study of how the brain transmits signals along the nerves to stimulate the body's immune system.

R

Radiesse Soft-tissue filler used for wrinkles, and an increase in facial volume. Also used in medical applications for incontinence, breast reconstruction, and vocal cord rehabilitation.

red light Light-emitting diode for use on clients to stimulate circulation and in collagen and elastin production.

reduction A risk management technique that takes measures the reduce the potential of loss. An example might be removing a marketing piece that may make a false claim.

reepithelialized Formation of new epidermis and dermis over an area of injury in which epithelial cells from the wound margin and the pilosebaceous units migrate to repair damage.

retention A risk management technique where the owner of a business assumes all of the risk rather than seeking outside help. This might be where a spa owner takes on the responsibility to replace a product or device if something goes wrong.

risorius Muscle of the mouth that draws the corner of the mouth out and back, as in grinning.

rhytides Wrinkles.

S

Sculptra Filler used for facial volume.

seborrheic keratosis Crusty-looking, slightly raised lesions in mature, sun-damaged skin. Often appearing in the cheekbone area, they may be black, brown, gray, or flesh-toned.

spasmodic dysphonia Voice disorder, often leading to a squeaky or high-pitched sound.

spatial intelligence Ability to arrange objects in space or to visualize a process before it takes place.

standard of care Necessary protocols that a practitioner must follow.

strabismus Eyes that are misaligned or crossed.

SWOT It is a business tool to use for analyzing one's competition. Often termed "SWOT" your business.

T

telangiectasias Small, dilated blood vessels; also called spider veins.

tinea barbae Also known as barber's itch; a superficial fungal infection that commonly affects the skin and is primarily limited to the bearded areas of the face and neck or around the scalp.

tinea corporis Fungus commonly known as ringworm.

tinea pedis Medical term for fungal infections of the feet; red, itchy rash of the skin on the bottom of the feet and/or in between the toes that is usually found between the fourth and fifth toes.

tinea versicolor Fungal infection which creates white patches where production of melanin has been compromised.

transfer A risk management technique where a business owner may transfer all if the risk to another party such as in purchasing an insurance policy.

Tretinoin Derived from vitamin A, also known as retinoic acid. Used to increase collagen and elastin production.

tyrosinase Enzyme that synthesizes tyrosine and L-dopa to create melanosomes.

Tyrosinase inhibitor A product or ingredient that inhibits the melanin producing enzyme tyrosinase.

U

U.S. Deparment of Labor and Bureau of Labor Statistics A government agency that produces economic data the reflects the state of the U.S. economy.

V

Vision board A visual accounting of ideas, hopes, and dreams of what we would like to have happen in our lives.

W

worker's compensation System of insurance that reimburses an employer for damages that must be paid to an employee for injury occurring in the course of employment.

Y

yellow light Light-emitting diode that aids in reducing inflammation and swelling.

Z

zygomatic bone Also known as malar bone or cheekbone.

zygomatics major and minor Muscles on both sides of the face that extend from the zygomatic bone to the angle of the mouth. These muscles elevate the lip and pull the mouth upward and backward in a laugh or smile.

Bibliography

Abrams, Rhonda. (2010). *Successful Business Plan: Secrets and Strategies*. Palo Alto, CA: The Planning Shop.

Allison, Rhonda. (2000, 2001). *Cooking with Acids: A Step-by-Step Peel Guide for the Professional Aesthetician*. Dallas, TX: Brown Books. www.brownbooks.com

Altman, Nathaniel. (1995, 1998). *Oxygen Healing Therapies: For Optimum Health & Vitality*. Rochester, Vermont: Healing Arts Press.

Banich, Marie T., and Compton, Rebecca, S. (2001, 2003). *Cognitive Neuroscience*, 3rd ed. Belmont, CA: Wadsworth/Cengage Learning. www.cengage.com/global

Becker, Robert O., and Selden, Gary. (1985). *The Body Electric: Electromagnetism and the Foundation of Life*. New York: William Morrow and Company.

Beckwith, Harry. (2011). *Unthinking: The Surprising Forces Behind What We Buy*. New York: Hachette Book Group. www.HachetteBookGroup.com

Buckingham, Marcus. (2008). *The Truth About You: Your Secret to Success*. Nashville, TN: Thomas Nelson, Inc. www.marcusbuckinghamc.com

Buckingham, Marcus, and Clifton, Donald O. (2001). *Now Discover Your Strengths*. New York: Free Press.

Cloud, Henry. (2006). *9 Things a Leader Must Do: Breaking Through to the Next Level*. Nashville, TN: Thomas Nelson, LLC.

Culp, Judith et al. (2010). *Milady's Standard Esthetics Advanced*. Clifton Park, NY: Cengage Learning. www.milady.cengage.com

D'Angelo, Janet. (2010). *Spa Business Strategies: A Plan for Success*, 2nd ed. Clifton Park, NY: Milady Cengage Learning.

D'Angelo, Janet, Deitz, Sallie, Lotz, Shelley, Frangie, Catherine M., and Halal, John. (2009). *Milady's Standard Esthetics Fundamentals*. Clifton Park, NY: Cengage Learning. www.delmar.cengage.com

D'Angelo, J., Deitz, S., and Lotz, S. (2010). *Milady's Standard Esthetics Fundamentals, Step-by-Step Procedures*. Clifton Park, NY: Delmar/Cengage Learning. www.milady.com

Davies, Juanita J. (2002). *A Quick Reference to Medical Terminology*. Clifton Park, NY: Milady Cengage Learning.

Dayan, Steven, and Wojak, Terri. (2009). *Mastering Medical Esthetics: A Guide to Estheticians Working in the Medical Field*. Chicago, IL: CCM Publishing. www.trueuniversityesthetics.com

de Bonvoisin, Ariane. (2008). *The First 30 Days: Your Guide to Making Any Change Easier*. New York: HarperCollins Publishers. www.first30days.com

Deitz, Sallie. (2004). *The Clinical Esthetician: An Insider's Guide to Succeeding in a Medical Office.* Clifton Park, NY: Milady Publishing.

Doidge, Norman. (2007). *The Brain That Changes Itself: Stories of Personal Triumph from the Frontiers of Brain Science.* New York: The Penguin Group. www.normandoidge.com

Eden, Donna, and Feinstein, David. (1998, 2008). *Energy Medicine: Balancing Your Body's Energies for Optimal Health, Joy, and Vitality.* New York: The Penguin Group. www.innersource.net

French, Ramona Moody. (2004). *Milady's Guide to Manual Lymph Drainage Massage.* Clifton Park, NY: Milady Cengage Learning.

Gardner, Howard. (1993). *Multiple Intelligences: The Theory in Practice.* New York: HarperCollins Publishers.

Goleman, Daniel. (2006). *Social Intelligence: The Revolutionary New Science of Human Relationships.* New York: Bantam Dell. www.bantamdell.com

Greive, Donald. (2001). *A Handbook for Adjunct/Part-Time Faculty and Teachers of Adults.* Elyria, OH: Info-Tec.

Hales, Diane. (2010, 2011). *An Invitation to Health,* Instructor's Edition. Belmont, CA: Cengage Learning. www.cengage.com/wadsworth

Hill, Pamela. (2006). *Milady's Aesthetician Series, Botox®, Dermal Fillers, and Sclerotherapy.* Clifton Park, NY: Milady Cengage Learning.

Hill, Pamela. (2006). *Milady's Aesthetician Series, Peels and Peeling Agents.* Clifton Park, NY: Milady Cengage Learning. www.milady.com

Hill, Pamela, and Bickmore, Helen R. (2008). *Milady's Aesthetician Series: Advanced Hair Removal.* Clifton Park, NY: Milady Cengage Learning. www.milady.com

Hill, Pamela, and Owens, Patricia. (2009). *Milady's Aesthetician Series Lasers and Light Theory.* Clifton Park, NY: Milady Cengage Learning. www.milady.com

Jablonski, Nina G. (2006). *Skin: A Natural History.* Berkeley and Los Angeles, CA: University of California Press.

Jarmey, Chris. (2003, 2008). *The Concise Book of Muscles,* 2nd ed. Chichester, UK: Lotus Publishing.

Jantz, Gregory L. (1998, 2008, 2009). *How to Destress Your Life.* Grand Rapids, MI: Revell, Baker Publishing Group. www.revellbooks.com

Layman, Dale. (2003). *Biology Demystified: A Self-Teaching Guide.* New York: McGraw-Hill.

Lees, Mark. (2007). *Skin Care Beyond the Basics,* 3rd ed. Clifton Park, NY: Milady Cengage Learning. www.milady.com

Lees, Mark. (2011). *The Skin Care Answer Book: Real-World Answers to 275 Most-Asked Skin Care Questions.* Clifton Park, NY: Milady Cengage Learning. www.milady.cengage.com

Lippincott Williams & Wilkins. (2005). *Anatomy and Physiology Made Incredibly Easy,* 2nd ed. Ambler, PA: Lippincott Williams & Wilkins.

Lipton, Bruce H. (2005). *The Biology of Belief: Unleashing the Power of Consciousness, Matter and Miracles.* Santa Rosa, CA: Elite Books. www.BruceLipton.com

Michalun, Natalia, and Michalun, M. Varinia. (2010, 2001, 1993). *Milady's Skin Care and Cosmetic Ingredients Dictionary,* 3rd ed. Clifton Park, NY: Milady Publishing.

Mitchell, Deborah. (2008). *Foods That Combat Aging: The Nutritional Way to Stay Healthy Longer.* New York: HarperCollins Publishers.

Northrup, Christiane. (2010, 2006, 1998, 1994). *Women's Bodies, Women's Wisdom: Creating Physical and Emotional Health and Healing.* New York: Random House Publishing Group.

Olpin, Michael, and Hesson, Margie. (2010). *Stress Management for Life: A Researched-Based, Experiential Approach.* New York: Cengage Learning.

Oz, Mehmet, and Roizen, Michael F. (2005). *You: The Owner's Manual: An Insider's Guide to the Body That Will Make You Healthier and Younger.* New York: HarperCollins Publishers. www.doctoroz.com

Parramon's Editorial Team. (2003). *Essential Atlas of Physics and Chemistry.* Barcelona, Spain: Parramon Ediciones, SA.

Pink, Daniel H. (2006). *A Whole New Mind: Why Right-Brainers Will Rule the Future.* New York: Riverhead Books, Penguin Group. www.danpink.com

Plonka, Lavinia. (2004). *What Are You Afraid Of? A Body/Mind Guide to Courageous Living.* New York: Penguin Group.

Pugliese, Peter T. (2005). *Advanced Professional Skin Care, Medical Edition.* Bernville, PA: The Topical Agent.

Rizzo, Donald. (2005, 2001). *Study Guide for Fundamentals of Anatomy and Physiology,* 2nd ed. Clifton Park, NY: Delmar Cengage Learning.

Rizzo, Donald C. (2006, 2001). *Fundamentals of Anatomy & Physiology,* 2nd ed. Clifton Park, NY: Milady Cengage Learning.

Rubin, Mark G. (1995). *Manual of Chemical Peels: Superficial and Medium Depth.* Philadelphia, PA: J.B. Lippincott Company.

Scott, Susan. (2002, 2004). *Fierce Conversations: Achieving Success at Work and in Life One Conversation at a Time.* New York: The Berkley Publishing Group.

Sharma, Robin. (2010). *The Leader Who Had No Title: A Modern Fable on Real Success in Business and in Life.* New York: Free Press.

Shipman, Claire, and Katty, Kay. (2009). *Womenomics: Write Your Own Rules for Success: How to Stop Juggling and Struggling and Finally Start Living and Working the Way You Really Want.* New York: HarperCollins Publishers.

Shiota, Michelle N., and Kalat, James W. (2012, 2007). *Emotion,* 2nd ed. Belmont, CA: Wadsworth Cengage Learning. www.cengage.com/wadsworth

Stewart, William B. (2009). *Deep Medicine: Harnessing the Source of Your Healing Power.* Oakland, CA: New Harbinger Publications and Noetics Books. www.newharbinger.com

Suzuki, David S. (2004, September). "Microcurrent's Coming of Age," *Professional Beauty UK* – February 2009, "Microcurrent's Coming of Age," *Cabines Espana* – February 2009, "Microcurrent's Coming of Age," *Les Nouvelles Esthetiques* – February 2009, "Microcurrent's Coming of Age," *China/Hong Kong Beauty.* February 2009.

Suzuki, David S. (2009, March). "Embracing Change; Re-Gaining Control of a Wandering Business," *Professional Beauty UK,* "Embracing Change; Re-Gaining Control of a Wandering Business," *Cabines Espana* – March 2009, "Embracing Change; Re-Gaining Control of a Wandering Business," *Les Nouvelles Esthetiques* – March 2009, "Embracing Change; Re-Gaining Control of a Wandering Business," *China/Hong Kong Beauty* – March 2009.

Suzuki, David S. (2011, July). "The Layers of Skin Rejuvenation," *Professional Beauty UK,* "The Layers of Skin Rejuvenation," *Professional Beauty Australia* – May/June 2011, "The Layers of Skin Rejuvenation," *Cabines Espana* – July 2011, "The Layers of Skin Rejuvenation," *Les Nouvelles Esthetiques,* July 2011, "The Layers of Skin Rejuvenation," *China/Hong Kong Beauty* – July 2011

Suzuki, David S. (2011, November). "Fair Pricing; A New Idea," *Professional Beauty UK,* "The Layers of Skin Rejuvenation,"

Les Nouvelles Esthetiques, "The Layers of Skin Rejuvenation," *China/Hong Kong Beauty –* November 2011, "The Layers of Skin Rejuvenation," *Les Nouvelles Esthetiques –* November 2011

Suzuki, David S. (2011, December). "Layers of Exfoliation," *Professional Beauty UK –* "Layers of Exfoliation," *Professional Beauty Australia –* January/February 2011, "Layers of Exfoliation," *Cabines Espana –* December 2011, "Layers of Exfoliation," *Les Nouvelles Esthetiques,* "Layers of Exfoliation," *China/Hong Kong Beauty –* December 2011, "Layers of Exfoliation," *Les Nouvelles Esthetiques –* December 2011.

Takemura, Masaharu. (2009). *The Manga Guide to Molecular Biology.* Toyko, Japan: No Starch Press and Ohmsha, Ltd. www.edumanga.me

Thornfeldt, Carl, and Krista Bourne. (2010). *The New Ideal in Skin Health: Separating Fact from Fiction.* Carol Stream, IL: Allured Books. www.allured.com/bookstore

Tierno, Philip M. (2001). *The Secret Lift of Germs, What They Are, Why We Need Them, and How We Can Protect Ourselves Against Them.* New York: Atria Books.

Tolle, Eckhart. (2005). *A New Earth: Awakening to Your Life's Purpose.* New York: Namaste Publishing, Penguin Group. www.eckharttolle.com

Underwood, Joseph, W. (2009). *Today I Made a Difference.* Avon, MA: Adams Media.

Wenborg, Craig. (2006). *The Esthetic Benefits of Oxygen Skin Care.* Carol Stream, IL: Skin Inc.

Wenborg, Craig. (2011). *Oxygen Facials: Red Carpet Services or Serious Skin Care?* Carol Stream, IL: Skin Inc.

Index

Note: page numbers followed by f or t refer to Figures or Tables

Microdermabrasion

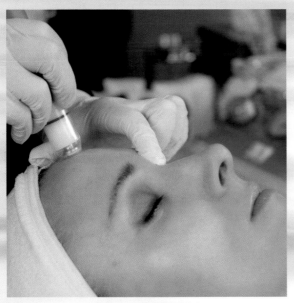

P5-1-09 With all types of devices (wet–dry, diamond tip, particle), use vertical strokes on the entire width of the forehead, starting at the center just above the eyebrow and working toward the hairline above the temple. (Refer to page 159 for corresponding content).

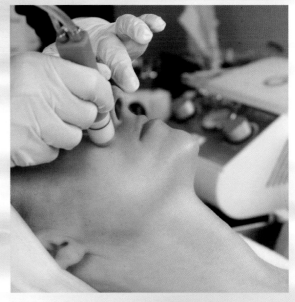

P5-1-11 Apply vertical applications to temples, around eyes, cheeks, upper lip and nasal areas. (Refer to page 159 for corresponding content).

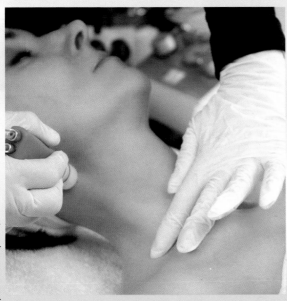

P5-1-13 Apply vertical applications on neck and decollete. (Refer to page 160 for corresponding content).

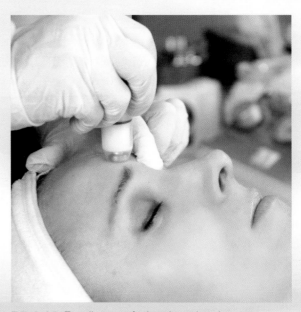

P5-1-16 For all types of microdermabrasion, start second pass on the forehead, working horizontally across forehead. (Refer to page 160 for corresponding content).

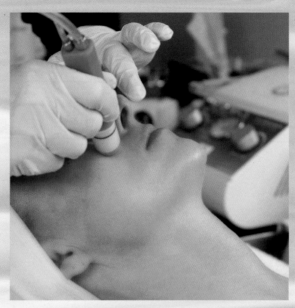

P5-1-19 Apply the horizontal application to temples, around eyes, cheeks upper lip and nasal areas. (Refer to page 161 for corresponding content).

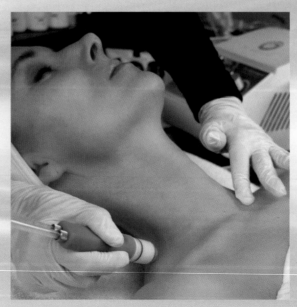

P5-1-20 Apply horizontal pass to neck and decollete. (Refer to page 161 for corresponding content).

Oxygen Therapy

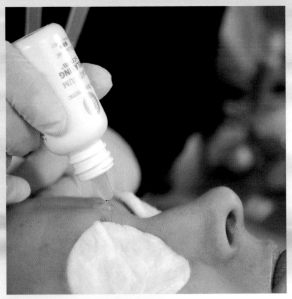

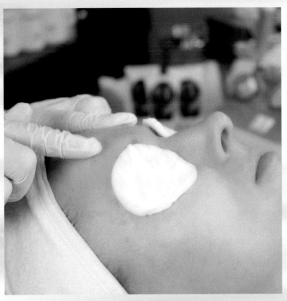

P5-2-5 Apply approrpriate serum to areas for infusion. (Refer to page 164 for corresponding content).

P5-2-6 Blend serum gently. (Refer to page 165 for corresponding content).

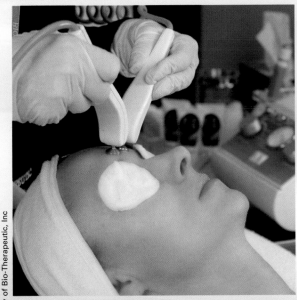

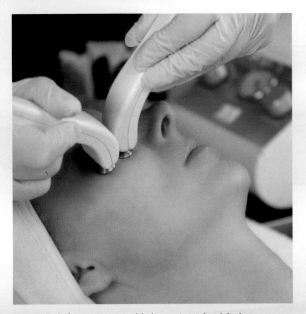

Courtesy of Bio-Therapeutic, Inc

P5-2-7 Infuse serum with jets. (Refer to page 165 for corresponding content).

P5-2-8 Infuse serum with jets at peri-orbital area. (Refer to page 165 for corresponding content).

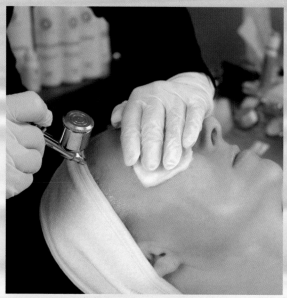

P5-2-9 Apply oxygenated product with wand. (Refer to page 166 for corresponding content).

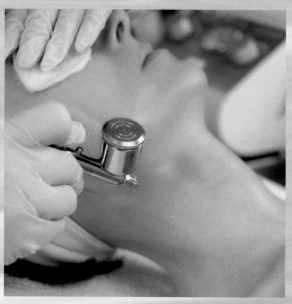

P5-2-10 Apply oxygenated product with wand to neck and decollete. (Refer to page 166 for corresponding content).

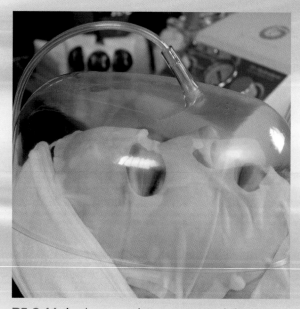

P5-2-11 Apply appropriate masque and dome. (Refer to page 166 for corresponding content).

Microcurrent

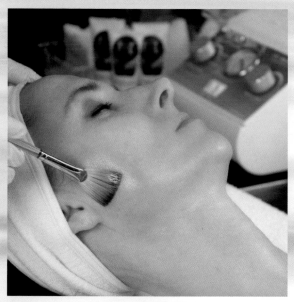

P5-3-4 Apply conductive solution. (Refer to page 170 for corresponding content).

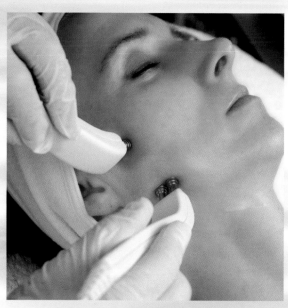

P5-3-8 Apply probes at masseter, lift and hold. (Refer to page 170 for corresponding content).

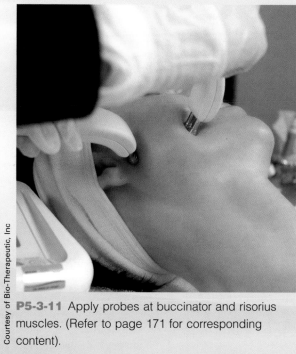

P5-3-11 Apply probes at buccinator and risorius muscles. (Refer to page 171 for corresponding content).

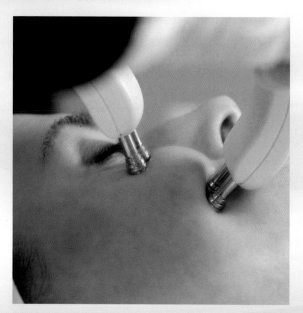

P5-3-12 Apply probes at zygomatic major insertion and pull up toward origin. (Refer to page 171 for corresponding content).

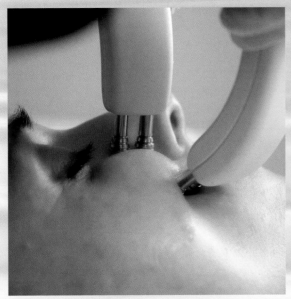

P5-3-13 Apply probes at levator labii superioris insertion and pull up toward the nasalis. (Refer to page 172 for corresponding content).

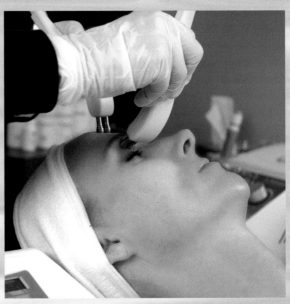

P5-3-14 Apply probes to orbicularius oculi and corrugator. (Refer to page 172 for corresponding content).

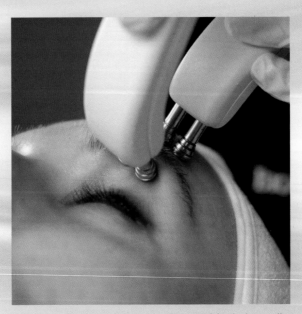

P5-3-15 Apply probes to the inner orbicularis oculi and lift up toward the frontalis. (Refer to page 172 for corresponding content).

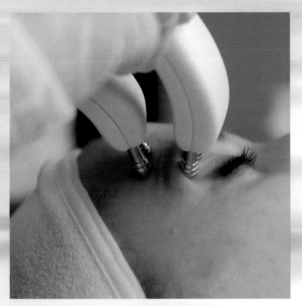

P5-3-16 Lifting orbicularis oculi toward the frontalis. (Refer to page 173 for corresponding content).

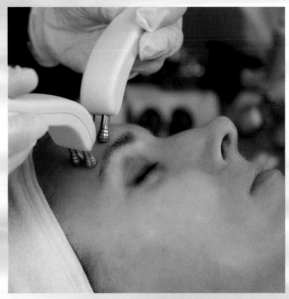

P5-3-18 Iontophoresis: product penetration. (Refer to page 173 for corresponding content).

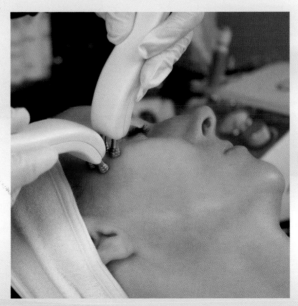

P5-3-20 Iontophoresis: product penetration all over face and throat. (Refer to page 173 for corresponding content).

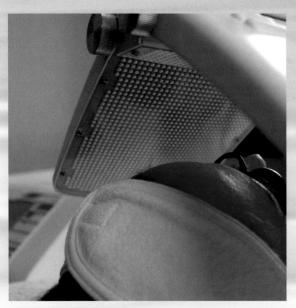

P5-4-8 Red light: anti-aging and healing. (Refer to page 177 for corresponding content).

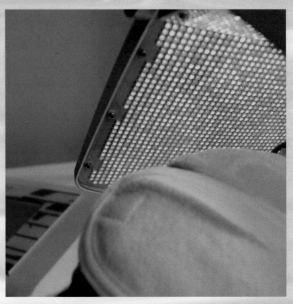

P5-4-9 Yellow light: anti-stress and anti-inflammatory. (Refer to page 177 for corresponding content).

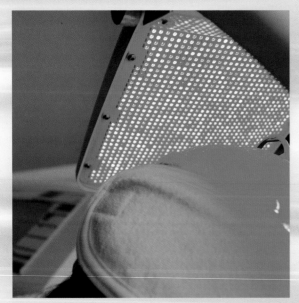

P5-4-10 Green light: for erythema and hyperpigmentation. (Refer to page 177 for corresponding content).

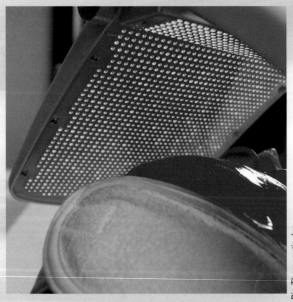

P5-4-11 Blue light for acne and rosacea. (Refer to page 178 for corresponding content).

Ultrasonic and Microcurrent

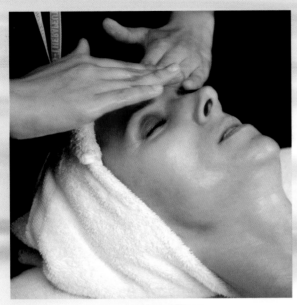

P5-5-3 Apply peel medium. (Refer to page 184 for corresponding content).

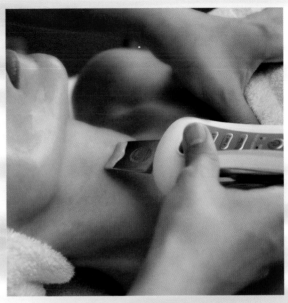

P5-5-5 Start at neck and peel upward. (Refer to page 185 for corresponding content).

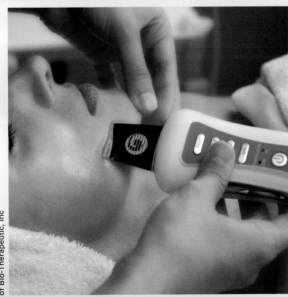

P5-5-6 Continue moving upward on face. (Refer to page 185 for corresponding content).

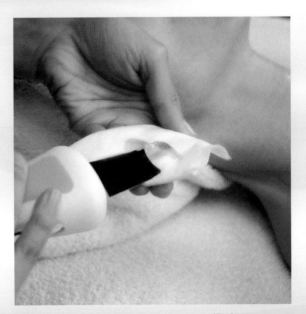

P5-5-7 Wipe device with each pass. (Refer to page 185 for corresponding content).

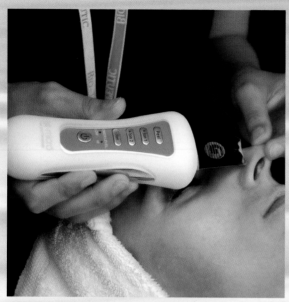

P5-5-8 Peel nasal region. (Refer to page 186 for corresponding content).

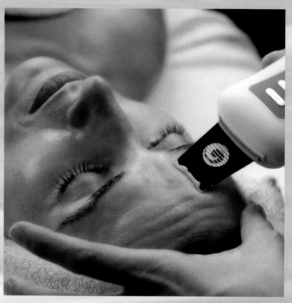

P5-5-9 Peeling foredhead. (Refer to page 186 for corresponding content).

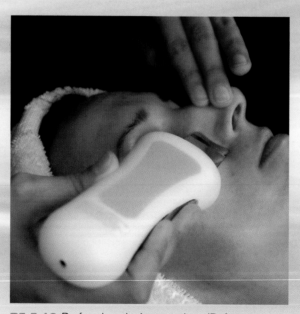

P5-5-12 Performing desincrustation. (Refer to page 186 for corresponding content).

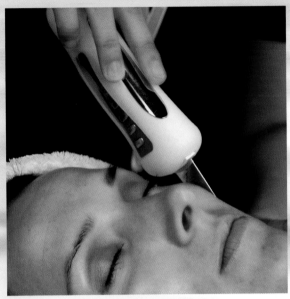

P5-5-15 Performing positive ionization with hydrating serum. (Refer to page 187 for corresponding content).

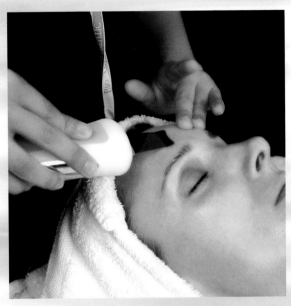

P5-5-17 Continue positive ionization. (Refer to page 187 for corresponding content).

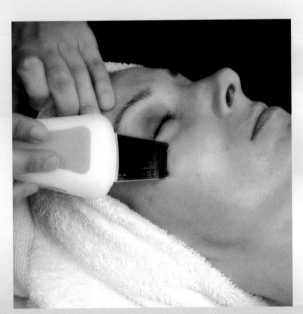

P5-5-18 Perform positive ionization with cream. (Refer to page 187 for corresponding content).

Pre and Post Op

BOTOX ▶

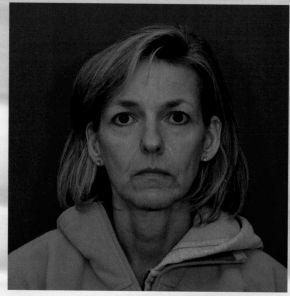

6-3 Patient Pre Botox. (Refer to page 216 for corresponding content).

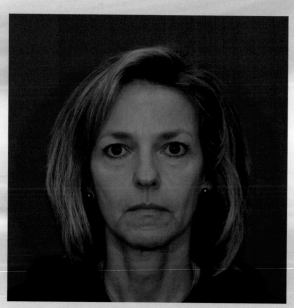

6-4 Patient Post Botox. (Refer to page 216 for corresponding content).

Hecht Aesthetic Center

SOFT TISSUE ▶
    FILLER

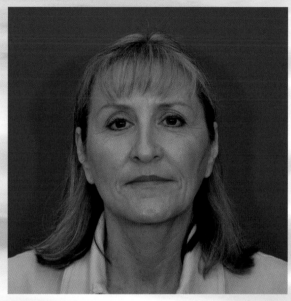

6-5 Patient Pre Soft Tissue Filler. (Refer to page 222 for corresponding content).

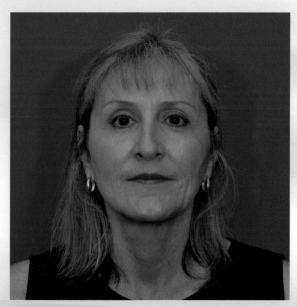

6-6 Patient Post Soft Tissue Filler. (Refer to page 222 for corresponding content).

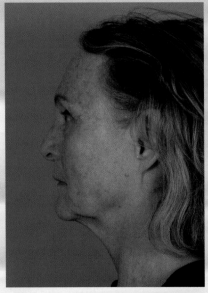

6-7 Patient Pre Skin Resurfacing
(Refer to page 226 for corresponding
content).

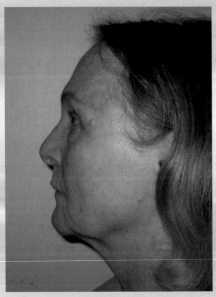

6-8 Patient Post Skin Resurfacing
(Refer to page 226 for corresponding
content).

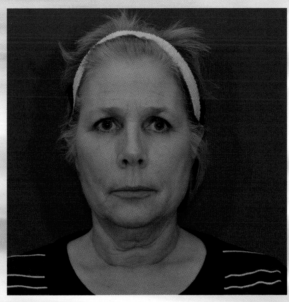

6-9 Patient Pre and Post Facelift Front view. (Refer to page 234 for corresponding content).

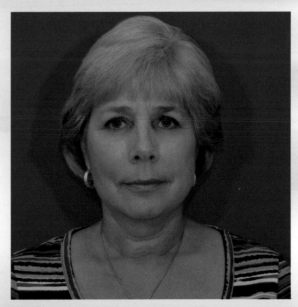

6-10 Patient Pre and Post Facelift Side View. (Refer to page 234 for corresponding content).

Hecht Aesthetic Center

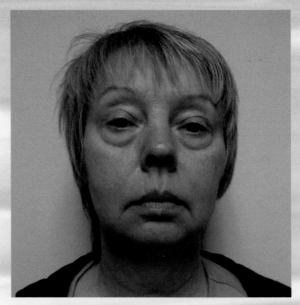

6-11 Pre Blepharoplasty. (Refer to page 241 for corresponding content).

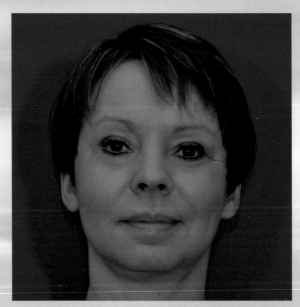

6-12 Post Blepharoplasty. (Refer to page 241 for corresponding content).

Hecht Aesthetic Center